Praise for
GORGEOUS FOR G

D0771676

"To be with Sophie is to be so caught up
in the thrill of potential Good."

— Julia Roberts

"Every page of *Gorgeous for Good* is full of eye-opening
(and eye-beautifying) information. And the beauty and pleasure
tips (like putting essential oil drops on clean washcloths) are
instantly applicable. I kept finding myself saying, 'Oh—I simply
must try this' over and over again as I read. *Gorgeous for Good*
is a pleasurable inspiration and cornucopia of solid health and
beauty information that will change you both from outside
and within. I highly recommend this treasure!"

— Christiane Northrup, M.D.,
author of *Goddesses Never Age*

"Sophie's transformational 30-day program works because
of her inside-out approach to beauty. It is unique because she
focuses on tending to our soul, as well as our skin . . . and
everything in between. Sophie is the real deal—she walks
the walk and is testament to her own philosophy."

— JJ Virgin, celebrity nutrition and fitness expert and *New York
Times* best-selling author of *The Virgin Diet* and *Sugar Impact Diet*

"Sophie's 30-day program thoroughly covers my favorite topics:
good nutrition and good skincare, and she does it with smarts
and a gigantic heart. If you're ready to feel great inside and out,
put the good back into gorgeous with this wonderful book."

— Kris Carr, *New York Times*
best-selling author of *Crazy Sexy Kitchen*

"Sophie Uliano is gorgeous from the inside out. I find
myself staring at her sometimes and marveling at her natural
beauty—and am so impressed by her boundless energy! I am
truly inspired by all the information she shares with us in this
book. It makes you think twice about how you treat your body.
More importantly, it will change your life."

— Cristina Ferrare, chef, *New York Times*
best-selling author, and host of Hallmark Channel's
Emmy-nominated *Home and Family*

GORGEOUS

FOR

GOOD

ALSO BY SOPHIE ULIANO

Gorgeously Green: 8 Simple Steps to an Earth-Friendly Life

The Gorgeously Green Diet

Do It Gorgeously: How to Make Less Toxic, Less Expensive, and More Beautiful Products

GORGEOUS
FOR
GOOD

A Simple 30-Day Program for Lasting Beauty— Inside and Out

Sophie Uliano

HAY HOUSE, INC.
Carlsbad, California • New York City
London • Sydney • Johannesburg
Vancouver • Hong Kong • New Delhi

Published and distributed in the United States by: Hay House, Inc.: www.hayhouse. com® • *Published and distributed in Australia by:* Hay House Australia Pty. Ltd.: www.hayhouse.com.au • *Published and distributed in the United Kingdom by:* Hay House UK, Ltd.: www.hayhouse.co.uk • *Published and distributed in the Republic of South Africa by:* Hay House SA (Pty), Ltd.: www.hayhouse.co.za • *Distributed in Canada by:* Raincoast Books: www.raincoast.com • *Published in India by:* Hay House Publishers India: www.hayhouse.co.in

Cover design: *Tricia Breidenthal* • Interior design: *Pamela Homan*
Interior illustrations: *Alexis Seabrook*

Credit for Logos:
Soil Association • *Soil Association*
NATRUE • *NATRUE www.natrue.org*
NPA Natural Seal • *Natural Products Association*
NSF International Logo • *NSF International*
Leaping Bunny Logo • *Coalition for Consumer Information on Cosmetics*
Fair Trade Certified™ Logo • *Fair Trade USA*

Library of Congress Cataloging-in-Publication Data

Uliano, Sophie.
  Gorgeous for good : a simple 30-day program for lasting beauty-inside and out / Sophie Uliano.
    pages cm
  ISBN 978-1-4019-4619-7 (paperback)
1. Beauty, Personal. 2. Women--Health and hygiene. I. Title.
RA778.U37 2015
646.7'2--dc23
                                     2015003380

Tradepaper ISBN: 978-1-4019-4619-7

10 9 8 7 6 5 4 3 2 1
1st edition, April 2015

Printed in the United States of America

SUSTAINABLE FORESTRY INITIATIVE
Certified Chain of Custody
Promoting Sustainable Forestry
www.sfiprogram.org
SFI-01268
SFI label applies to the text stock

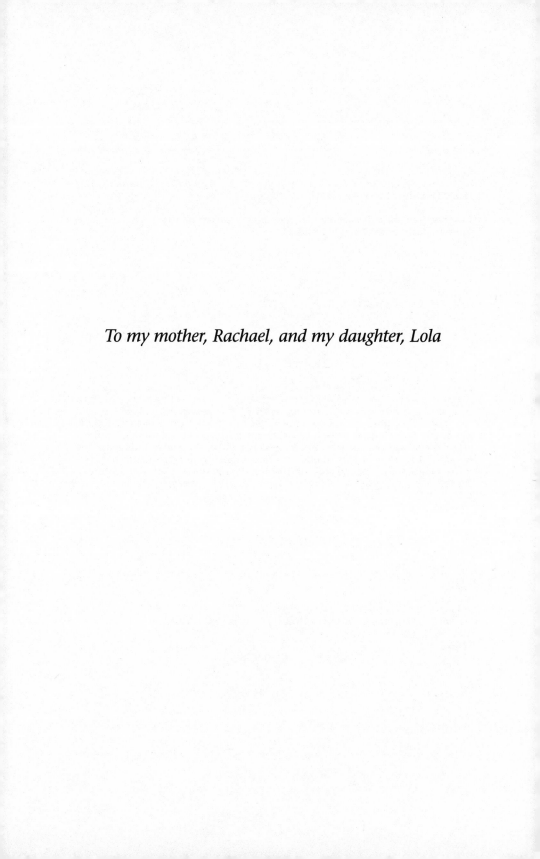

To my mother, Rachael, and my daughter, Lola

CONTENTS

INTRODUCTION

Do you ever catch a glimpse of yourself in the mirror and see someone you barely recognize? Do you trash almost every selfie you take because . . . well . . . you're just not as gorgeous as you should be these days? Have you tried and failed to change something about your physical appearance? Do you sometimes feel as if you are fighting a losing battle in your quest to look younger and/ or more beautiful? If you've answered affirmatively to one or two of the above questions, then join the club! And let me welcome you to Gorgeous for Good, a community of women who not only feel the same way as you but want you to join with us in creating a new consciousness—a paradigm shift in the way we think about ourselves that will transform not only the way we look but also the way we feel about our lives.

Let's face it, the mere attempt to look younger or different from what we really are can be extremely stressful. The new information flooding into our inboxes daily is mind-numbing. How on earth can we keep up with all these cutting-edge products and procedures that will miraculously bestow a youthful glow on us, when there's a new one every week? The panic about downing enough antioxidant-infused juice, folding into hundreds of spasm-inducing squats, and coughing up cash for laughably expensive facial peels and fillers—well, that in and of itself is stressful enough to deepen those fine lines that we're hell-bent on erasing.

I picked up a magazine the other day that has a strong focus on cosmetic surgery. Each glossy page showed another grinning plastic surgeon explaining how he or she can completely fix a woman's face and/or body with a couple of simple surgeries. Although I'm not against a few cosmetic tweaks, the whole magazine left me feeling empty, less-than, and afraid. Maybe I should have the bump in my nose shaved off, or get a brow, knee, stomach, or butt lift? But, honestly, aside from the fact that I can't afford most of these invasive procedures, I'm terrified of them. What if it all went wrong and I came out looking completely bizarre? Or, even worse, what if I went to sleep in the operating room . . . forever? As I dumped the magazine in the trash (I didn't want my 13-year-old daughter to see all the lurid before-and-after images), I reminded myself that reading content that focuses almost entirely on *fixing* a woman's physical imperfections is not the most positive use of my precious time. Besides, I rather like most of my "imperfections"; I've gotten to know them (dare I say *love* them?) because they make me who I am.

The good news is that the tide is turning against skin that's stretched as tight as Saran Wrap. No one wants to look like a robotic Barbie. The ubiquitous term "antiaging" has become boring and meaningless. Instead of attempting to look like something we're not, we now simply want to look and feel like more revitalized versions of ourselves.

The truth is that we all want to *be* natural. The problem is that many of us have a slight problem with *looking* natural if it means saggy jowls and deep wrinkles. So, what can we put in place of the laughably expensive products and procedures that could make us look like weird versions of our original selves? Oh, sure, a lifetime of SPF 50, yoga, and an organic, vegan diet will do it, but for most of us, that ship sailed long ago!

What we really need is a daily beauty regimen that is practical, easy, and doable and that will not only stop time in its tracks but also maybe rewind it. We need a holistic plan that partners the "miraculous cures" of the latest scientific discoveries with the healing powers of nature so that we can age naturally and gorgeously—despite the pressures of our busy lives and polluted atmosphere. Impossible, right? Wrong, because this is exactly what I'm going to show you how to do. I'm excited to share my program with you because it's what I have figured out works really well for me. From years of trial and error and intensive up-till-three-in-the-morning research, I've discovered a whole-life program that seems to work like a charm for everyone who has trusted me enough to give it a go.

And, by the way, I know that while many of us care about the environment—separating our recyclables and even growing our own greens—there aren't many of us who are prepared to compromise, even a little bit, when it comes to beauty. Eco-consciousness often flies out the window in the face of a woman who wants to maintain her allure. The reality is that many of us don't care what's in our skin cream as long as it works. What we all want are results—good ones, and *now*. But I want to let you know that there is a way to look beautiful and not throw out all of your environmental cares—because true beauty is an inside job. Nothing looks as good as healthy, and healthy generally works for both you and the earth.

Don't worry—I'm not going to tell you to give up the products and procedures you love. I am a beauty flexitarian with a foot in both the enhancement camp and the one nature intended. By firmly taking a stand for the middle ground, I have learned to own my own beauty while taking charge of the future of my face and body.

My Beauty Revolution

The revolution in my approach to beauty came about through understanding that a gorgeous woman is an *authentic* woman. An authentic woman is a happier woman. Authentic + Happy = GORGEOUS. Every woman in my life who is breathtakingly gorgeous is absolutely *herself*: she doesn't attempt to be anything other than who she is.

I believe that our purpose in life is to express who we truly are while supporting others to do the same. When we express our unique inner truth, we shine. This is way easier said than done, which is why part of the 30-day Gorgeous for Good program is a journey of uncovering, discovering, and discarding who you are *not* in order to find out who you really *are*.

Media and advertising are almost wholly responsible for perpetuating the myth that to be happy, loved, accepted, and sexy, we need to look like airbrushed 15-year-olds. Foundation and moisturizer commercials promise us "flawless" skin. But this is ridiculous, because attempting to get even close to flawless *anything* sets us up for crashing failure. When we realize that our hair, skin, nails, personality, and pretty much every single thing about us are so far from flawless that it doesn't even warrant the effort, we slink away with our tails between our legs because we feel we must have gotten something wrong: maybe we haven't caught on to the beauty secret that "they" all know. But the truth is that it's our imperfections that make us truly gorgeous.

Think of your best girlfriends: the ones you laugh with until you almost pee your pants, the ones you've been through everything with—they've seen your suffering, and you've seen theirs. Think of why you love these women. Think of why everyone else loves them. It's not because they have even skin tones, immaculate hair, and perfect bodies; it's not even because they're successful—*no!* It's because they have beautiful flaws and personalities that have most likely been shaped by adversity. So the first thing that I want to address in my "beauty" book is that flawless is *out*. It's old-school, and any woman over the age of 20 who wants to look "perfect" is in for a big disappointment, because there's no such thing. Contrary to what we've been led to believe, vulnerability is beautiful. It takes great courage to be vulnerable—to allow ourselves to be who we really are, warts and all. However, the prize for that courage is a deep connection to the world and especially to those we love—something that money cannot buy.

I'm afraid I must visit the "French women don't . . ." conversation here: we know they supposedly don't get fat, don't age, and probably don't fart, but the real difference is that they don't seem to want to change their natural characteristics. Look at French movies and you'll see actresses who aren't afraid of high-def close-ups, even after a certain age. The reason is that French culture celebrates individuality rather than cookie-cutter perfection. The white teeth, turned-up nose, and glossy tan of the American starlet are not considered beautiful in France. The French like interesting faces with features that are unique. This could mean asymmetry, a large nose, or even deep wrinkles. Our European friends are certainly not strangers to the plastic surgeon's office, but speak to any Parisian plastic surgeon and he'll scoff at what his peers are doing in the U.S. because he believes in keeping character in a face rather than obliterating it.

My husband asked me the other day how I felt about turning 50, which at the time of this writing is just around the corner. "I'm thrilled," I replied. He looked at me quizzically. "Really?" he asked, raising an eyebrow. "Yes!" I said, looking him straight in the eye. "Why wouldn't I be thrilled that here I am, nearly fifty years old, and have so much to be thankful for: I have had almost fifty years of living with good health on this beautiful planet. I have garnered (albeit sometimes through suffering) an enormous amount of wisdom. I'm excited almost every morning when I wake up about what the day might bring. Why wouldn't I be ecstatic about where I am in my life right now?" With that, we toasted each other and got on with the rather more serious business of ordering our sushi rolls.

My viewpoint on this matter is why I've decided that it's so important to reframe or rename the concept of "antiaging." Although it's hard to avoid, I'm bit fed up with that term. Since aging is a natural process that happens to every single one of us, to be against it is ridiculous. Getting older brings so many benefits; why not look at the cup as half full rather than half empty? The beauty industry's marketing engine has banged the antiaging drum so hard that it's beginning to wear a bit thin. I prefer to think of a treatment, product, or lifestyle change as being proactive rather than antiaging. If we choose to drink green smoothies, exercise, and use incredibly effective skin-rejuvenating products, we are taking powerful steps toward looking and feeling the way we want to. I will say it once more: I am *not* against aging. All of my role models are women who are over 70, so why would I be against who they are and what they have to offer?

Aging is an honor. Let's not deny what's both natural and inevitable. Rather, let's enjoy every day that we have gained a little more life experience and wisdom. Only a century ago, the life expectancy of most women was 50 years. Modern medicine and lifestyles have allowed us to enjoy long, pain-free lives. I love that as we age, we can leave the neurosis of our youths behind and move into a life of deeper creativity and love . . . and look simply gorgeous!

It's Now!

The Gorgeous for Good program is not a "when" program, it's a "now" program. It's all about what you can achieve *today*. When you set long-term goals such as "I hope to lose 30 pounds in 30 days," you so easily set yourself up to fail. Moreover, 30 days is an entire day-counting month away. Do you really want to spend the next month just waiting for that moment when you can perhaps stand on the scale and potentially find happiness? The flaw in this approach is that you are keeping happiness right out there in front of you, just out of your grasp. Why not find fulfillment, strength, and contentment today? This is what the Gorgeous for Good program is all about: How can you challenge yourself *today?* What can you learn *today?* What proactive action can you take *today?* What fear can you face *today?* And what can you do to your skin today that will make it look fantastic? Whatever proactive steps you can take *today* will inevitably create a better tomorrow.

So, how does the program work?

I like to start from the micro and then move in toward the macro. When it comes to gorgeousness, the *macro* is your mind, body, and spirit—it's the big-picture stuff. The *micro* is your skin, hair, and nails. I like to think of concentric circles around the body: The outermost circle, the most superficial level, is the skin and hair. This is the first area that I address, because it's where you can perform quick fixes. Moreover, I always feel 100 percent better when I'm beautifully made up. And let's face it, it's easier to purchase a different lipstick than it is to shift your diet and start meditating, so why not start somewhere easy? After that, I move inward to what I put into my body and how I move through the world. And finally, I go deeper—to the innermost circles of mind and spirit.

After teaching you all about these things, I lay out a simple 30-day program that helps you bring together everything you've learned. I lay out step-by-step beauty, nutrition, movement, and self-care exercises to do each day. It's an easy, doable way to jump-start your more gorgeous life—no matter how busy you are.

I hope you enjoy your 30-day program as much as I've enjoyed putting it together for you. It's an absolute honor to have you trust me enough to try it out and become part of my valued community. Because my philosophy is about making lifestyle changes that will keep us looking and feeling gorgeous forever, I encourage you stay as connected with me and my community as possible. If you suddenly stop following the program on day 31 and slowly return to your old habits, you'll be doing yourself a massive disservice. The great thing about the Internet is that it's now easy for us all to stay connected. We need to continue to cheer each other on, to help and support each other, and to discover what we can add to what we already know.

My commitment to you is that I will always stay on top of the latest advances in holistic nutrition and skin care and that I will constantly update you with exactly what you need to stay gorgeous for good. Suffice it to say, it would be hugely helpful if you sign up for my newsletter—or, at the least, check out my website, www.sophieuliano.com, as often as you can. Also, after you read the skin care chapter, you will want (and need) actual product recommendations. I've chosen not to include those in the book because companies and products change, and you might still be reading this book decades from now, so all my recommendations will live on my website. Okay—now that I've got that bit of housekeeping over (I promise that I'll never mention it again), it's time to get down to business.

Part One

BEGINNING ON THE OUTSIDE . . .

Chapter 1

My Philosophy of External Beauty

Do you consider yourself to be beautiful? If your answer is a definitive *no*, then you're not alone—in a 2004 Harvard study commissioned by Dove, less than 2 percent of women across the globe used the word *beautiful* to describe themselves. Well, it's time for us to take back our power from popular culture and media and own the definition. To identify with the word *beautiful* is a wonderful thing—but, admittedly, it's not easy.

For most of us, it's almost impossible to feel beautiful because we only see what we think is wrong with us physically. Pimples, dark circles, uneven features, and our wobbly bits all play into the "I'm not beautiful" lie that we tell ourselves every day. The other day, I was having my hair blown out by a lovely stylist named Gabrielle. As soon as we met, I was enchanted by her gigantic smile and throaty laugh. As she fired up the hairdryer, we began chatting and somehow got onto the subject of "fake" beauty. We began ruminating on whether either of us would ever consider dramatic plastic surgery. She admitted to me that she had been considering a nose job for years. "Why?" I asked, astonished.

"Because I've always hated my nose," she said. "My brothers used to tease me about it being big when I was a kid, and I've always wanted a smaller one." I just couldn't believe what she was saying, because to me, she had a beautiful nose—granted, it wasn't tiny or turned up, but it was absolutely perfect on her face.

"Don't!" I begged her.

She turned the dryer off, looked me in the eyes, and implored me to be brutally honest with her. "Wouldn't it look better if I just had it thinned out a bit?" she asked, pointing to an area that she thought was too fat.

"No!" I yelled, almost jumping out of the chair. I made her promise that she would never, ever do anything to her nose, because if it became thinner and smaller, it just wouldn't match the rest of her face.

She thought about it for a moment while observing herself in the giant mirror. "I guess you're right," she said, gently touching the nose that she'd hated for years. "Maybe I can learn to live with it." I told her that I hoped she'd learn to do more than that—that she'd learn to *love* it.

Gabrielle isn't alone. Many women obsess about one area or feature of their faces or bodies, thinking that if it were made "perfect," they could then be loved and appreciated by others. But the insanity is that others don't even notice the very things we want to change. Men and women see us as whole, integrated people where not only our features but also our energy and spirit contribute to who we are. Besides, when you change one feature, it's like buying a new, expensive dress: you can't stop there, because you need the shoes, jacket, and jewelry to go with it.

But the real issue is that if we try to change something about our physical appearance in the hopes of dulling the ache of not feeling good enough, in time, we'll find other features that need fixing, too. Sure, a good nose job could give a woman tremendous confidence, but it still doesn't fix the fear within. The truth is that if you look *into your eyes* in the mirror and tell yourself (as you would tell a little girl) that you are indeed a beautiful spirit, you will be better able to connect with your *true* beauty.

So, can we start off *Gorgeous for Good* with the simple, albeit incredibly embarrassing, action of standing in front of the mirror right now? Go on, put down the book and tell yourself the truth about who you really are. Even if you don't feel valuable or like a good person deep down, I assure you that underneath whatever is happening in your life and your psyche at this moment, there is a beautiful woman waiting to be discovered.

Creating a Gorgeous Exterior

Ironically, feeling like a beautiful person within makes me want to take care of the "outside" even more—probably because I feel that I *deserve* to use gorgeous products. I used to think that it was a bit shallow and vain, not to mention wasteful, to spend more than five minutes a day taking care of my physical appearance. I believed that wearing little to no makeup and allowing my hair to naturally frizz (as it does in the absence of a high-speed hairdryer) was virtuous. After all, I should be focusing on more important things, right? But I've learned that taking care of my outer beauty is a wonderful thing, too. I feel enormously better about myself when, instead of lounging around in my sweats when I get up, I throw myself in the shower and get going with my head-to-toe beauty business.

So, what have I learned about sprucing up the outside since I made this shift? Basically, I've learned that there's a lot of confusion, shaming, and scaremongering when it comes to making ourselves beautiful. We tweak here and there to get rid of our "imperfections." We do everything we can to fix different parts of our bodies—from dark under-eye circles to cracked heels, we desperately try to rectify whatever seems unattractive. However, the problem is that we regard the parts of our bodies as separate entities rather than as members of an integrated whole.

Our approach to health care is similar, right? "Conventional" medicine treats the symptom, not the cause, while "alternative" medicine focuses on the underlying problem—but doesn't necessarily bring relief as quickly. Most of us today have our feet in both the conventional and the alternative camps when it comes to our health. We've evolved to understand that treating the symptom is just the tip of the iceberg. We also now know that treating the symptom is a short-term solution at best.

In much the same way, conventional beauty treats symptoms: If you have a skin condition, you'll make an appointment with a dermatologist and get a treatment or drug to try to get rid of it. Even wrinkles are treated like a disease: "Here, slather on this acid peel, and you might see your wrinkles disappear." The flaw in this approach is that the skin is only part of the whole. In treating our skin, hair, and nails, we have to treat the whole person. This is "holistic" beauty, and it's the beauty of the future. The black-and-white thinking of past decades no longer serves us.

I do understand, however, that "holistic" skin care frightens some of us because it seems to imply that we'll have to give up our antiaging chemicals and fillers for oatmeal scrubs. This couldn't be further from the truth. The reality for me is that the most potent ingredients for sustainable beauty are those that are fresh, active, and healthy. I also know that treating the symptom can seriously improve your life while you're waiting for the underlying health outcomes to show. So my focus for making you glow takes both conventional and alternative approaches into account. I like products that make me beautiful but also healthy.

Picking Your Products

Having worked in the "green" space for almost a decade, I've come across many "organic beauty" zealots who won't allow any chemical products near their skin and want what they think is "natural." I understand that this misunderstanding comes from fear and can be exacerbated by erroneous and hysterical Internet hype based on disproven scientific studies, but let's get one thing clear: every compound, whether natural or synthetic, is a chemical.

Many natural botanicals can be really toxic: poison ivy is an obvious example, but there are many more. Moreover, many people are allergic to certain pure essential oils such as lavender. On the other hand, it's also important that we don't shove everything that's made in a lab into the "toxic" camp. After all, some of the most potent and effective skin care ingredients in "green" beauty formulations are made in labs: vitamin C and retinol are some prime examples.

Rather than vilify specific ingredients based on their perceived origins, it's more helpful to look at all the ingredients that make up a formulation as a whole and consider how they work synergistically. It's even more important to consider the manufacturing process of the company you are buying from: What is the shelf life of their products? Where and how are the formulations made? Who created the formulation, and what is the scientific thinking it's based on? And, most important, what are the company's values in terms of sustainability, ingredient transparency, and giving back?

Forgive me for sounding a bit New Agey here, but I do believe that everything has an "energy" to it. How a product is sourced, manufactured, and sold is part of a long creative process involving many people. I prefer to buy my products from companies that have my best interests at heart: they want me to feel good, they want me to see results, and ultimately, they want me to be healthy. I also love to purchase from companies that treat the earth and their employees well. It all feeds into the concept of "good" energy.

I invite you to become super conscious about each and every personal-care product you use. To be mindful of what you are putting on your skin, eyes, hair, and nails is a beautiful thing. It feels good to know that you are nourishing yourself with gorgeous, healthy ingredients that smell and feel delicious. This doesn't mean you have to walk around with a huge magnifying glass, prepared to read every ingredient label in sight. It means that you can take charge of your beauty by empowering yourself with a few basic truths.

My mission in this chapter is to equip you with enough information so that you can fearlessly shop for what you want and need rather than having to trawl the Internet for reviews and information (much of which may be bogus), trying to make sense of the plethora of scaremongering and marketing agendas.

Kale and Ice Cream!

Many people are surprised when I admit to having highlights in my hair or occasionally allowing a makeup artist to use a totally nonnatural foundation on my face before going on TV. But I'm not a zealot about green beauty, because I understand what I *really* need to avoid—and what's best to simply minimize—in terms of toxic ingredients. Given that there are now toxic chemicals lurking in every area of our lives 24/7, it doesn't make sense to get hysterical about every single beauty product in our bathroom cabinets. However, it's smart to educate ourselves on the basics so that we can keep our bodies and our bank balances as healthy as possible.

I've always been passionate about educating myself to make the smartest choices I can. It's all about living mindfully in every area of my life. My approach to using nontoxic beauty products is similar to the way I eat: I employ the 80/20 rule. This means that 80 percent of the time, I am super-duper healthy (meat-, dairy-, sugar-, and gluten-free). But occasionally, I like a bowl of ice cream after my kale salad, and other times, I just *need* to have a deep-crust pizza, or a huge bowl of salty fries. For the most part, I'm really healthy, so when I take part in a few transgressions, I can easily get away with it. It's the same with my beauty regimen: my everyday, go-to products are really clean and healthy, but every now and again I'll use a few products that may not be perfect.

Here's the deal: ingredients such as parabens and phthalates, which I try to avoid, are all around us—they are in our food, water, cars, homes, airplane seats, malls, and offices. In our modern-day world, we are literally surrounded by thousands of chemicals that didn't even exist a hundred years ago, and many of them were never adequately tested for human safety. We've mercifully been designed with a complex immune system that can handle much of this toxic assault, but it can't keep up if we inundate it with ever more of the chemicals it's trying to get rid of. That's why I focus on limiting my exposure rather than tyrannical, hysterical avoidance. (This is also why an important part of any holistic beauty program is to strengthen our own immune systems—but we'll get to that later.)

The other day on set, a new producer came up to me and mentioned that she'd love for me to help her get a bit more natural with all her beauty products. "But," she said with wide-open eyes, "you won't take my Chanel foundation away, will you?" I laughed because I think this is how many women feel. There are certain products that we love because they work for us. I told her that it's more important to concern ourselves with the products that we use on larger areas of the body, such as body lotion and shampoo. She was relieved.

And that's really what this program is all about: balance and smart choices. In being mindful of what we apply to our skin, we can minimize our daily exposure to a multitude of toxins, but stressing out about it too much is way more unhealthy and can lead to problems that a botanical shampoo and natural foundation can never cure.

Your Body Burden

There's no getting away from it—we all have a body burden. Toxic chemicals, both naturally occurring and man-made, get into our bodies. We might inhale them, swallow them, or absorb them through our skin. A pregnant woman may pass them to her developing fetus through the placenta. The term "body burden" refers to the total amount of these chemicals that is present in a person at a given point in time.

Some chemicals lodge in our bodies for only a short while before being excreted, but continuous exposure to such chemicals can create a persistent body burden. Other chemicals, however, are not easily excreted and can remain for years in our blood, adipose (fat) tissue, muscle, bone, brain tissue, or other organs. Of the approximately 80,000 chemicals that are used in the U.S., we do not know how many can become a part of our chemical body burden, but we do know that several hundred of these chemicals have been measured in people's bodies around the world.

Your Healthy Beauty Starting Place

How on earth do we begin to choose a skin care or makeup brand that is not only going to be good for our skin and our health, but is also going to deliver outstanding results? It can be very confusing, because most of the reviews you read in magazines and on blogs only focus on the performance aspects, and those, of course, are very subjective. What may work beautifully on a 23-year-old beauty editor might be a terrible waste of money for you.

Here are some questions I like to ask myself as I search for new products:

- **Does the brand have a healthy track record?** Is it known for more natural formulations? This shouldn't be hard to figure out, because if the company's focus is on healthier ingredients, it will make that very clear on its website.

- **Does the company share my values?** This is very important for me because I want to purchase from a company that embraces strong ethical and sustainable principles.

- **Does the company disclose a full ingredient list?** This is imperative. I don't trust any brand that doesn't fully disclose every single ingredient it uses (unless they have a very good reason). I don't want to have to don my Sherlock Holmes hat to find out.

- **Does the brand offer samples?** This is important if the company is not carried in a large beauty chain store (where you can always get samples). You always need to get samples when it comes to primers, BB creams, and foundations.

- **What is the company's return policy?** The good news about buying from a large beauty chain is that usually you can always return an item, even if it's been opened. This also holds true for many department stores. If you buy online, check to see if the company has a return policy that works for you should the product not perform as advertised.

While these questions won't necessarily tell you how well the product will work for you, they can ensure that you start on the right track. Also, remember that these are questions *I* like to ask myself. You might decide that not all of them are important for you. (But my hunch is that since you're reading this book, they likely will be.)

Now let's get a little deeper into exploring the ins and outs of product judgment.

Are the Ingredients Good for You?

If I'm going to slather a product all over my face and body every day, it better contain ingredients that are actually going to be good for my skin and body. Unfortunately, many skin care and cosmetics companies don't care about the health of your skin as much as you do. Therefore, it's important that you purchase with as much knowledge as possible—which means knowing something about the ingredients in the products.

As you move into this space, I'll warn you—it's much easier to read an ingredient list on a *skin care* product than on a *cosmetic* product. Most skin care companies have awakened to the fact that consumers now want transparency. More and more women are eschewing parabens, and others are on high alert for any possible allergens and/or "toxic" ingredients that they've read about. But how do we actually find out what's in the products we love or are thinking of purchasing?

Some products make the label-reading process easier than others. When I go shopping for a night cream or body lotion, the ingredients are almost always clearly listed on the container or outer box. However, it's a different story with cosmetic items such as foundations or mascaras, because they list so many ingredients I don't recognize, and the print is ridiculously tiny. The reason I recommend doing a bit of research before you buy anything is that many of those complicated-sounding ingredients are irritants, skin sensitizers, and possible hormone disruptors.

Natural Versus Synthetic

I would love to imagine that the ingredients in all of my products come from wild botanicals grown in the Swiss Alps rather than from a lab in an industrial park. It makes sense to me that ingredients that are as "natural" as possible are going to be way better for my health and my skin. However, it's a bit more complicated than it seems at first blush. The term *natural* doesn't mean much because in the food, skin care, and cosmetics industries, the term is not adequately regulated or quantifiable. Anyone can slap the label "natural" on a box or jar and hope we won't bother to read the actual ingredient list, which may be chock full of synthetic additives, preservatives, and other lab-made ingredients that our skin won't love.

To assist you in getting ready for some product selection, I want to lay out some definitions here that can help guide you. The terms *natural, organic, raw, farm-to-face,* and *synthetic* all imply certain things—but these implications aren't necessarily true. Many of our perceptions are sculpted by myth and hearsay, so I want to make clear what each of these terms can mean.

Natural

The first definition of *natural* in the dictionary is "existing in, or formed by, nature." So, when I think about the ingredients in my beauty products, it seems to make sense that something that sprouted straight from the earth will be healthier than a laboratory concoction. This is why my heart sings when I see that a product contains aloe vera and/or organic, cold-pressed plant oils. Keep in mind, though, that no matter how natural the ingredient, it's highly unlikely to have jumped straight from the farm or forest into its recyclable container. There's always a degree of physical processing, which may include heating and the addition of other not-so-natural ingredients. So, unless you're pulling the plants up from your own yard and mashing them with a pestle and mortar to smear on your face, the meaning of the word *natural* can get a bit muddy!

Organic

Organic is another term that has become a bit problematic because it's really hard to quantify. The first thing is not to confuse "organic chemistry" with "organic plants and foods" (as in those that are grown without synthetic herbicides or pesticides). Organic chemistry is the science of substances that contain both carbon and hydrogen, and many are made in the lab as molecularly exact matches for original ingredients that were pulled up from the earth.

Why does a skin care ingredient need to be "organic"? In fact, truth be told, you are not necessarily smearing pesticides on your skin if your ingredients aren't organic—the processing involved in getting an ingredient into a formulation has likely removed every last trace of pesticide. However, I will say that if a company takes the trouble to source organic ingredients, then you can be pretty sure that it is concerned with quality. Another reason that I love to buy formulations from companies that use at least some organic ingredients is that I like to support organic farming.

If a food or agricultural product is certified to be organic, it should be:

- Produced without synthetic fertilizers, herbicides, or pesticides
- Non-GMO
- Nonirradiated
- Not fertilized with sewage sludge

If it's important to you to purchase skin care products made with organic ingredients, you need to make sure that a bona fide organic certificate is involved. In the U.S., the FDA does not define or regulate the term *organic* as it applies to beauty or personal-care products; however, it does regulate the use of the term *organic* when it comes to agricultural products with a USDA-certified organic seal. The facility that produces the agricultural ingredient(s) needs to be certified by a USDA-accredited organic certifying agent.

Once certified, a product might be eligible for one of the four following categories:

1. **100% organic:** Every ingredient (except water and salt) is organically produced.

2. **Organic:** Contains at least 95 percent organically produced ingredients.

3. **Made with organic ingredients:** Contains at least 70 percent organically produced ingredients. The product label may list up to three of these ingredients on the principal display panel (for example: "Made with organic lavender, chamomile, and rosemary").

4. **Less than 70 percent organic ingredients:** This product cannot use the term *organic* anywhere on the principal display panel, but it can identify specific ingredients that are organically produced on the information panel.

Raw Beauty

Because the terms *organic* and *natural* can be rather misleading in the beauty space, the term *raw* skin care has mercifully appeared, and it much better describes what many of us are after. A *raw* product's ingredients haven't been treated with any kind of heat. This is very important when assessing the efficacy of many ingredients, especially pure plant oils, which lose many of their nutrients when they are exposed to heat. Just as a raw food diet provides valuable enzymes that would have been destroyed during cooking, a raw skin care product retains its basic nutrients. Almost all raw beauty products are vegan—and preservative free, so unless they're in dry powder form, you need to keep them in the fridge.

Farm-to-Face

There are a couple of companies in the U.S. that really are literally farm-to-face and totally walk the walk. One of these companies, Tata Harper, is based at owner Tata's farm in Vermont, where most of the plants and botanicals for her formulas are grown. All the manufacturing, from planting the seeds to packaging, is done on the farm, and the results are exquisite. Another wonderful farm-to-face company is Farmaesthetics, where owner Brenda Brock sources all the herbs and plants she uses in her formulations from American family farms. If something says *farm-to-face*, you can be sure that the ingredients are pure and that the product has gone through little processing. When owners care enough to plant, harvest, and package everything themselves, you know there's a whole lot of integrity behind their products.

Synthetic

What about synthetic ingredients? Surely an ingredient that's made in the lab is worse than one that comes straight from nature. Not necessarily. Some synthetic ingredients can be safer and way more effective than their natural counterparts. This is where I take off my natural-ingredient-zealot hat. An example of a good synthetic is L-ascorbic acid (aka vitamin C). You know that white, powdery vitamin C that you can buy in a jar at the health-food store? It's a form that's made in a lab and therefore far from natural—bit of a shocker, right? As far as skin care is concerned, L-ascorbic acid is a potent antiaging ingredient, but it must be in a stable form when added to formulations, or it will oxidize and lose its efficacy. The stable forms that are used in skin care (and I'm talking natural skin care) are almost always synthetic. So when it comes to the term *synthetic*, all I want to make you aware of is that it isn't inherently bad. Don't count something out entirely because it contains these ingredients—it simply means that there's more to learn.

Gorgeously Green

Now, let's address the argument that we should always use natural, organic, raw ingredients to help protect the earth. While this is a wonderful idea, as with most things, there's a bigger picture to be considered here. Botanicals straight from nature can sometimes require a lot more energy than synthetics to process and manufacture, especially "super ingredients" such as camu camu, exotic African butters, and certain oils. Now the question becomes, "How green is it to fly in botanicals from the rainforest (or elsewhere)?" Or, how much of nature had to be demolished to bring us that amazing natural ingredient?

Açai sounds great sitting in a skin care product in the "green" section of a beauty store, but think about the energy required for the transport and processing of that little berry. Moreover, if the demand for these popular super ingredients increases, where are they going to come from? Remember, we used to think that palm oil was a good thing until we found out that swaths of rainforest were being hacked down to grow the stuff. When you consider that it takes 60,000 roses to make just one ounce of rose absolute essential oil, you begin to understand that there are only so many botanicals to go around.

The solution is to focus on companies that are invested in either sustainable harvesting of their ingredients and/or "green chemistry." The concept of green chemistry was created by the EPA, and the 12 principles of green chemistry it drew up are centered around any number of issues that are really important to me: waste prevention, eliminating hazardous substances, preventing pollution, and increasing energy efficiency. I think we're going to see this field growing exponentially over the next few decades.

The Real Deal

If you want proof that the ingredients in your product are organic or natural, you'll need to look for some kind of a certification stamp. A number of organizations work very hard to make it easier for consumers to find the products they're looking for. They do the research so you don't have to.

Here are the most trusted labels to look for:

NSF

ORganic
certified
skin care

NSF/ANSI 305

NSF International is a public health and safety organization that develops standards, tests and certifies products to ensure they meet very strict regulatory standards in specific fields. Due to the explosion of the natural and organic skin care industry, they created an American national standard that specifies labeling and marketing requirements for the term "contains organic ingredients." Here's the thing: if a skin care or cosmetic product claims it is made with 95 to 100 percent organic ingredients, it can apply for the USDA organic certification, which is usually granted to food products only. Very few products meet the requirement, so NSF International came up with this certification, which considers the intricacy of skin care product formulations. With the NSF/ANSI 305 label, you can be assured that the product contains at least 70 percent organic ingredients. This also means that the product avoids a plethora of petroleum-based functional ingredients, such as preservatives.

NPA (The Natural Products Association)

This nonprofit organization has been around for years, and it certifies personal-care products that are 95 percent natural, allowing for only synthetic ingredients that are eco-friendly. You can visit their website at www.npainfo.org/NPA/NaturalSealCertification/NPANaturalStandardforPersonalCareProducts.aspx to find a list of ingredients they allow in products with their seal.

NATRUE

NATRUE (www.natrue.org/our-label) is a not for profit international organization. The NATRUE label offers three levels of certification, which include both natural and organic personal-care products. Their strict criteria specify that no petroleum or silicone-derived products can be used, and all ingredients must be non-GMO.

Soil Association

The UK's Soil Association encourages independent endorsement, providing companies with an organic seal if their products and ingredients are truly organic. The Soil Association logo is respected and trusted worldwide.

COSMOS
NATURAL

COSMOS Organic and Natural Standards

This is the newest cosmetic certification and it differs from the others in that the inspectors take a global approach, considering both the environmental and the human impact of the product. The COSMOS seal is internationally recognizable for natural and organic cosmetics, which is great because up until now the certifications in Europe have been quite different (and often more rigorous) from those in other countries. To get an organic certification, 95 percent of the ingredients must be organic. To get the natural certification, 100 percent of the ingredients must be of natural origin.

Do these labels mean the product with a certification is better than the one without? Again—not necessarily! In fact, many of my favorite companies don't use these certifications. It's useful to compare skin care companies to food companies in this respect. Just like beauty product producers, there are many food producers who use sustainable and responsible farming practices but don't have an organic certification. The reason might be that the certification process is too costly for the farmer or that the farm is focusing more effort on sustainability rather than on jumping through loopholes.

On the other hand, there are mega food companies that have purchased smaller organic companies and gotten them into mono-farming so they can drive down prices for big-box stores. This process may be cost-efficient, but it depletes the soil of valuable minerals and can lead to other negative impacts for the land. Would I rather buy lettuce from the latter company, which may not be thinking of the health of the soil, or from the dude at my farmers' market, who hand-picked his muddy, sustainably produced lettuces at 3 A.M. that day? It takes a bit more washing, but my farmers' market guy's lettuces taste like . . . well . . . lettuce. I make a similar comparison between some of the smaller skin care companies that focus all their budgets and attention on formulating outstanding products and those that fork out big dollars for packaging and marketing or use cheap ingredients to compete in big-box stores.

The takeaway is always to think of quality above everything else. Just like with food, you should buy the freshest, best skin care you can afford.

Protecting Our Furry Friends, Our Farmers, and Our Planet

Another set of labels will give you information on how many of your favorite products are manufactured and packaged. Again, you have to figure out if these considerations are important to you. And just like with the information about the ingredients earlier, just because a company doesn't have a seal on its products, it doesn't mean that they don't fit a seal's standards. The seals are simply easy ways to know if certain products match up with your values.

Leaping Bunny

I always look for cruelty-free certifications. I'm an animal lover, and it doesn't make sense to me to beautify myself with ingredients that have caused a furry friend to suffer in any way, shape, or form. I often visit the website of People for the Ethical Treatment of animals (www.peta.com) to see which companies have signed PETA's statement of assurance. PETA suggests that if a company you like is not on its list, you write or e-mail that company to ask the following questions:

- Does the company test its products, ingredients, or formulations on animals?

- Does it contract with an outside laboratory to conduct animal testing?

- If it does not use animal tests, does this decision reflect a permanent commitment to use only humane alternatives?

You can also look for the Leaping Bunny logo, which is the official stamp of approval from www.leapingbunny.org. This organization is composed of eight animal protection groups that have formed the Coalition for Consumer Information because they understand how hard it is to figure out if a product is cruelty-free or not. Thousands of products in the U.S. and Europe have the Leaping Bunny logo on their packaging, which assures no new animal testing on ingredients, formulations, or finished products.

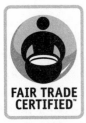

Fair Trade

I like to try to purchase from companies that use ingredients that are fair trade, meaning that the farmers who grow and harvest the crops are fairly compensated for their labor and that their working conditions meet certain basic standards. This certification often encompasses taking care of the environment, too. Ingredients such as shea butter, coconut oil, and red palm oil most often do not qualify for the Fair Trade Certified seal, so look for companies that are invested in taking care of their producers. Alaffia (www.alaffia.com), for example, was one of the first skin care companies to pledge that all its ingredients are fair trade, and it has continued to be an industry leader.

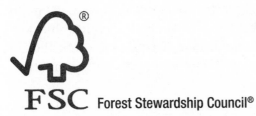

FSC Forest Stewardship Council®

I always look for paper packaging that carries the FSC® certification, because this means that the company uses paper from sustainably managed forests. Since skin care is, by and large, overpackaged, the least we can do is to vote with our dollars for companies that choose FSC-certified paper for their outer boxes and paper inserts.

Going Deeper into the Ingredients

Now that we've discussed some of the general ideas about ingredients and things you need to know about their classifications, I want to empower you with an even deeper level of information. And let me prepare you for the hard reality: it's really tricky to figure out what to avoid in skin care products, because for most of the ingredients involved, there is no clear-cut conclusion as to whether they are toxic or not—especially in the concentrations that are used in personal-care products.

Obviously, if an ingredient (such as formaldehyde) has been officially classed as a *known* carcinogen, I put it on the top of my "avoid" list, but most of the other ingredients, many of which have been vilified across the Internet (watch out for scaremongers), fall into more of a gray area.

I've realized that choosing which ingredients to avoid and which to allow is very personal and that there's no one right answer. Where some women might decide to use nothing other than plant oils and butters to avoid synthetic chemicals at all costs, others may want more "transitional" products. What I mean by this is that they want to avoid the worst offenders but don't mind some of the other ingredients that pose little to no health risk as far as peer-reviewed scientific studies have found—even though there are ample warnings out there from purists who don't trust any scientific studies.

Having spent years researching, often knee-deep in conflicting peer-reviewed studies and medical journals, I've put together a list of ingredients that I *try* to avoid in all my beauty products because they *might* combine with other ingredients to form possible carcinogens, or they may be endocrine disruptors. Notice that I use the word *might,* because there is a great deal of controversy about whether or not many of these chemicals are safe. I choose to adhere to the precautionary principle, which means that I try to avoid ingredients unless they have been, without any doubt, proven to be 100 percent safe when used long term.

It's important, however, to realize that one or two applications of products containing these ingredients is extremely unlikely to harm you; it's more about the cumulative effect from years of use. Moreover, many of them aren't kind to Mother Earth because they're not biodegradable, meaning that, like plastic, they hang around in the environment (polluting air, soil, and water) for hundreds of years.

What's an Endocrine Disruptor?

An *endocrine disruptor* is a synthetic chemical compound that mimics the hormone estrogen and is sometimes referred to as a "xenohormone" or a "xenoestrogen." Your endocrine system is a complex network of glands and hormones that regulate your bodily functions. Your endocrine glands release carefully measured amounts of hormones into your bloodstream that act as chemical messengers to make sure all of your body's organs operate as nature intended them to. Miraculous, right? Indeed. But an endocrine disruptor can mimic or block the natural activity of your own hormones and therefore disrupt your body's normal functions.

John Lee, M.D., coined the term *estrogen dominance* and was the first to bring this important issue to mainstream America. In his book *Dr. John Lee's Hormone Balance Made Simple,* he explains that estrogen imbalance is the main issue when we're talking about hormone imbalance. When there is too much estrogen in your system, you might become progesterone-deficient, which is a problem. Christiane Northrup, M.D., recognizes the following symptoms as signs of estrogen dominance: decreased sex drive, irregular periods, bloating, breast tenderness, fibrocystic breasts, mood swings, weight gain, cold hands and feet, hair loss, thyroid dysfunction, sluggish metabolism, foggy thinking or memory loss, fatigue, insomnia, and PMS. She also believes that estrogen dominance is linked to allergies, autoimmune disorders, breast and uterine cancer, ovarian cysts, and increased blood clotting.

So where do these xenoestrogens come from? Pretty much everywhere. Since World War II, more than 100,000 synthetic chemicals have been introduced into a hitherto more natural environment. Most are industrial chemicals that include fire retardants, pesticides, and herbicides. They get into our bodies in many different ways: from our food, our cleaning supplies, household chemicals and pesticides, and personal-care products. Unfortunately, we can't avoid them, but we can minimize our exposure by:

possible sources of endocrine disruptors

- Making sure the meat and dairy products we eat are organic
- Reducing or eliminating meat and dairy in our diets
- Switching to green cleaning and laundry products
- Avoiding pesticides in our foods, homes, and yards
- Avoiding non-BPA-free plastics
- Using paraben- and phthalate-free cosmetics
- Eating loads of fiber, because estrogen is excreted through our bowels

However, I am far from perfect in all of my choices. There's been many a time when I've used a shampoo, foundation, or volumizing mascara that contains less than desirable ingredients. When I do this, I remind myself that one or two applications won't strike me down. I also remind myself that I slathered nasty chemical formulations, including a foul-smelling body spray and hair lacquer that made my '80s hairdo as bulletproof as wire wool, all over my body through my teens and 20s—and I'm still living to tell the tale. So, again, be kind to yourself. No beating yourself over the head if you buy a product that doesn't meet all of your standards. No stressing so much about finding the perfect product that you either lose your mind or give up. Just do the best you can.

Unfortunately, there's no catchall list for ingredients you should absolutely avoid, since there's so much speculation involved. However, the following list names some of the ingredients I avoid or try to minimize. You will see instances where certain ingredients *could* combine with others to form possible carcinogens. In other cases, certain ingredients *could* be endocrine disruptors. However, many medical journals consider these combinations to be perfectly safe in the trace amounts in which they are added to personal-care products. Luckily, there are now hundreds, if not thousands, of companies that eliminate most of these risky ingredients, so we mercifully have choices.

- **BHA/BHT (butylated hydroxyanisole/butylated hydroxytoluene):** These two chemicals are synthetic antioxidants that are used to stabilize and help

24

preserve all kinds of food and cosmetic materials. There is a lot of controversy about whether or not BHA is a possible carcinogen, so I choose to avoid both of them. They can also cause allergic reactions. (Don't confuse this BHA with the valuable Beta Hydroxy Acids [BHAs] that I address later.)

- **Bismuth oxychloride:** This is a drying skin irritant that is often used in mineral powder makeup. I often wondered why my skin felt itchy and dry when I tried some well-known mineral powder makeups. I now understand that it was probably because of the bismuth, so I avoid it.

- **Coal tar dyes:** Coal tar dyes are synthetic and derived from petroleum. Many of them can be contaminated with heavy metals. (More information on heavy metals follows.) Where possible, I try to avoid D & C Red 2, 3, 4, 8, 10, 17, 19, and 33; Green 3 and 5; Orange 17; FD & C Blue 1, 2, and 4; Red 4 and 40; and Yellow 5 and 6.

- **DEA (diethanolamine), cocamide DEA, lauramide DEA, ETA (ethanolamine), MEA (monoethanolamine), and TEA (triethanolamine):** These ingredients are added to creams and foamy products to make sure they don't separate. They also adjust the pH in a product. The problem is that these ingredients can combine with nitrites in the formulation, which in turn creates carcinogenic nitrosamines. Also, cocamide DEA itself is a possible human carcinogen.

- **Formaldehyde-releasing chemicals including DMDM hydantoin, diazolidinyl urea, imidazolidinyl urea, methenamine, and quaternium-15:** These are preservatives that can interact with other chemicals to release formaldehyde, a known carcinogen and neurotoxin.

Although the amounts released are considered by many to be negligible, I play it safe because there are so many great alternatives.

- **Fragrance/parfum that includes DBP, DMP, or DEP:** Unless it's clearly stated that a formulation is fragranced with pure essential oils, it's likely that the fragrance cocktail, which is often made of hundreds of chemicals, will contain a class of hormone-disrupting chemicals called phthalates. DBP, DMP, and DEP are all phthalates and are sometimes listed as ingredients. If you adore the fragrance of a particular product, just pop the company an e-mail asking if its products are phthalate free. If they know their stuff, they should be able to tell you. Obviously, a mildly scented foundation or face cream isn't going to kill you, but it's better to look for products that are fragranced with pure essential oils instead.

- **Heavy metals (lead acetate, chromium, thimerosal, and sodium hexametaphosphate):** Heavy metals are generally found in makeup such as lipsticks and eye shadows, and they are a worry because they can be neurotoxins and hormone disruptors. I don't fancy the idea of these on my skin, however stunning the result of the products might be. Products containing hydrogenated cottonseed oil may also be contaminated with heavy metals.

- **Hydroquinone:** Found in skin lighteners and facial moisturizers, hydroquinone can cause irritation and has been restricted in Europe and Japan because it is a possible carcinogen.

- **Isopropyl alcohol:** This ingredient can be very drying, which means that it ages your skin more quickly and it can lead to irritation.

- **Nanoparticles:** These uniquely engineered, über-tiny ber-tiny particles may pose a health risk when brought into your body, either through inhalation or through application to the skin. Little is known about the long-term health effects of nanoparticles, as they're a relatively new science, so to err on the side of caution, avoid them where possible. If in doubt, ask a company if its products contain them.

- **Parabens (methyl-, ethyl-, propyl-, butyl-, and isobutylparaben):** You've probably heard of parabens, because they are now the most widely recognized endocrine disruptor. Some people also warn against these as carcinogenic; however, there is no conclusive scientific evidence to date that provides a causal link between parabens and any kind of cancer. What has been shown is that they most likely have weak estrogenic effects on humans.

- **Propylene and butylene glycols (also listed as "mineral oil"):** These are forms of mineral oil made from petroleum, which are used in foods, cleaning products, industrial products, and some skin care products. These mineral oil derivatives are effective at preventing moisture loss, and they make the product feel smooth (think of Vaseline, which is pure petroleum jelly). Aside from possible contamination with carcinogenic by-products, mineral oils can be comedogenic, meaning that they can clog up your pores. There are so many beautiful cold-pressed plant oils that do a better and healthier job, it makes no sense to buy products containing these cheap ingredients.

- **PVP/VA copolymer:** This film-forming chemical is found in hairspray. If you use it repeatedly (especially daily—hairstylists, watch out!), you could be putting yourself at risk of developing lung disease as a result of the propellants.

- **Siloxanes (cyclomethicone) and ingredients ending in "-siloxane":** These synthetic chemicals (cyclotetrasiloxane, for example) are used in moisturizers and hair products to soften, smooth, and moisten. They may be endocrine disruptors.

- **SLSs (sodium lauryl sulfate and sodium laureth sulfate):** These are foaming ingredients that may cause dryness and irritation and may also be endocrine disruptors. The biggest thing to note with these is that they can easily be contaminated with 1, 4-dioxane, which is a known carcinogen.

- **Stearalkonium chloride:** This chemical was developed by the fabric industry as a fabric softener, but it is now used in hair conditioners to impart a soft feel. I prefer to use botanicals and proteins that actually nourish my hair instead of a chemical that sits on top of it, masking dryness.

- **Talc:** There's a lot of scaremongering about the dangers of talc. These fears largely arose in response to the finding of tiny asbestos fibers in mined talc. However, today's laws require that any toxic metals be completely removed from all cosmetic talc. Some also believe there is a connection between talc and cancer (specifically lung and ovarian), but it is *extremely* controversial. Although the cancer connection has not been scientifically substantiated, you may wish to go talc free because a bunch of companies now offer wonderful, talc-free formulations. You also may want to ditch makeup with talc because it tends to block pores and just sit on top of your skin, which looks cakey.

- **Toluene:** This is a VOC (volatile organic compound), a compound that can "off-gas" toxic chemicals as it breaks down. Nail polish contains it unless otherwise stated.

- **Triclosan:** This little guy is found in deodorants, cleansers, and most antibacterial products such as hand and dish soap. It could be an endocrine disruptor and in some cases is irritating to the skin. The biggest worry for me is that the ubiquity of this ingredient in products across the board will contribute to an increase in superbugs (strains of bacteria that are resistant to antibiotics).

What's Up with Nanoparticles and Micronized Minerals?

There's a huge debate about the nanoparticles that may be lurking in your makeup and skin care and whether or not they can harm your health. Nanoparticles were developed for powder mineral makeup because the finer the particle, the silkier the finish.

A nanoparticle is defined as a particle between 1 and 100 nanometers (billionths of a meter) in diameter. Minerals are pulverized into particles that small. Nanoparticles, though, are different from the *micronized* minerals often found in "natural" sun protection, which are bigger—these measure between 100 and 300 nanometers.

There are two main health concerns when it comes to nanoparticles: The first is that they are so tiny that they could be absorbed into your skin, making their way into your bloodstream and causing internal damage. There is no evidence to date that micronized minerals can actually get beyond the layers of your skin. However, this particle technology is relatively new, so to err on the side of caution, you may want to avoid them. The second concern is that you can easily inhale both sizes of tiny particles. My common sense tells me that this is probably true. If you ever swirl a brush around in powder mineral makeup, you have to take great care that it doesn't dust more than just your face—those particles fly everywhere.

What about PEGs?

There's so much confusing information about PEG (polyethylene glycol). While some "experts" think of PEGs as the devil incarnate, much of the serious scientific research that I've uncovered leads me to understand that there is a big "it depends" here. PEGs are found in about 80 percent of beauty products. They act as emollients, emulsifiers, and penetration enhancers, and they always come with a number after them that shows their particular molecular weight. Typically, the lower the number (which ranges from 1 to 100), the better the product can be absorbed into your skin.

The main concern with respect to PEGs is their possible contamination with measurable amounts of 1,4-dioxane, which is a known carcinogen. However, dioxanes can be (and often are) removed in manufacturing. A company with a good, healthy track record tests the PEGs it uses to ensure that they are 1,4-dioxane free.

Another concern about PEGs is that they can help other ingredients drive deeper into your skin. This is only an issue, of course, if those "other" ingredients are harmful.

Finally, PEGs can irritate skin, but this is typically only a concern if your skin is highly sensitive or broken. My trusty peer-reviewed studies concluded that PEGs are safe for use in cosmetics but shouldn't be used on "damaged" skin (such as that of a burn victim). Actually, I would say that 90 percent of ingredients shouldn't be applied to burned or otherwise damaged skin.

There are a handful of incredibly good, clean formulations that contain PEGs, and the companies that make them have likely removed any contaminants. It's really your call on whether or not you choose to avoid them. I apply the 80/20 rule as far as PEGs are concerned: I avoid them wherever possible, choosing one product over another if it is PEG-free. However, if there is an occasional product that I am in love with, if the company has proven to me that it has a good, healthy track record, I may decide to buy/use the product in question.

The takeaway from all of this is that if you don't have broken skin and if the company has a really good track record of concern for consumer health, a few PEGs aren't going to harm you. If you're a purist, you can stay away; moreover, PEGs aren't necessary anymore. There are plenty of less risky and more effective ingredients that do the same job.

Different Place, Different Regulations

The European Union is way more safety conscious, cosmetically speaking, than the U.S. In the U.S., the FDA requires skin care companies to ensure that their products are safe but doesn't require any premarket testing. This means that the safety of your skin-lightening potion (or whatever) lies with the Cosmetic Ingredient Review (CIR) panel. This panel has found only 11 ingredients to be unsafe in cosmetic formulations, whereas the EU has banned 1,342 ingredients because of their links to cancer, birth defects, and reproductive harm. So, if you buy your cosmetics in the U.S., you've got to don your Sherlock Holmes hat and do a bit of research.

And What about Preservatives?

common preservative

Common preservatives in skin care products were the first ingredients to raise the red flag that all might not be well with our lotions and potions. Parabens were the first culprits to be dragged into the limelight for public scrutiny. A 2004 study found parabens in breast tumors; however, since then, no scientific proof has connected parabens with any kind of cancer. There is also a great deal of concern that some parabens might be xenoestrogens. Many argue that the minuscule amount of these compounds in our skin care products has a negligible effect, and they may be right. Although more research is needed, studies have found parabens to elevate estrogen levels, so I always play super safe with them. This is not to say that I freak out if a paraben comes into contact with my skin. Many of us have been using them for years with no ill effects, but as with most of these suspect chemicals, it's all about cumulative damage.

Beauty products must have really good preservatives or they'll go bad. Parabens are used in 90 percent of personal-care products because a very small amount prohibits the growth of mold, fungus, and bacteria. Parabens are added at very low concentrations and are popular because of the broad spectrum of microorganisms they cover. Conversely, a more natural preservative such as vitamin E may only affect as few as one type of microorganism, making it a bit dicey.

Many natural skin care companies now use a preservative called phenoxyethanol in place of parabens. There's a spirited debate among purists as to whether or not this preservative is safe. Here's my take: all your formulations need a really effective preservative, especially if you don't keep them in the fridge. If our skin care products are improperly preserved, bacteria, mold, and fungus can easily grow in them, and these organisms can cause your skin to become irritated or even infected. When phenoxyethanol is added to a formulation at one percent or less, scientific and toxicology reports deem it perfectly safe. Even the strict European Union has given it the thumbs-up. Remember: it's the dose that makes the poison.

The healthiest choice is to look for carefully formulated blends of essential oils, which will drive up the price of the product because they are way more expensive than broad-spectrum synthetics such as parabens. It's smart to ask a company whose products you are considering what blend they use, and more important, you should ask if all its products have been subject to preservative and stability challenge tests. Finally, they should be able to tell you the exact shelf life of each product both before and after opening. You can also inquire if the company recommends any specific storage specs to keep the products fresh for longer. I keep all of my skin care products in a mini-fridge in my bathroom (which my husband thinks is beyond bizarre) because it extends the shelf life considerably.

Yikes! Should I Stop Using Everything Now?

I've had so many e-mails from women freaking out about certain ingredients in their cosmetics, terrified that with a few more applications, they'll be struck down with a terrible disease. There's a lively and healthy debate about what we should avoid in our skin care products, but I have to emphasize again that you are not going to be in danger from one or two applications of any one ingredient.

When I wrote my first book, *Gorgeously Green*, in 2008, even the idea of unsafe ingredients in our skin care products was new and pretty shocking to most women. Since then, the knowledge has become commonplace; however, searching the Internet for information about what to avoid can be confusing and overwhelming—and the "information" is often wrong. Moreover, we now have well-intentioned guides, apps, and databases springing up that often supply outdated or inaccurate information. If you do find scaremongering information on the Internet, be on high alert, because the "research" behind it might be coming from a skin care company that's trying to frighten you as part of a sales pitch, or from a database that needs updating.

There is a good reason that many companies use certain ingredients that I might not love. For example, parabens are very effective broad-spectrum preservatives that are ostensibly safe at the low concentrations found in cosmetics and skin care products. Parabens and ingredients such as mineral oils are also cheaper than pure essential oil blends and cold-pressed plant oils used as preservatives. So, one downside to choosing fewer synthetic ingredients is that products cost more.

One of the scariest words linked to certain personal-care ingredients is *carcinogen*, right? It doesn't matter whether it's a "possible," "probable," or "known" carcinogen—if there's any link, however tiny, I don't want it near my bathroom cabinet. However, in my research, I've come to understand that there is a huge difference between *possible* carcinogens and *known* carcinogens. To put the point in perspective, the World Health Organization has determined that electromagnetic fields, including those connected with cell phones, are *possible* carcinogens. Does this concern me? Heck, yes! Am I going to stop using my cell phone anytime soon? No! Not until the threat is upgraded to the "probable" category . . . and even then, I'll still use the phone, but I will be religious about using that hollow, tubular earpiece device currently hiding in the bottom of my horrendously messy kitchen drawer. So, in short, you need to look at the spectrum of concern. Don't jump to conclusions when you hear the word *carcinogen* unless you want to avoid a solid portion of all products on earth.

It's useful to evaluate how much of a purist you want to be before you decide what to change about your beauty regimen. Over the years, I've realized that I have friends on one end of the scale who don't really care what's in a skin care product as long as it works, and I have friends on the other end who freak out at the mere mention of anything that isn't a cold-pressed plant oil. I stand somewhere in the middle, embracing the amazing advances of science while being hugely mindful of my health and the environment. I'm also acutely aware that some women have very good reason to be über-vigilant about ingredients in their personal-care products. Many of my readers have had to make big changes in their beauty routines because of their health. They may have had a scary diagnosis, a compromised immune system, or a growing sensitivity to chemicals. Incidentally, many women (including myself) get more sensitive to chemicals as we age. If you are facing a health challenge right now or if you are pregnant, I suggest you err on the side of caution and follow my suggestions of what to avoid to the T.

Ingredient List Tip

Always check out the ingredient list of any cosmetic on the company's website before you head to the store. If there isn't one there, a little Internet research should pull up a full list. Yep, thank goodness for all those obsessive beauty bloggers who snap photos of ingredient lists on the backs of boxes for us all to see.

How to Read an Ingredient List

I wish shopping for beauty products were as simple as deciding to be vegan and never going near a piece of meat ever again, but it's way more complicated—largely due to the fact that we are subject to the health-washing and green-washing marketing tactics of giant cosmetic companies with their myriad "proprietary" formulas. If a product has a fancy, proprietary formula with a fancy trademarked name, you'll rarely be able to find out which ingredients make up the concoction, because it's a trade secret.

It's also not as simple as declaring that you won't eat anything or apply anything to your skin that you can't pronounce. I can't easily recognize or pronounce 80 percent of skin care ingredients that I love. For example, acetyl hexapeptide and magnesium ascorbyl phosphate are both beautiful, proactive ingredients found in some of my favorite formulas. This is why I think it's simpler to look at the company or brand as a whole rather than try to decipher *every individual* ingredient, the effort of which will drive you crazy. The most important thing is that the company's website provide you with a *full* ingredient list. Many companies just show us their "key" ingredients, which I don't love. I want full exposure so I can make an informed choice by going through my checklists before purchasing.

If you work by the guidelines below and look into the company making the products, you'll be on solid footing.

Red Flag Ingredients: If I spot any of these on a label, the formulation probably won't do me any favors.

- DEA, TEA, MEA
- BHA/BHT
- DMDM hydantoin
- Triclosan
- Coal tar dyes: D & C Red 2, 3, 4, 8, 10, 17, 19, and 33; Green 3 and 5; Orange 17; FD & C Blue 1, 2, and 4; Red 4 and 40; and Yellow 5 and 6

- Lead acetate, chromium, thimerosal, sodium hexametaphosphate (heavy metals—which can even be found in hydrogenated cottonseed oil)

- Aluminum (heavy metal)

- Quaternium-15, bronopol, imidazolidinyl or diazolidinyl urea, germall II or 115.

- Stearalkonium chloride (in hair conditioner and some creams)

- PVP/VA copolymer (in hairspray)

- Hydroquinone (in skin-lightening products)

- Nanoparticles (typically used in antiaging products, sunscreens, and mineral makeup)

Orange Flag Ingredients: I try to avoid these where possible because I know that, although they won't harm me short term, years of repetitive application could pose a health risk that I'd rather not take.

- Fragrance/Parfum (unless confirmed phthalate free)

- Propylene and butylene glycols (also listed as mineral oil, liquidum paraffinum, paraffin wax, paraffin oil, petrolatum)*

- Parabens (methyl-, ethyl-, propyl-, butyl-, and isobutylparabens)

- PEGs

try to avoid

Yellow Flag Ingredients: I use or avoid these on a case-by-case basis. If the company has a good track record of watching out for consumer health, I figure that its use of these ingredients is unlikely to harm me. Are there better alternatives? Absolutely! But if an otherwise great formulation has a sprinkling of one or two of these ingredients in it, it doesn't unduly concern me. My caveat is that if you have broken or inflamed skin, I recommend steering away from these ingredients, too.

- Dimethicone*
- Phenyoxyethanol (preservative)*
- Isopropyl alcohol

* Green Purist: If you are a green purist—and kudos to you if you are—you should avoid all of the ingredients on the red, orange, and yellow lists, particularly the ones that I've marked with a star, because these are not biodegradable and thus not great for the environment.

Green Light Ingredients: If I spot these in a product, I'm probably on to a good thing. Note that this is only a partial list. You will find much more detailed lists of ingredients to look for on pages 96 and 102–103.

- Aloe vera leaf
- Coconut oil
- Shea, mango, and cocoa butter
- Rose hip seed, borage, carrot seed, and sea buckthorn oil
- Vegetable glycerin
- Oat beta glucan
- Green or white tea
- Zinc oxide

Other Label Reading Tips

Now that you know a bit more about some ingredients to avoid, I want to give you just a few hints about other things to think about when you're looking over a label. You'll see that some companies can be very sneaky about what's actually in their products. But you're smarter than them!

Check the Order *FIRST 3 ingredients = 90-95% of product*

Once you find the ingredient list, it's key to look at the order in which the ingredients are listed—this way, you can be sure that you are getting enough of the good stuff. Know that the first three or four ingredients make up 90 to 95 percent of the entire product. The midsection of the list (which is often composed of a bunch of emulsifiers, surfactants, binders, softeners, and fillers) is roughly 5 to 8 percent of the product, and the last five or so ingredients make up the remaining 1 to 3 percent.

Let's look at this ingredient list for an organic, antiaging moisturizer that I love:

> Water, Mangifera indica (Mango) butter, Aloe barbadensis leaf juice*, Carthamus tinctorius (Safflower) oleosomes*, Caprylic/Capric Triglyceride (derived from coconut), Olea europea (Olive) oil*, Glycerin, Hamamelis virginiana (Witch Hazel) distillate, Oryza sativa (Rice) extract*, Rosa damascena flower water*, Simmondsia chinensis (Jojoba) seed oil*, Cetearyl olivate (derived from olives), Leuconostoc ferment filtrate (radish root extract), Raw honey, Sodium hyaluronate, Theobroma cacao (Cocoa) butter, Menyanthes trifoliata (Buckbean) flower extract, Salix alba (Willow) bark extract*, Medicago sativa (Alfalfa) flower*, Borago officinalis flower*, Calendula officinalis flower*, Filipendula ulnaria leaf & flower*, Tilia europaea (Linden) leaf & flower*, Lavandula stoechas (Spanish Lavender) extract, Arnica montana flower*, Aloe barbadensis leaf juice powder*, Galactoarabinan (gum derived from larch tree), Sclerotium gum (derived from root vegetables & corn), Sorbitan olivate (wax derived from olives), Cetyl palmitate (wax derived from olives), Sorbitan palmitate (wax derived from soy), Soy peroxidase (derived from soy), Superoxide dismutase (derived from horseradish root), Essential oil blend from clinical grade essential oils: Benzyl salicylate, Citronellol, Eugenol, Farnesol, Geraniol, Limonene, Linalool. ***organic ingredients**

As you can see, the ingredient is listed by its International Nomenclature of Cosmetic Ingredients (INCI) name first and then its more commonly recognized form in parentheses. In the above label, the first six ingredients—water, mango butter, aloe leaf juice, safflower, coconut, and olive oil—make up the lion's share of the formulation. The last ingredients on a list (for instance, the essential oil blend, here made up of the last seven ingredients) are added in very small (and in some cases trace) amounts.

Here's an ingredient list for a leading drugstore brand's antiaging cream:

> Water, Glycerin, Isohexadecane, Niacinamide*, Isopropyl Isostearate, Aluminum Starch Octenylsuccinate, Nylon-12, Dimethicone, Panthenol**, Tocopheryl Acetate***, Sodium Hyaluronate, Palmitoyl Pentapeptide-4^, Camellia Sinensis Leaf Extract^^, Aloe Barbadensis Leaf Juice^^^, Allantoin, Stearyl Alcohol, Polyethylene, Cetyl Alcohol, Sodium Acrylates Copolymer, Behenyl Alcohol, Benzyl Alcohol, Acrylamide/Sodium Acryloyldimethyltaurate Copolymer, Dimethiconol, Sodium Peg-7 Olive Oil Carboxylate, Peucedanum Graveolens (Dill) Extract, Peg-100 Stearate, Stearic Acid, Disodium Edta, Cetearyl Glucoside, Cetearyl Alcohol, Citric Acid, C12-13 Pareth-3, Laureth-7, C13-14 Isoparaffin, Sodium Hydroxide, Caprylic/Capric Triglyceride, Ethylparaben, Methylparaben, Propylparaben, Fragrance, Titanium Dioxide, Mica. ***Vitamin B3, **Pro-Vitamin B5, ***Vitamin E, ^Amino-Peptide, ^^Green Tea, ^^^Aloe Vera**

As you can see, the first three ingredients are: water, glycerin, and isohexadecane (a petroleum-derived ingredient that makes the formulation feel creamy). The fourth ingredient, aluminum starch octenylsuccinate, is a thickening and anticaking agent. Although there's nothing that would kill you in this formulation, it won't nourish your skin in the same way as the previous product. Also note that the green tea, which is near the end of the list, is in only a teeny amount, which is a shame, because green tea is a powerful antioxidant. And this brings me to my next hint.

Look Out for Fairy Dusting

"Fairy dusting" is a sneaky little trick that many personal-care companies try to hoodwink us with. They "dust" the ingredient list with a few great-sounding ingredients such as green tea and aloe vera, but we are talking about a few *negligible* sprinkles. As a general rule of thumb, see what ingredients make up the lower third of the label; anything in it is likely to appear in only minuscule amounts, yet the company may tout these ingredients as "key" or focus all its marketing efforts around it. It may extol the "benefits of green tea!" or whatever other ridiculously negligible antioxidant amount they've thrown in there.

Don't Be Fooled by the Front of the Label

I despise having to look at the small print on anything now because it necessitates a pair of reading glasses, which I never have on hand. So, if you're just picking up something and hoping for the best, at least don't be hoodwinked by the verbiage on the front of the container.

These are terms like I mentioned at the beginning of the chapter, *natural* being the biggest offender for misleading consumers. There are no regulations associated with this particular term. Also watch out for any company that uses the word *organic* in the name of a product. Any maker is well within its rights to call a company or product "Organic Heaven" or "Organic Elixirs," but the product might include only two minuscule organic ingredients in a sea of junk.

Putting It All Together

I know I've given you a lot of information in this chapter, so I wanted to pull it all together at the end in a crib sheet of how to choose a product.

Here are the considerations I recommend:

- **Health:** Is this product healthy, or could it harm me?
- **Effectiveness:** Do the product's ingredients deeply nourish my skin, or do they just make my skin *feel* good for a few minutes?

- **Freshness:** Are the vitamins and antioxidants still good (is the product fresh)? I always check to see if the company mass-produces and ships internationally (which requires a super-long shelf life), or if the product is more locally produced in small batches.

- **Environment:** Is the manufacture of this product good or bad for the environment? I pay attention to the packaging, making sure that it's as minimal and as eco as possible.

- **Ethics:** Does the company I'm considering buying from have good, ethical practices? Does it treat its workers well and pay them a fair wage? Does it give back in any way? Are the products cruelty-free?

- **Finance:** Does the product seem reasonably priced? If it's expensive, do the high-quality/specialized ingredients justify the cost? Is it within my budget to splurge?

Some of us might only consider the cost of an item, whereas others may take a firm stand for the environment or their personal health. Having established what is important to you, you can then zoom in to product specifics:

- First, scan for **ingredients to avoid**. You can refer to my checklists of those I don't love. If you spot one or two to avoid, you might want to move on to another brand.

- If you're satisfied that the product is on the right track, it's time to look at its **full list of ingredients**. A list of "key" ingredients isn't enough information. You need the whole list, and if it's not included on the package or website, move on.

- Be mindful of **fairy dusting** when reading the ingredient list. You want to see if the brand is trying to hoodwink you by dusting in a few good-sounding ingredients at the *end* of the list.

- Check the **preservative system** of the product. The best choice is a blend of pure essential oils.

- Check for a **sell-by date** and/or any information about when the product might expire after opening.

The Good News

We've covered a lot here—good and bad. Hopefully, you feel a bit more prepared to choose products that are good for you and the environment. The good news is that thanks to market pressures and informed consumers, we can now buy and make beauty products that are not only healthy and nourishing for our skin, but also extremely effective. Although there is no miracle antiaging lotion or potion to date, we can combine the best of what science and nature offer to renew and revitalize our skin, hair, and nails.

The even better news is that if you continue to affirm that you are a beautiful, empowered woman, with or without lotions and potions, the rest is just the icing on the cake—and I'm never averse to a generous dollop of creamy frosting, especially if it's healthy and organic.

Chapter 2

Gorgeously Clean Makeup

(Foundation, Concealer, Powder, Eyes)

I absolutely adore makeup. It always makes me feel better about myself, and I make no apologies for this. Although we're told that women cover up their insecurities with makeup, I think the opposite is often true: a woman who feels bad about herself gives up on taking care of herself. She doesn't feel that she's worth spending time or money on. I think the perfect balance is to be able to look into your eyes and see the beautiful person that you really are *and* to enjoy making that beautiful person look even more gorgeous by way of some serious primping. It's all about simply making the best of what you've got.

Women have been accentuating their features for thousands of years. The Egyptians were the first to use kohl, a thick eyeliner, to make their eyes pop. Other cultures paint their faces with stripes or incredible patterns. A study by Richard Russell at Gettysburg College found that women look younger and more attractive when their features are differentiated from the rest of their faces; in particular, when their eyes are made darker and their lips redder. Hmmm, I look terrible in red lipstick . . . but that's probably because I'm very fair, and I'm not 20 anymore. However, I think we can all agree that no matter the shades you choose, accentuating lips, eyes, and cheekbones is never a bad thing.

As I've already mentioned, when I take the time to style my hair and apply makeup, I feel about 200 percent better about myself, and way more ready to face the day. Conversely, on a day when I lounge around in my sweats and stick my hair into a messy ponytail, it makes me feel lethargic, and I want to hibernate rather than hurl myself into the flow of life. I'm a firm believer that if I take an action the polar opposite of what I *feel* like doing, the rest will follow. On those mornings when I feel a bit off, if I wash my hair and apply beautiful makeup, it can completely alter my mood. I so agree with makeup doyenne Bobbi Brown, founder of her namesake cosmetic line, when she says about using makeup, "We are able to transform ourselves, not only how we are perceived, but how we feel."

Beauty as Skin Care

Before I jump into the specifics of how to choose and apply products to beautify your exterior, I want to talk about a huge change that I've seen gradually evolve over the last decade or so. Nowadays, companies are realizing that women want cosmetics that are good for our skin. We no longer want to use products that are like toxic paint. Jane Iredale, who was one of the first to come up with the concept of makeup that's good for your skin, created her mineral makeup line over two decades ago. Having worked for years in the entertainment industry, she woke up one night and realized that this was the way forward—that models, actresses, and regular women shouldn't be plastering their skin with unhealthy ingredients in order to look gorgeous. Iredale Mineral Cosmetics now sells its ever-expanding line in 48 countries across the globe.

Many others have followed in Iredale's path, and now there are more "healthy" mineral makeup companies than I could ever keep up with. This is why I bring up the shift in ingredient interest: now you have more options than ever for finding the perfect products for you. However, you still have to be a little wary about whom you buy from; the "contains nourishing ingredients" marketing ploy can mislead consumers even of mineral makeup.

I was in a department store the other day, and as an experiment, I asked the sales assistant of a very well-known brand what was in its "age defying with organic botanicals" foundation formulation. She assured me that the product was chock full of natural antiaging ingredients, including shea butter. When her back was turned, I whipped out my readers and scrutinized the ingredient list to see exactly what all these antiaging ingredients might be, and I can assure you that the minuscule amount of shea butter floated in a sea of toxic and inflammatory ingredients. There was nothing antiaging about this formulation whatsoever.

Hero Products

In my almost ten years as a natural-beauty editor, I've discovered one thing to be true: it's best to pick different products from different companies. I very rarely get *all* my products from a single company, because they all have their strengths and weaknesses. I've made the mistake before of assuming that because lipsticks from a certain company are fantastic, their foundations will also be awesome. Not so!

Prepping for Beauty

Before we jump into discussing makeup itself, I want to talk about something that I feel is essential for applying makeup well: brushes. If you are going to invest in any cosmetic item, it should be a good-quality brush—or, really, brushes. Though there is a huge price discrepancy between drugstore makeup brushes and those you can find in a high-end department store or beauty supply shop, more expensive doesn't always mean better. However, I have consistently found that not only do the really cheap ones perform poorly, but they also almost always fall apart, leaving large, black hairs stuck to my makeup. So, while you don't have to spend oodles of money on brushes, go perhaps a step up from the cheapest versions.

I always buy vegan brushes at a medium price point. I really don't want to pay what I'd spend on a pair of shoes for an eyeliner brush, but I do understand that a good-quality brush will last me for up to ten years if I take care of it.

The ten most important brushes to invest in are:

1. A foundation-blending brush

2. A big, soft, silky powder brush

3. A blush brush

4. A flat eye shadow brush

5. An angled eye shadow contouring brush

6. A flat, angled eyeliner brush

7. A soft, silky eye shadow blending brush

8. A Kabuki brush (if you use powder mineral makeup)

9. An under-eye concealer brush

10. A duo eyebrow and shadow brush with a spoolie brush on the other end (to brush out your lashes and brows). I like to purchase a two-in-one brush, for ease of use, and it's great when I travel.

How to Care for Your Brushes

Once you've made the investment in good brushes, it's really important to care for them properly. You should clean, condition, and sanitize your brushes every week. I have tried many different DIY recipes with varying results. Ironically, the most important brush to clean is your foundation brush. But it's often the hardest to clean because of the oils in the foundation.

Here are some of my favorite cleaning tips for foundation and concealer brushes:

- Put a dab of liquid Castile soap in a cup of warm water. Soap up the brush, rinse well, and leave it to air dry.

- Some people like to use a little vegetable oil because it helps to pull the oils out of the brush, but I don't love the residue it leaves.

- To sanitize the brush, try using rubbing alcohol. Pour a little onto a paper towel and swirl your brush over it.

- For a stronger solution, look for a nontoxic brush cleaner such as Mona Lisa Pink Soap.

All your other cosmetic brushes should be way easier to clean than your foundation or concealer brushes, because most shadows, blushes, powders, and bronzers do not contain oil or water, which is where the bacteria can take hold. A simple weekly wash with warm water and some Mona Lisa Pink Soap should do the trick for those.

I also keep a square of recycled paper towel next to me when I am doing my makeup and dust off each brush after use.

Bacteria-Prevention Tip for Lipsticks and Lip and Eye Pencils

Keep a bottle of rubbing alcohol in your bathroom cabinet. Every now and again, soak a sheet of paper towel in the alcohol and wipe off the tops of eyeliner and lip pencils. You can also wipe off the tips of lipsticks. The alcohol will kill any bacteria that might be hanging around.

Creating Your Base

The first step in making yourself up is to create the perfect base. You can't paint a masterpiece on an uneven canvas—and the same holds true for your makeup efforts. To create a smooth base, most women reach for a tinted moisturizer, a tinted sunblock, or a BB cream even before they pull out their foundation brush. Do you really need to prime your skin with any of these formulas before you get to the covering-up stage? It depends on what you want to achieve. For some women, it may be a polished, beautifully made-up look; for others, it may be just a sun-kissed glow. You now have a plethora of choices available so you can create exactly what you want.

Here's some information about the most popular prefoundation steps you could choose to use:

Primer: Do you really need a primer under your base? It's totally a matter of preference. Contrary to what many sales assistants would have you believe, your makeup will not cake into your wrinkles or slide off your face if you don't use a primer. However, the silicones in most of them can create a velvety base for foundation. Some purists don't like silicones because they ostensibly coat your skin, sealing in bacteria. However, many women love the silky feel, and silicone products don't seem to break them out. I personally think there's a place for silicones in primers and foundations, and I use them as needed. I will say, however, that I don't love 99 percent of the ingredients in most popular primers. So, when considering one, check its ingredients against my lists.

Tinted Moisturizer: Many women love to use a tinted moisturizer in place of a foundation. Typically, tinted moisturizers contain a little pigment for color, and in some cases, a sprinkling of light-reflecting minerals. Formulas vary so much in moisture, coverage, and color that you really do need to experiment to find one that works well for you. You can also use a good tinted moisturizer as a primer to give you just a bit of color before you apply your foundation.

BB Balm/Cream: The concept of BB (aka blemish or beauty balm) cream came from Korea, and it's ingenious. It's typically a five-in-one product that contains moisturizer, blemish treatment, primer, sunscreen, and foundation. Many women love BB cream because it dramatically cuts down on the steps in their morning routine. However, as with all cosmetics, not all BB creams or balms are created equal, so do your research.

- **The Good:** A healthy-formula BB cream can be a super-efficient single product. Some of my favorite formulas contain hyaluronic acid, blemish-controlling essential oils, light-reflecting mineral pigments, and a physical, mineral sunblock.

- **The Bad:** Don't assume that a so-called treatment balm contains all healthy ingredients. I'm horrified by the ingredients in many mainstream BB cream brands. Be extra vigilant about your label-reading. If this one product is going to take the place of five other products, you need to be sure that it's all good.

CC Cream: CC cream arrived hot on the heels of BB cream. CC means "color correcting," and in theory it's a smart idea; however, for the most part, it's just a marketing ploy to get you to try yet another product. Color-correcting pigment in makeup is not a new concept. There are green pigments in some foundations to counteract redness, orange pigments to counteract hyperpigmentation, and lavender or violet to correct dull or sallow complexions. These color correctors are also used in primers and concealers. Many top makeup artists agree that you can't just color correct with one do-all product—we need multiple makeup products, techniques, and tools to create the desired effect because we don't all need the same corrections.

- On a similar note, many companies are trying to cash in on the BB and CC trend with "DD" ("do"-all) creams. Goodness knows what other abbreviations are coming down the pike. Just be extremely wary of fads and marketing hype and save your money. It seems good in theory to have one product that does it all, but I'm skeptical, especially if a product tells me that I literally don't need anything else. The other problem with these "multifunctional" products is that they seem to assume that we all have the same skin. Most of us need to cherry-pick products to suit our particular concerns.

Choosing Your Foundation

Foundation has come a long way since Max Factor introduced the concept in the 1930s. Up until then, only actresses of stage and screen used foundation. In silent movies, it was greasepaint. When Technicolor film arrived, the actresses were appalled to see that greasepaint makeup looked terrible under its lights. Thus, Max Factor invented his matte Pan-Cake makeup, which he subsequently marketed to the public, telling people that they, too, could look like movie stars. Pan-Cake was the fastest-selling product in the cosmetics industry. Max Factor also coined the word *makeup* for products that up until that point had just been called cosmetics.

Pan-Cake and all the foundations that evolved over the next five to six decades weren't particularly good for the skin, and many contained toxic, aging ingredients. It's only in the past couple of decades, starting with visionaries like Jane Iredale, that foundations have taken a turn for the good. A few decades ago, we didn't really care. Foundation was foundation, and it didn't need to have any function other than to create a blank canvas that would helpfully smooth out imperfections. Now we want our foundation to be good for our skin, too.

As formulas have become more and more sophisticated, building in not only light-reflecting pigments but also antioxidants and sunscreen, we have been able to achieve a much more natural-looking effect while taking care of our skin at the same time. The line is blurring between foundations and BB creams as more and more companies add all kinds of functional ingredients to foundation formulas.

Choosing a foundation is something of a science, and I highly recommend you take the time to make sure you get exactly what you want before you commit.

Here are the questions you need to ask yourself when choosing a foundation:

- What is my skin type? Is it oily, combination, or dry/mature?
- What kind of coverage do I want?
- What's my shade?
- How much time do I want to spend on my makeup?
- Do I prefer a liquid, stick, cream, or mineral powder?

Let's examine each of these questions in detail.

What's my shade? This is almost the most important question, because the wrong shade can obviously be a disaster.

Your best bet is to visit the beauty store with a large magnifying mirror in your purse. Apply a dab of foundation to your jawline, and use a little cosmetic wedge to blend it into your neck. Walk outside the store into natural daylight and inspect the shade in your mirror. If it seems to be the right shade, apply it to your whole face. This is important, because we sometimes go for a lighter shade that matches our necks, but when we do full makeup, it ends up looking way too pale. I often decide to go one shade darker than I've tested when I've seen my whole face made up, because I like a bit of warmth.

Buying foundation online is obviously more challenging with respect to shade. Definitely ask for samples.

What's my skin type? This is the first question that you'll be asked at the beauty counter, and it is important because you'll be guided to either an oil-free or a moisturizing foundation. However, it's actually more important to know what look you are trying to achieve.

For example, I have dry skin, but the kind of super-hydrating formula I'm likely to be guided toward is often too creamy for TV, and I don't want a foundation that I have to heavily powder to dull its shine. So, although my skin type should be taken into account, I always start with the end result I'm looking for: a natural-looking base that will moisturize my skin without adding too much oil.

Conversely, if you have oily skin, you may want to avoid a foundation that has too matte a finish and leaves you looking dry and powdery. Most large companies offer a few different foundation types (for oily or dry skin, for example) to cover their bases, while smaller companies may only offer a single kind. In either case, it's vital to sample a foundation. Leave it on for a full day so that you can see if it winds up making you look too powdery or oily.

What kind of coverage do I want? You may need two different foundations: one for a natural, daytime look, and one for going out. Sales assistants will tell you that you can always "build" a foundation for extra coverage, which means that you can add another layer on top of the one that you've just applied, but I prefer to use two different foundations: a lighter one for day and a heavier one for evening.

Many lines carry long-lasting foundations, which are designed to go from day to night. These formulas tend to be much thicker or heavier, so you need to apply them sparingly to avoid a Kabuki-actor look.

How much time do I want to spend on my makeup? If you are a low-maintenance girl, you might want to use a BB cream in place of a foundation. Or choose a foundation with a high SPF (25 or beyond) so that you can skip at least one separate step.

Do I prefer a liquid, stick, cream, or mineral powder? Your lifestyle and skin type will determine which form of foundation you use. For example, if you are always on the road, you might choose a stick, a cream compact, or a pressed mineral foundation. However, if you like to do a full makeover in your bathroom every morning and have drier skin, you might be better off with a liquid mineral foundation.

Less Is More

As we get older, we often think we need a heavier foundation to cover irregularities and brown spots; however, thicker foundations can make us look way older than we are. If you have deep wrinkles, a lighter-bodied foundation plus a concealer to even out your skin tone where needed is the best way to go.

The Myth of Mineral Makeup

Before I jump into discussing the pros and cons of different types of foundations, I want to take a moment to debunk a common perception of one popular variation: mineral makeup.

Almost all makeup can technically be called "mineral" makeup because it is likely to contain minerals such as titanium dioxide, zinc oxide, mica, iron oxides, and bismuth oxychloride. *Mineral makeup* is a marketing term that leads consumers to believe the makeup they're purchasing is probably healthier, but it's simply not true. There can be a massive difference between mineral makeups: some have healthy ingredients, but others are full of potential toxins and irritants.

Take a look at the two ingredient lists below, which are from the bottles of different liquid mineral foundations:

Water, Cyclopentasiloxane, Butylene Glycol, Cetyl Peg/ Ppg-10/1/Dimethicone, Squalane, Triethylhexanoin, Isononyl

Isononanoate, Polyglyceryl-4 Isostearate, Caprylic/Capric Triglyceride, Peg-32, Dimethicone/Vinyl Dimethicone Crosspolymer, Disteardimonium Hectorite, Methicone, Polymethyl Methacrylate, Propylene Glycol, Retinyl Palmitate, Tocopheryl Acetate, Disodium Edta, Sodium Dehydroacetate, Phenoxyethanol, Methylparaben, Ethylparaben, Propylparaben, Butylparaben. (May Contain: Titanium Dioxide, Iron Oxides.)

Aqua/Water/Eau, Titanium Dioxide (Ci 77891), Glycerin, Algae, Sodium Hyaluronate, Avena Sativa (Oat) Kernel Extract, Glyceryl Polymethacrylate, Salix Nigra (Willow) Bark Extract, Calendula Officinalis Flower Oil, Camellia Sinensis (White Tea) Leaf Extract, Aloe Barbadensis Leaf Juice, Raphanus Sativus (Radish) Root Extract, Chondrus Crispus (Carrageenan) Extract, Hyaluronic Acid, Magnesium Ascorbyl Phosphate (Vitamin C), Squalane, Ubiquinone (Coenzyme Q10), Boron Nitride, Stearic Acid. [+/- (May Contain) Mica, Iron Oxides (Ci 77489, Ci 77491, Ci 77492, Ci 77499), Chromium Oxide Greens (Ci 77288)]

The first list contains loads of cheap, unhealthy mineral oils and preservatives. The second contains all kinds of healthy and nourishing ingredients, including algae, hyaluronic acid, calendula, and so on.

Although it's not going to kill you to use the foundation with the first ingredient list, it would be way better for the health of your skin to go for the ingredients in the second.

Also, watch out for an ingredient in many mineral foundations called bismuth oxychloride, which is not a naturally occurring mineral. It's very popular in makeup because it imparts a shimmery glow to the skin, but it can also cause itchiness and skin irritation.

Comparing Foundations

To help you choose the best foundation for you, I want to discuss a little bit about each of the four most common forms of foundation: mineral powder, liquid, cream, and stick. Figuring out what works best for you is often just a process of trial and error, but the information here will give you a good place to start.

Pros of Mineral Powder Makeup: If you find a good brand that doesn't contain bismuth oxychloride or the nanoparticles we discussed in the last chapter, mineral powder could be a great choice for you if you have acne, rosacea, or very sensitive skin. Because of the dry formulation, a pure mineral makeup will likely not contain preservatives, propylene glycol (which is petroleum derived), mineral oil, dye, or fragrance. Many women who break out or who are way too sensitive for liquid and cream foundations love a mineral powder.

You will find mineral powder foundation in either a pressed compact or a loose-powder shaker jar. One is not better than the other; it's just a matter of personal preference. Mineral powder makeup also contains titanium dioxide and zinc oxide, which provide a physical sunblock. The SPF is debatable (usually around 15 to 20), so it's fine for running errands, but if you are going to be in full sun, you will still need a full-spectrum sunscreen underneath.

Cons of Mineral Powder Makeup: Unless you apply it very carefully, you can inhale the airborne particles of mineral powder. Even if they are non-nano, these particles can irritate your respiratory system. If you're wondering whether or not the product you're interested in has nanoparticles, you can always ask the company. Another concern about powder mineral makeup is that it can be too drying for women with dry or mature skin. Some companies offer a hydrating setting mist, which can help a lot with the finish, but if you have dry or mature skin, you may be better off with a liquid or cream formula.

Pros of Liquid Foundation: Liquid foundation is often the best choice for a beautiful, finished look. It is buildable, so you can choose your level of coverage from medium to full. You will always be able to find the perfect shade, consistency, and finish for your particular skin because there is such a huge choice in this foundation category. Good liquid foundations are also formulated with great antiaging ingredients, so you'll know that they don't harm your skin—hopefully, they're even doing some good. Liquid *stop from skin Vu drying out.*

foundations can also contain highly moisturizing ingredients such as hyaluronic acid, which will stop your skin from drying out.

Cons of Liquid Foundation: It can be tricky to find a formulation that works for you in terms of the exact right coverage, shade, and texture in one brand, so samples are definitely required. You need a brush or sponge to apply your foundation, which can add a bit of work to your beauty routine because you'll need to wash the brush regularly or switch out the sponge. Foundation bottles can be a bit messy, so they aren't great for travel.

Pros of Cream Foundation: Most cream foundations come in a refillable compact or a stick. You will also find that many are cream-to-powder foundations, meaning that they go on as a cream and dry to a soft, velvety powder. The coverage tends to be light to medium. Cream foundations are great for makeup touch ups and perfect for travel, especially when they come in a stick. I like some of the ingredients that I'm beginning to see in cream foundations, such as shea butter and various antioxidants, which make them double as a skin treat.

Cons of Cream Foundation: You generally don't get as good or precise a coverage as you would with a liquid foundation. Some of the "moisturizing" cream foundations tend to be a bit greasy, and the cream-to-powder can end up being too dry for mature skin.

Nano Labeling

In the U.S., there is currently no mandatory labeling for the use of nanoparticles in a formulation. Conversely, in the EU, every product is subject to a safety assessment before it's allowed on the market, and if it's found to contain nanoparticles, this must be clearly stated. This tells me that it's a good sign if the particular mineral brand you're looking at is also sold in Europe, because you can check on the European website to see how it's been labeled. If it's sold only in the U.S., write to the company and ask for detailed info about their stance on nanoparticles.

Best Way to Apply Foundation

According to green celebrity makeup artist Geoffrey Rodriguez, the key to foundation application is to prepare your base properly. Make sure your skin is beautifully hydrated. Before an important event, drink loads of filtered water, and then prep your skin with a moisturizer that contains hyaluronic acid. Then use the simple guidelines below, depending on which form of foundation you're using.

Liquid Foundation or BB Cream: Squeeze a little onto the back of your hand and then apply with your fingers. This way, you don't waste a ton of foundation by soaking a sponge or brush with it. Using this technique, you can also easily mix two different shades. I often use a lighter shade for winter and a darker one for summer, but in the in-between months, I mix the two. Once you've evenly applied the foundation over your entire face, use a good foundation brush to smooth it out and blend it onto your neck.

Mineral Powder: If you use a loose powder foundation, it usually comes in a shaker jar. You can tap a little into the lid of the jar and pick it up with a flat-top Kabuki brush. A pressed powder generally comes in a compact, and you apply it similarly. A Kabuki brush picks up more powder and concentrates it on its flat surface. Carefully swirl the Kabuki brush around the jar lid or over the pressed powder, and then gently swirl it onto your face. Spritzing your brush before picking up the powder with a little antioxidant mist can also really help minimize the powder puffing up, and it helps to set your makeup.

Cream Compact or Stick: I always apply a stick foundation with my fingers because it should be warmed up a bit before application. A cream compact often comes with a little sponge, which actually works pretty well, although you must wash it regularly so that bacteria don't grow in it. You can also apply stick or cream compact foundation with a small foundation brush.

Hiding Blemishes and Dark Circles

The next step in a makeup regimen is to apply concealer to hide any blemishes or to mask those dark circles under your eyes—the top concern of most women I know. Whether to apply your concealers before or after your foundation is really a matter of choice; however, it usually works best to apply under-eye concealer *before* your foundation and blemish concealer *after.*

Shopping for a concealer can be very confusing, and it's important that you choose exactly the right kind for your specific concern. If you have dark circles and blemishes to cover, you will probably need two different concealers because the shade for under your eyes is likely too light to work for blemishes.

Check out the notes below to help you choose your best type(s) of concealer:

Choosing the Right Concealer Shade

Dark Circles: Choose a shade one or two shades lighter than your foundation.

Blemishes: Choose a shade as close to your foundation shade as possible.

Liquid Concealer: This kind of concealer usually comes in a tiny tube or bottle. It's the most versatile of all concealers and is easy to apply with your finger or a small concealer brush. It's the best choice for wrinkled under-eye skin because it's less likely to crease; however, you need to gently powder it to prevent slippage. I also like liquid concealer for blemishes because it's less likely to cake. Some liquid concealers for under the eyes contain illuminating pigments, which can impart a pretty glow. However, you may prefer to use an illuminating pen on top of your concealer. I have found a number of liquid concealer pens that double as illuminators—these work well on their own, but only if your dark circles are very light.

Stick Concealer: This comes in a semisolid form and generally has a thicker, creamier texture that a liquid concealer. It tends to be quite rich in pigment, so it's perfect for dotting onto blemishes. However, remember than whenever you dot or smear over a blemish, it's imperative that you blend really well.

Cream Concealer: This comes in a tiny pot, compact, or palette and is thicker than other concealers. This kind of concealer delivers full coverage, so it's best for severe discolorations such as birthmarks, melasma, or bruising. It's very important to choose a shade that is the same as your foundation and to blend with your foundation brush.

I asked Geoffrey Rodriguez how he deals with dark under-eye circles, and he said,

> Hydration is absolutely crucial for any concealer to look smooth when applied. First, start by using a good eye cream. Massage the under-eye area (and lids) with the eye cream and allow it to thoroughly absorb. Secondly, always choose a creamy, blendable textured concealer. Apply a few small dots of concealer on the darker areas and in gentle circular, patting motions. Blend from the outer corner of the eye inward (counterclockwise), ideally exactly in the same direction that you would apply an eye cream. Try to avoid being too heavy-handed by pulling or tugging the skin when you are applying your concealer, as this can actually result in accentuating the lines around your eyes, which is sadly a common mistake. To apply, a small, nylon-bristled brush works well, as does the amazing blending sponge. If you choose to use your fingers, use the ring finger for the least amount of pressure.

Another way to deal with dark circles is to use what's called an under-eye illuminator, which is designed to lighten an area such as the inner corner of your eyes or the outer folds of your nostrils. These products contain light-reflecting pigments, which will not only lighten but also soften grooves that become deeper with age. I asked Geoffrey if he feels that an under-eye illuminator is a must-have product in every woman's makeup bag, and he said: "I actually love (under-eye) illuminators and think they are the quickest and most convenient way to look refreshed and awake. In fact, I think that under-eye illuminators are among the most essential beauty items to have, and in terms of modern 'minimalist' beauty—absolutely key!" There you have it: let's all rush out and buy one.

Concealing Tip

The area directly underneath your lower lashes tends to darken as you age, so make sure you bring your under-eye concealer or illuminator right up to this lash line with a small, soft brush.

Setting with Powder

The purpose of powder is to set the lovely base you've just created to help make it last longer by preventing slippage and to minimize oiliness and shine. However, if you are using an oil-free or matte foundation, you really don't need to use powder unless you tend to get shiny no matter what you use. I prefer to use little to no powder for my day-to-day makeup, but I definitely have to use it for TV and videos because of the crazy shine from the lights. Less is more when it comes to powder, and for reducing oiliness and shine, my first line of defense is always blotting papers. Then, if I still have shine, I'll use a finely milled powder.

There are two main decisions you have to make before you choose a powder, and both are truly a matter of preference:

1. **Do I want pressed or loose powder?** Many makeup artists prefer loose powder because they can pile it on to eliminate any sheen on the face. The advantage of a loose powder is that you can create a sheerer finish

because the powder is finely milled and fluffy (much like the cornstarch in your kitchen) and can be easily dusted onto shiny areas; but the con is that it is messy and thus not great for travel or popping into your purse. Pressed powder is simply the same thing, with added waxes and emollients to keep it in solid form. It's less messy, but it also delivers a less natural finish.

2. **Do I want translucent or colored powder?**
Translucent (uncolored) foundation is the best choice for setting and/or blending foundation and blush. A colored powder will add a little more pigment to your foundation, so make sure you go for one shade lighter than your foundation itself. This will help further blend your foundation across your jawline and onto your neck. If in doubt, choose translucent, because there's no risk of getting the shade wrong. Choosing the perfect powder shade to enhance your foundation requires a little more work.

Be Careful of Overpowdering

However finely milled your powder is, it will add some dryness to your skin because its function is to soak up oil. Too much powder can be seriously aging. Unless I'm going on TV or having photographs taken, I lightly powder my T-zone *only*. I prefer for the rest of my skin to look slightly dewy.

A great alternative to powder is blotting paper. Do, however, carefully read the ingredients, because many brands load up their papers with synthetic chemicals.

Adding Color and Style

Now that you've created the perfect canvas on which to paint, so to speak, it's time to move on to the most fun part of makeup—adding color and style. This is where you really get to show your personality. And remember, you don't have to pick just one style and stick with it. You can play with different moods for different occasions—or simply different days!

Blush

If there's one thing I can never have too many of (shoes aside), it would be shades of blush. Maybe it's because the subtle shade differences in even a single line all look good and all belong in my cosmetic purse! After all, one day I might feel like a soft peach glow, and on another day I might want to pump it up with a bubblegum pink.

I love watching makeup artists dip their brushes into multiple shades to create the perfect one for somebody, but since I'm not a makeup artist and don't have much time to fiddle around in the morning, I have a couple of favorite, go-to blushes.

Your choices of blush types are as follows:

Cream Blush: This is pretty because it can make you look almost as if you are blushing from within. It's also great because it's easy to apply and blend with your fingers. A cream blush often comes in a stick form, and a lot of brands offer a multifunctional stick that ostensibly works for your eyes, cheeks, and lips. I've never been a huge fan of a do-it-all stick because I prefer to use totally different shades on my lips and cheeks. But for travel, it's a good option.

Powder Blush: I always use a powder blush when I'm getting really made up, either for TV or the evening, and also when I plan to apply powder bronzer or face powder, because it's easier to blend when all the textures are the same. I also love how powder blush is beautifully buildable. And, if I've been a bit overzealous with my blush brush, I can always powder over a color to minimize the clown effect! I recommend investing in a good blush brush for this specific task.

Shimmer Blush: Many mineral blushes contain shimmery pigments, which are sometimes lovely for highlighting the apple of your cheeks. Shimmery pigments, however, can accentuate wrinkles, so be careful to go easy around areas where you notice fine wrinkles. I recommend playing it safe and only using shimmer on the areas of your face that would naturally glow if you were 15 years old!

Bronzer

I'm obsessed with bronzers because of the warmth they can give me when I'm feeling a bit pasty and tired. Bronzers can also be used for contouring areas of your face where you want to create dimension. A clever makeup artist uses a bronzer or contouring powder to minimize features such as a nose, jawline, or forehead that they want to make appear smaller.

You have the same choices in a bronzer as you have in a blush:

Liquid/Cream Bronzer: This will give you an all-over glow and is best applied with your fingers. You can also add a drop or two to your foundation for added glow.

Powder Bronzer: You will usually find powder bronzer in a pressed form, although some mineral makeup companies make loose powder bronzer. I prefer pressed because it is way less messy and easier to control. I recommend using a bronzer brush and always tapping off excess pigment before you apply.

How to Apply Bronzer

Using a soft, silky bronzer brush, begin by sweeping it across your forehead near your hairline. Then bring the brush around the base of your cheeks, and finally, dust just under your jawline, making sure there are no harsh lines between where the bronzer ends and your neck. Finally, gently sweep the brush down over your nose. If you feel you have overdone it a bit (a common mistake), you can blend a soft powder brush over it with (or without) a little translucent powder.

Eye Shadow Primer

Some women can't live without their eye shadow primer. While I don't think it's absolutely necessary, it's a fantastic addition if your shadow tends to clump or stick and/or if you have discoloration on your eyelids. Most primers contain silicone derivatives to impart a slick, silky feel, and some have a very subtle shimmer. If you have a lot of discoloration, which is normal for mature skin, you might want to consider a primer that contains a little pigment, because it will help cover to create an even base for your shadow. Some of the new eye primers also contain an SPF, which is a big bonus because we typically leave out our eyelids when we apply sunscreen.

Eye Shadow

I get very excited about using my eye shadow palettes because it's like painting—I get to create whatever look I want. When I shop for eye shadow in large beauty stores, I'm like a kid in a candy store. I can waste way too much time diddling around trying to find the perfect combo that, after a few strokes of a velvety brush, will transform me into Kate Moss. But the quest is always so much fun.

From my experience doing quite a bit of TV, where I get to see my handiwork in high def on a large screen (yikes—what on earth made me think peacock blue would ever work?), I've realized, once again, that less is more, especially for the over 40s.

Well-blended, neutral shades can both soften and accentuate your own beautiful eye color. It's always good to start with a "nude" or "natural" palette because the colors are buildable, meaning that you can add more if you are going out at night. You can also add singles of certain on-trend colors to your collection, but you'll be happy to always have a go-to "natural" palette.

Eyeliner

You now have myriad choices of eyeliner to make your eyes pop. The type of liner you choose is mostly a matter of preference, but in considering the product and method of lining, you need to take your skill level into account.

Here are your choices:

Liquid Eyeliner: You need a very steady hand to apply liquid eyeliner without ending up looking bizarre. Liquid eyeliner can give a dramatic, sexy line to your eye, but it may be a little too harsh for women over 50, who benefit from a softer look.

Gel or Cream Eyeliner: This usually comes in a little pot and is applied with a brush. The big advantage is that it is moveable for a few minutes until it sets—so if you make a mistake or want to smudge it for a smoky eye, it might be a good choice. It's also a great choice if you like to line your waterline, as it might be the only kind that will stay in place for you, minimizing any problem with watery eyes.

Blended Beauty

I cannot overestimate the importance of blending. Every time I walk onto a set, having applied my own makeup, and see the makeup artist squinting at my face (because, clearly, something is off), it's because I wasn't as vigorous with my blending brush as I needed to be.

You can not only blend away mistakes, but if, like me, you experiment with, let's say . . . some *interesting* shades, rather than having to erase the whole thing and start over, that blending brush can turn a clownish mistake into a rather . . . well . . . smoky, sexy eye.

As we get older, blending becomes even more important because shadow and eyeliner, whether cream or powder, do tend to accumulate in those wrinkles and pesky folds.

Pencil (Kohl): Pencil liner is one of the most inexpensive items of makeup you can buy; however, a good pencil needs to be hard enough to draw a solid line but soft enough not to drag on the skin—a combo that's not so easy to find! If you use a pencil, it needs to be very sharp to create a clean line. A pencil is obviously a good eyeliner choice for travel.

Shadow Eyeliner: I nearly always use a shadow liner because it's the only way that I can create a soft line that I can easily blend. Because of my age and because I'm very fair, I look better in the daytime with a very soft line. You need to invest in a good, angled eyeliner brush for this. You can pick up more color and/or create a sharper line if you dampen the bristles first. One of the best ways to look more natural is to actually use powdered eye shadow as eyeliner. It creates a softer line that can be easily blended. A harder pencil line (especially with a liquid pencil) might work on a younger woman, but over a certain age, it's prudent to stay away from anything too harsh.

Mascara

The final step in creating fabulous eyes is enhancing your lashes, which for most people means applying mascara. Keep in mind that there is so much marketing nonsense when it comes to mascaras: each one is ostensibly going to endow you with insanely long, full, unclumped eyelashes. But the only real choice you need to make is between a waterproof and a nonwaterproof formula.

Waterproof: Although you might want to use waterproof mascaras once in a while, be mindful that they are harder on your eyes because they contain waxes and mineral oils, which coat your lashes. Waterproof mascara is also much harder to remove.

Nonwaterproof: Regular mascara formulas are oil free and typically less toxic. They can be washed off with a soft, hydrating cleanser. For day-to-day use, I definitely recommend these.

False Eyelashes

Fake lashes are another option if you want something a bit more dramatic than mascara can likely provide. They give any girl a bit of instant glamour, but remember to keep these points in mind:

- Lash adhesive can contain formaldehyde, which is a known carcinogen. Look for an eco-friendly brand that openly declares that it does not use this ingredient.

- The adhesive is likely to contain latex, so if you suspect you have a latex allergy, you'll have to look for a latex-free adhesive. (You'll probably know already if you have this allergy because of how you react to latex Band-Aids.)

- Always use vegan-friendly false lashes.

- Do not use false lashes every day, because they will pull out your natural lashes. Plus, you don't want to cover your lash line with adhesive on a daily basis.

Lash Extensions

I used to be horrified by lash extensions until I met a wonderful lash expert in Los Angeles who not only created her own line of nontoxic lash extension products but also explained that extensions can be healthier than full false lashes because you don't rip them off. If you rip off regular false lashes often enough, it can eventually really thin out your natural lashes.

Many women who have lost lashes due to chemotherapy can enjoy thicker-looking eyelashes with a little extension help. What are these fake lashes made of? There are a few choices:

- **Synthetic (sometimes called "faux mink"):** These are made from nylon or polyester. They vary greatly in quality; I've seen some that look and feel like doll lashes and others that are as soft and silky as real hair.

- **Silk lashes:** These lashes are often shinier and stiffer than synthetic lashes because they are treated with a chemical to help them hold their shape.

- **Real mink:** These obviously come from real, furry animals. Most companies who offer real mink lashes proclaim that they are completely cruelty free. The hair is just combed off the animals and then cleaned and sterilized. Real mink is the most expensive option, but most eyelash extension technicians I've spoken to don't love real mink because, they say, it's too flimsy.

Whichever kind of lash extension you decide to try, there are some very important things to know:

- The adhesive should be formaldehyde free. You can always ask for a copy of their MSDS (Material Safety Data Sheet) to double-check, because a lot of technicians will tell you something is formaldehyde free when they don't really know for sure.

- You absolutely need a good, highly experienced technician. As with all things beauty, many "technicians" have learned their craft from a quick YouTube video. Ask to see photographs of their work. Even better, get a personal recommendation.

- Your lash extensions will last from three to four weeks, depending on the natural growth cycle of your eyelashes. As your lashes fall out, the extensions will go with them. But don't worry about all of them falling out at once; they'll fall out randomly.

- You need to clean your extended lashes regularly with an oil-free solution. Try mixing a little aloe vera gel with water in a cup and cleaning your lashes off with a cotton swab dipped in this gentle solution. After cleaning, it's a great idea to brush out your lashes with a clean eyelash brush.

- Because oil can dissolve lash extension adhesive, you will need to use oil-free mascara, oil-free cleanser (around your eyes), and oil-free eye makeup remover.

- You will need to be very mindful not to rub your eyes. One or two unconscious rubs could pull a few lashes out.

Lash-Lengthening Solutions

Touted as a "lash miracle in a tube," lash-lengthening solutions are selling like crazy, but users have experienced a number of side effects with these popular products. Some of the more worrying include:

- Iris discoloration

- Eyelid discoloration

- Eye irritation

- Hair growth outside of treatment area

- Swelling

To be a little safer, look for a product that is bimatoprost- and prostaglandin free. Most of the best, safest lash-lengthening products contain peptides and amino acids, which can be extremely effective in helping to lengthen and thicken your lashes.

Lipsticks and Lip Gloss

Lipsticks and lip glosses can add that final shine to a soft look or a bit of wow if you're going for something more dramatic. And for lipstick, it's all about finding the right color for you.

I would like to make a note about ingredients here, too—even though I haven't talked much about it for other makeup products. But it's imperative that all your lip products are non-toxic—you'd be amazed by how much of the goop you actually ingest. The main concern with lipsticks and lip gloss is that studies have found many of them to contain heavy metals including lead, cadmium, chromium, manganese, and aluminum. With the exception of aluminum, these heavy metals are by-products of pigment and base material manufacturing. Because they are not considered "ingredients" in and of themselves, they don't have to be tested for or listed. (Aluminum, however, is added as a stabilizer and keeps color from bleeding, so you will definitely find it in the ingredients.)

In studies, the trace amounts of heavy metals that were actually detected were deemed safe by the FDA; however, the regularity of application was not taken into account. Women reapply lip products an average of 20 times per day, and since lead accumulates in the body, it is definitely a concern if it's in your lipstick.

It's very tough to find out if the lipstick you like is contaminated. I recommend asking the company you love if their lip products have been tested for heavy metals. Also, look for lip products that are colored with fruit pigments.

Eyebrows

Beautifully shaped and shaded brows can completely alter a face—but these take a bit more to style than simply applying some makeup. Eyebrows need constant upkeep to be their most gorgeous.

I only started really taking care of my brows when I took possession of a mega-magnifying mirror that lights up and shows me every little stray hair poking out of them. It's a terrible time-waster, that mirror, because I whittle away a good 30 minutes with my tweezers in hand. (My mother was horrified when she came to visit me, because she'd never seen her face magnified to that degree—I literally heard shrieking from the bathroom. She wonders why any woman would ever put herself through the torture of having to stare at enlarged pores and strange markings that are absolutely invisible in a "normal" mirror.)

In our efforts to shape our brows, many of us have tried plucking, threading, waxing, and shaving under them. Really, brow grooming is just a matter of personal preference.

Plucking: This is the easiest method of brow maintenance because you can do it on your own. If you're thinking of shaping your eyebrows into a look that isn't their natural shape, I recommend that you first go to a skilled threading or waxing technician. Once you have the shape you want, you can pluck as upkeep.

SOOTHING EYEBROW GEL

I always keep a little bottle of this gel handy to apply post threading, plucking, or waxing.

one 2-ounce plastic bottle
1 ounce aloe vera gel
1 teaspoon sweet almond oil
5 drops tea tree essential oil
5 drops lavender essential oil

Simply mix the ingredients together in a small bowl, then use a funnel to transfer the mixture to your bottle. Store it in the fridge for up to six months.

Threading: In threading, synthetic or cotton threads are twisted into a double strand that is used to remove a line of hair. The technique originated in India and became popular in the West because women loved the crisp eyebrow definition they saw on Indian movie stars. It's kinder to the skin than waxing because you don't get a layer of skin ripped off in the process. However, make sure that your technician is really well trained. Ask to see plenty of photographs and get personal recommendations. Also, you need to be very clear about the shape you are looking to achieve before you get into the chair.

Waxing: Most nail salons perform a simple eyebrow wax that is usually combined with plucking. I love to wax because it gets rid of the fuzz and leaves me with a really clean brow on which to apply makeup. I sometimes use tiny waxing strips at home. I never get quite as good a result as in a salon, but they're great in a pinch.

And, bonus: you can now get eco-friendly wax strips made with natural waxes and oils.

Shaving: This method necessitates some caution; those little eyebrow-shaving tools can too easily cut little nicks in your skin, which can become infected. If you do get cuts or nicks, dab a drop of tea tree oil or lavender essential oil directly on the cut. These oils are antibacterial and will help to prevent infection.

Another thing to take into consideration about beautiful brows is that as we age, our eyebrows tend to thin out. This usually becomes more evident at their outer edges; in essence, they shorten. This is where shading with a soft eyebrow pencil or shadow is magical.

I go back and forth between pencil and shadow, but my trusted TV makeup artist, Laci, thinks that you can get a better shape using *both*. She likes to establish the shape by creating an outline with a soft pencil and then fills in with a shadow.

Getting the shade right can be a bit tricky. When you shop for an eyebrow shadow or pencil, I highly recommend that you try it on in the store and then as you walk about, try to catch sight of yourself in various mirrors along the way. What looked great in the beauty store might look like a Groucho Marx impression in broad daylight. Most makeup artists recommend using products one or two shades lighter than your natural eyebrow color, regardless of your skin tone.

Keeping Your Products Fresh

Most personal-care and cosmetic products are marked with some indication of freshness such as an expiration date, an icon showing how long to use it after opening, or a batch code.

Note that if a product's shelf life is considered to be three years or more, the company is not required to include an expiration date on the packaging. I try not to buy from any company with a three-or-more-year shelf life because I know that the product is likely chock full of synthetic preservatives.

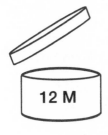

- **Icon:** The icon shows a number followed by the letter M; this indicates that you can use the product for 12 months after you open it.

- **Batch code:** Usually printed on the bottom of the container, a batch code can tell you a date of manufacture and expiration date of an item. Go to www.checkcosmetic.net and enter the product name and batch code. If the brand is supported by this excellent database, the exact expiration date will be revealed to you.

All of this information is great, but I also want to give you some general guidelines. As a rule of thumb, you can assume that the following formulations last this long:

- Powders (including powder blush, eye shadows): 1 to 3 years
- Liquid or cream foundation: 6 to 12 months
- Lipstick, lip gloss: 1 year
- Pencil (eye or lip): about 1 year
- Solid eyeliner and eyebrow pencils: 6 to 8 months
- Bronzer: 1 year
- Mascara: 3 to 6 months
- Liquid eyeliner: 3 to 4 months

The most important hint, however, is to use your own eyes, nose, and common sense. If a product starts to smell strange, discolor, or separate, it's time to get rid of it.

DIY Shelf-Life Marker

Remembering when you purchased and/or opened a product can be challenging. I keep a permanent marker handy, so as soon as I open a product, I note the date with my marker on the bottle, tube, or bottom of the jar—this takes the guesswork out of it.

Moving On

Now that you know the basics of creating a beautiful face, it's time to shift our focus to some features that can really enhance your overall gorgeousness—your hair, nails, teeth, and perfume. Let's face it, a movie with an amazingly talented lead but horrible background players just isn't all that it could be.

Chapter 3

Stunning Supporting Players

(Hair, Nails, Teeth, and Perfume)

I have to admit that a bad hair day doesn't work for me. I *wish* I was one of those women who look a bit Kate Moss-ish with unwashed hair scraped back into a messy ponytail, but I'm just not! On those days when I'm feeling hideously vulnerable, a good blowout or a pretty mani-pedi can go a long way toward helping an otherwise dire situation in the confidence department. So, my hair, nails, and teeth are not always *supporting* players—sometimes they just need to take center stage.

Hair

"Natural" hair products have often been my sticking point. My hair is subject to a fair amount of daily abuse from my high-powered hairdryer and numerous styling tools in the TV makeup trailer, and honestly, most health-food-store hair products haven't been man enough for the job of moisturizing and protecting my frazzled locks. Things are improving in this space, and I've recently found a small handful of shampoos and conditioners in the health-food store that I'll use.

When I first tried switching from my petroleum-laden hair products to "healthier" versions a few years ago, I was appalled at the results. My hair, which tends to be pretty dry anyway, wound up feeling (and, according to my husband, *looking*) like wire wool. I now know that it was because most of those fossil-fuel-derived products were able to impart a slithery shine to almost any hair type regardless of its level of damage. They coat the hair shaft with a wax-like residue that does a great job of masking the wreckage.

I only pray that the hairstyle I sported in the mid-'80s will never come back into vogue. It was commonly agreed among friends that I looked like a cross between Madonna in *Desperately Seeking Susan* and a troll doll. I backcombed my hair within an inch of its life into a huge cotton-candy creation and then flat-ironed the bangs. This laborious process necessitated half a can of mousse and almost an entire can of toxic hairspray.

Anyway, I'm now confident in reporting that despite the dyeing and daily styling, my hair is in stellar condition—so much so that I've been able to grow it quite long. I keep telling my stylist that she's got to let me know if/when I'm too old for super-long hair, and she's assured me that if it's in good condition and cut regularly, I'm good.

Choosing hair products can sometimes be overwhelming because there are so many options. In addition to the ingredients we talked about in Chapter 1, there are some very important hair-care specifics to look out for. In shampoo and conditioner, there are a number of ingredients that you are better off avoiding for both health and performance reasons.

First off, let's deconstruct a conventional drugstore shampoo and compare it with a healthier one.

Here's an ingredient list for a typical drugstore brand shampoo:

1101617 Pt1 Ingredients: Aqua/Water/Eau, Sodium Laureth Sulfate, Cocamidopropyl Betaine, Sodium Lauryl Sulfate, Glycol Distearate, Sodium Chloride, Amodimethicone, Ppg-5-ceteth-20, Parfum/Fragrance, Sodium Benzoate, Salicylic Acid, Guar Hydroxypropyltrimonium Chloride, Trideceth-6, Carbomer, Lactic Acid, Linalool, Hexyl Cinnamal, Arginine, Glutamic Acid, Benzyl Salicylate, Benzyl Alcohol, Limonene, Serine, Hydroxy-propyltrimonium Hydrolyzed Wheat Protein, Cetrimonium Chloride, Amyl Cinnamal, Citronellol, 2-oleamido-1,3-octa-decanediol, Alphaisomethyl Ionone, Sodium Hydroxide, Citric Acid. F.I.L. D163546/1 US Patents: 5,618,523; 5,661,118

And here's a list for a healthy, "natural" shampoo:

Aloe barbadensis (aloe vera) leaf juice, aqua (water), babas-suamidopropyl betaine, decyl glucoside, sodium cocoampho-diacetate, panthenol (vitamin B5), avena sativa kernel protein, hydrolyzed rice protein, sorbitol, hydrolyzed rodophicea ex-tract, carageenan, citrus aurantium bergamia (bergamot) fruit oil, chondrus crispus (irish moss) extract, hydrolyzed soy pro-tein, borago officinalis (borage) seed oil, helianthus annuus (sunflower) seed oil, soy lecithin, linum usitatissimum (flax) seed oil, mel (honey), potassium sorbate, simmondsia chinen-sis (jojoba) seed oil, sodium benzoate, sodium chloride, soy tocopherols, triticum vulgare (wheat) germ oil, guar hydroxy-propyltrimonium chloride, sodium hyaluronate, citrus grandis (grapefruit) peel oil, hibiscus rosa sinensis (hibiscus) flower fex-tract, copernicia cerifera cera, sulfur, limonene, linalool

Both of these lists come from reparative shampoos for "ex-tremely damaged" hair.

Four ingredients in the first product give me pause. In addition to the sodium lauryl sulfate (SLS) and parfum/fragrance, which we've covered before (see pages 26–28), the drugstore shampoo lists water as the first ingredient. This tells me that water is the main ingredient, whereas in the second shampoo, the first ingre-dient is aloe vera. Aloe vera is obviously way more moisturizing than just water.

The drugstore brand also contains sodium chloride, which is just salt. There is no reason that this should be in a reparative shampoo—salt strips your hair of its natural oils, color, and smoothing treatments. So, when you're choosing a shampoo—especially one for moisturizing—look out for water and sodium chloride.

Sulfate Free?

Nowadays, you'll see a lot of shampoos labeled as "sulfate-free." Why this sudden trend? Is it just another marketing ploy? It is a trend, and yes, a great marketing tool. It came about because consumers caught on to the fact that their beloved foamy shampoo was doing more harm than good. Sodium lauryl sulfate (SLS) and "sulfate" are one and the same. The problem with SLS is not only cosmetic (it makes your hair dryer and strips it of [expensive] color), but it can also be really irritating to your eyes, scalp, and skin; cause allergic reactions; and be contaminated with rather worrying chemical compounds. The other reason that even women who hate "natural" products eschew it is because it strips any hair-straightening treatments right out. A friend of mine who risks the most toxic "smoothing" treatment because she'd rather die than face her frizzy hair (yes, I've pleaded with her) was disgusted when her SLS-laden shampoo turned a $200 "smoothing" treatment into a frizzy mess. Finally, SLS strips the natural oils out of your hair, which can make you feel you have to wash your hair more often.

Will Dyeing My Hair Give Me Cancer?

There is still a really lively debate about whether or not permanent and semipermanent hair dyes increase one's risk for bladder cancer or a blood cancer such as leukemia or non-Hodgkin's lymphoma. The jury is still out. It seems that many studies on this, especially with regard to bladder cancer, concluded that hairdressers exposed daily to these chemicals were indeed at risk. However, there have also been plenty of peer-reviewed studies that don't substantiate any link between bladder cancer and hair dye.

My take is that there are more than 5,000 different chemicals used in permanent and semipermanent hair dyes, some of which have been found to be possible carcinogens, endocrine disruptors, and skin sensitizers. Since hair dyes can be absorbed right through the scalp, I prefer, especially for a single-process color, to use a dye that doesn't contain any of the following ingredients: PPD, PTD, "amines," ammonia, resorcinol, or parabens.

There are now a handful of fantastic hair dyes that don't contain these ingredients; however, you may need to experiment if you are making the switch to a more natural brand. Many good colorists insist that you need ammonia, bleach, and peroxide to get very bright highlights. One of my eco-sins is occasional bleach highlights; however, when it comes to a single process, which I sometimes use, especially in the winter months, I get my colorist all set up with the more natural stuff.

How do you find a safer hair dye? I recommend going online. They'll state right up front if they don't use PPD, PTD, or resorcinol in their formulations.

Skin Sensitizers: Are They *That* Bad?

A skin sensitizer can be pretty problematic. Such a substance can cause a serious allergic reaction. Here's how it usually works: If you are susceptible to a certain chemical in, for example, hair dye, you might notice a little discomfort when it's first applied to your scalp. This could include burning, itching, or watering eyes and nose. "Okay," you might say, "that lasted for all of twenty minutes, and now that I'm walking out of the salon with my lustrous locks swinging in the wind, I'm fine." However, your immune system has taken note, and the next time that same dye is applied, it's going to mount a serious attack because it's sensitive to the chemical that burned you. The second attack might cause such a major allergic reaction that it might be impossible for you to use the dye again without experiencing severe contact dermatitis or even chronic respiratory conditions. So, if you feel a bit off when your single-process color is burning into your scalp, you might want to give your immune system a break by using a product that you know is free of the bad guys.

The Worst Hair Offender

As you already know, if I had to choose one single ingredient out of every personal-care and beauty product to avoid, it would be formaldehyde, because it is one of the few that is actually known to be a carcinogen. Formaldehyde can be found all around your home in things like particleboard furniture and toxic cleaners from which it may slowly off-gas (that is, release small amounts of toxic gas). However, in the case of hair-smoothing or hair-straightening treatments, it gets really gnarly because the action of hot tools causes a huge amount of toxic gas to be released. Moreover, the fumes are on and around your head!

I spoke to a hairstylist who had continued to perform keratin treatments despite the risks, because it was a great source of revenue for him—at $200 a pop, he couldn't afford to say no. But he admitted to me that his nose had started running 24/7, and on closer inspection, he'd realized that the hairs on the inside of his nose had been burned off! Other stylists have reported nosebleeds and severe respiratory issues. But it's not just these uncomfortable symptoms that the stylists have to worry about; it's more that with the cumulative exposure over time, they could develop cancer.

Many brands will tell you that they are now formaldehyde free, but in order to completely flatten the hair follicle for the necessary length of time, much like the chemical cocktail used in permanent-press clothing, there's almost always a need for at least *some* formaldehyde in the formula.

If you absolutely cannot go without having your hair straightened, I beg you to find a stylist who'll do the treatment outside for you, because however well ventilated the salon may be, you're still going to be exposed to a lot of fumes. Or you can opt to wear a mask. Another stylist I know wears a mask whenever one of the other stylists in the salon performs a toxic blowout.

Hairstyling Products

I am an absolute hairstyling product junkie—every time I go to the salon and have a different styling spray spritzed through my locks, I have to own it. Even though I know that the shininess of my gorgeous new style has way more to do with my stylist's expert blowout skills, I still have hope that I might get a similar effect from a product. (I never do.)

Hairstyling products are a bit of a racket because they are so expensive, and for the most part, they're filled with the same old toxic cocktail of ingredients we've seen before. Hairsprays are the absolute worst, followed by leave-in-conditioning sprays, and then the rest.

Before you buy any hair product, go to the company's website and you'll very quickly find out if it uses clean and natural ingredients or not. If it does, that will be the marketing slant, and the company will explain in great detail what it doesn't use. If a company uses toxic ingredients (most big-name brands do), there'll be no mention of ingredients on the website.

There are now so many excellent brands that carry truly natural, healthy styling products that you don't need to compromise to get the hold, texture, or shine that you're looking for. You can also make a lot of effective hair products at home. Check out my lustrous Hair Food Balm (page 388) for one deep-conditioning product that is all natural and healthy.

Beware of So-Called Healthy Oils

Hair salons and beauty supply stores now boast an enormous choice of oil or dry-oil serums that will supposedly transform your frizz into a lustrous mane in seconds. They are marketed as healthy and frankly sound like it, but beware—very few of these oils are pure. They are mixed with all kinds of chemicals, including synthetic fragrances. You can save a lot of money by purchasing a small bottle of sweet almond oil or argan oil and rubbing a couple of drops between your fingers before applying to the ends of your hair. Unlike adulterated store-bought "argan" oil serums that contain all kinds of other ingredients, this oil is very rich and concentrated, and unlike the store versions, a little goes a long way.

Nails

Next up in our cast of supporting players are nails. And here's the scoop with them: an unpolished nail is obviously healthier than a polished one. If you love to get your nails polished regularly, try to go the odd month without. It takes at least a month for your nail bed to return to optimal health. I try to leave my toenails unpolished during the winter months when I won't be wearing open-toed shoes. I also like my nails to be naked when I go on a beach vacation because the sand and the water help to clean and buff them to natural, pink perfection.

When you do polish your nails, luckily you have good choices for some healthier polishes. Healthy-beauty advocates have put enough pressure on big cosmetic companies to get them to remove some of the worst ingredient offenders. Look for polishes that don't contain the following toxic ingredients: formaldehyde, toluene, DBP, camphor, and parabens. (You can read specifics about these ingredients in Chapter 1.) They are often marketed as either "3-Free" or "5-Free."

- 3-Free: Does not contain formaldehyde, toluene, or DBP.

- 5-Free: Does not contain formaldehyde, toluene, DBP, camphor, or parabens.

Water-based polishes are a good, healthier option, especially if you are sensitive to chemicals, because the oil-based solvents are replaced with water—so you don't have to worry about these containing the toxic chemicals that many polishes do. These polishes don't last as long in my experience, but the advantage is that it's really easy to remove them with rubbing alcohol or vodka. They also don't smell nail-polishy at all.

Gel polishes are another popular option, and I'm not surprised—to have a chip-free polish for three weeks seems miraculous. However, there are some health issues with these.

- It's tough to find a brand of gel polish that is 5-free. Fortunately, this is changing rather quickly.

- Gel polish can absolutely ruin your nail bed if it's removed improperly. The only salons I've found that remove it properly are the Japanese salons, which makes sense because gels originated in Japan and they've had years to perfect this service. If anyone soaks off your gel polish for less than 15 minutes and uses a metal tool to scrape off the polish, you should jump out of the chair because you are about to have your nail beds ruined for months. A salon should never scrape your nail bed. Your nails should be soaked long enough so that the polish can be gently eased off with a wooden orange stick.

- UV lights are used to cure and harden each layer of gel polish, which can be horrible for your skin. Make sure the mini-sun bed is an LED light, which not only cures your nails faster but also emits much fewer UV rays. It's also a good idea to protect your hands with anti-UV gloves so only the tips of your fingers poke out.

If you do most of your nail upkeep at home, remember that nail polish lasts for about one year after opening, so don't keep your polishes forever. And, just like with makeup, I recommend that you note right on the polish the date you opened it—just to avoid confusion.

What about Acetone?

Acetone is the smelly chemical solvent used to remove most polishes, both regular and gels. I've never fancied the idea of soaking my fingers in a chemical solvent, but that is what gel manicures require. For regular polish, you can look for an acetone-free remover, which uses ethyl acetate—it's still a chemical solvent but is a little less drying than acetone. The only get-around is to use a water-based nail polish in the first place. There are also a few brands I love that offer a "soy" based polish remover.

Manicure Tips

- If you file your nails yourself, never file back and forth. You will get a much smoother finish and a better shape if you file in one direction only.
- Never let a nail salon clip your cuticles. This can lead to them peeling, bleeding, and even becoming infected. In a healthy, properly performed manicure, your cuticles should be gently pushed back with an orange stick. The snipping implement should only be used for hangnails.
- To help clean and whiten your nails at home, soak them in a solution of equal parts hydrogen peroxide and warm water for ten minutes.
- Take a bottle of tea tree oil with you to the salon and add ten drops to the footbath and/or three drops to the hand-soaking bowl.

Teeth

Who doesn't want a gorgeous smile? Coming from the U.K., where dentistry still lags behind that in the U.S., I really understand how important beautiful teeth are. When I visit the U.K. every summer, I'm always surprised by how little attention men and women pay to their teeth and their oral health. They'll fork out huge amounts of money for facials and fillers, but teeth, and to some extent nails, are last on the list.

Whitening Your Smile

The first thing that I notice when I visit the U.K. is that everyone's teeth are some shade of yellow. The Brits drink a lot of tea, which is a serious tooth-staining agent, and without the kind of dedication that we have to bleaching in the U.S., those yellow teeth are honestly . . . rather aging. But is bleaching our teeth safe?

I spoke with Dr. David Keen, D.D.S., M.S., one of the top cosmetic dentists (prosthodontics specialists) in the U.S. He believes that bleaching is safe, but only when the directions on the package are followed. He says that it's a good idea to have a chat with your dentist before you start bleaching, because you may have certain gum and tooth conditions that need to be taken into consideration before you go crazy with the strips or blue-light gizmos.

For example, some of us get gum recession as we age, which can be caused by a number of things such as periodontal disease, teeth grinding, hormonal changes, and overzealous brushing. The first sign that you might have gum recession is that you experience that awful nerve pain after drinking very hot or cold beverages. Your teeth also might start to look longer. (Have you heard the expression, "She's a bit long in the tooth"? That's where it comes from.) Anyway, Dr. Keen explained that when the gum becomes separated from the tooth, the root structure is exposed (eek), and instead of the glossy white enamel of a regular tooth, we start to see the more yellowy shade of the dentin layer. Dentin is softer and more porous than enamel and doesn't respond as well to bleaching as the rest of the tooth. Also, dentin's porosity causes teeth to become sensitive to bleaching. Dr. Keen explained that gum recession can be corrected by filling the recessed area with a bonding agent; however, the bonded areas also don't respond to whitening as well as nonbonded parts of the tooth. Does this mean that you'll have two-tone teeth? Maybe, but it won't be obvious because for most of us, our lips hide these not-so-attractive regions. Artistic bonding *after* you whiten your teeth is the best method to develop the ideal color match.

If you establish that you are a good candidate for bleaching, which is the most effective method? Dr. Keen says that most bleaching products (trays, gels, or over-the-counter products) use varying concentrations of hydrogen peroxide or carbamide peroxide, which in and of themselves are perfectly safe. You'll pay more for all the "mega" whitening strip products, but this is just because a higher percentage of hydrogen peroxide has been thrown in. People are moving away from laser whitening treatments because they're so expensive and deliver similar results to at-home bleaching products (if you use the strips or trays consistently). Depending on the shade of your teeth, you may opt to bleach more frequently (every other day for 14 days) for shorter times (20 to 30 minutes). Once you've achieved the desired result, you can top up with a whitening once a month to maintain your new dazzling smile.

Creating a Healthy Look

After we finished talking about bleaching, I asked Dr. Keen if our teeth get more crooked as we age, because I've noticed a lot of women around my age going in for orthodontic braces. He reassured me that our teeth don't suddenly get crooked; it's more that if you had your teeth straightened by way of orthodontic braces when you were a kid and haven't worn a retainer for years, they may well migrate back to their original positions. Interestingly, teeth have memory for this.

What about our tooth enamel thinning—or even worse, our teeth shrinking, like the rest of our skeletons? Again, Dr. Keen reassured me that our teeth do not shrink and that the only thing that can happen is that tooth enamel can get thinner as it's exposed to the elements. Apparently, one way that we can mitigate this is to stay away from acidic foods. You have to be careful about drinking beverages with lemon in them all day, because Dr. Keen said that in the oral cavity, lemon is acidic and over time can eat away at tooth enamel. I drink my lemon water in the morning and rinse my mouth with water afterward—I'm not going to give up my lemon water, because it's so good for my body and skin. That said, I don't add it to any other beverages, especially tea.

Finally, what about veneers? Again, I've noticed women of my age forking out small fortunes to give their teeth total makeovers. And I must admit that a lot of people who have veneers don't get a great result. I've seen some women wind up with huge, tombstone chompers that look oddly uniform and out of place in their faces. Maybe this is because it looks unnatural for an older woman to have perfectly uniform teeth. Dr. Keen feels that porcelain veneers can be an excellent method to enhance smiles for some patients, but he says they're not the only way to create a gorgeous smile. In fact, he often opts to be a little more conservative by closing spaces and remedying irregularities with artistic "dental bonding" instead.

Dr. Keen feels strongly that some patients are good candidates for veneers and some are not. And since everyone's teeth are different and have different needs, the key to success is to find a dentist who will listen to what you want and who will study your smile and face with digital photographs taken from all angles. Then, he or she can develop a treatment plan to conservatively and comprehensively enhance your smile, fully incorporating what you want and also what you need.

Dr. Keen's Rx for Maintaining a Gorgeous, Healthy Smile

- Brush your teeth with a fluoridated* toothpaste as soon as you get out of bed and before breakfast, because without brushing before you eat, the bacteria in your mouth will stick to the particles of food you ingest, and it's the bacteria that cause cavities.
- Brush your teeth after breakfast, too.
- Brush consistently, but not too aggressively.
- Enjoy a lot of water throughout your day. Water is neutral in pH, lubricates the gums, and dilutes acids on your teeth and in your mouth.
- Avoid acidic beverages such as highly concentrated lemon in water or tea, and carbonated soda drinks. (Note: Even carbonated water contains carbonic acid, which is acidic.)
- Floss morning and evening.
- Consider a night guard if your teeth are chipping and becoming worn or if your dentist suspects that you have gum recession caused by grinding.
- Consider a technique Dr. Keen refers to as "dry brushing." Brush gently for about 30 seconds with a moist toothbrush *before* you brush with toothpaste. This will help remove plaque and stains from your teeth.

*If you wish to avoid fluoride in your toothpaste, Dr. Keen advises that you be extra vigilant about avoiding sugar-containing foods and acidic beverages. Fluoride helps to build the enamel, which is eroded by these foods and drinks.

Gum and Mouth Health

Dr. Keen's suggestions are pretty well accepted by the majority of people, but if you're looking for a little something more, you can try out these ancient Indian Ayurvedic recommendations, which I love:

- Use a tongue scraper every morning to remove bacteria from the back of your tongue.

- Use an oil-pulling mouth rinse in place of your usual mouthwash. This helps remove bacteria and treats your oral cavity with healing and antibacterial essential oils.

- Use toothpaste that contains an herb called *neem*.

. . . .

OIL-PULLING RECIPE

1 cup raw virgin coconut oil
5 drops clove essential oil
5 drops peppermint essential oil

Place the coconut oil in a small Mason jar. Gently heat the jar in a bowl of very hot water so that the oil liquefies. Add the essential oils. When you are ready to use it, swirl 1 tablespoon of the oil around your mouth for at least 60 seconds and then spit it out.

If the ambient temperature is cool, your oil will harden when stored, so you may need to stand it in a sink or bowl of hot water before use each time.

. . . .

If you stick with regular mouthwash, I recommend being very mindful about which kind you use. Most drugstore mouthwashes contain cocktails of harsh and sometimes toxic chemicals. If I'm not using the oil-pulling recipe above, I always use a homemade mouthwash, because then I know for sure that it's healthy.

Perfume

Over the years, I have become increasingly sensitive to synthetic chemicals in the environment. The first time I noticed this was when I was exposed to the stench of strong, synthetic perfume. I was in a car in the U.K. It was freezing outside, so all the windows were closed, and the driver had drenched herself in a designer perfume. I began to feel dizzy, light-headed, and nauseous—it was terrible. I put it down to possible motion sickness until it happened again: I was in an elevator in LA, and a woman walked in who had clearly sprayed herself within an inch of her life. The same nauseated feeling came over me. I took the elevator back down and staggered outside for some fresh air.

And it's no wonder I felt so terrible: 95 percent of chemicals used in fragrances are synthetic compounds derived from petroleum. They include phthalates, benzene derivatives, aldehydes, and many other known toxics and sensitizers capable of causing cancer, birth defects, central nervous system disorders, and allergic reactions.

These chemicals are so prevalent in our society that we've become sensitized to them, which means that we can no longer tolerate them. They are in every product that contains "fragrance" or "parfum," which could be anything from candles to cleaning supplies. And in a perfume, they are used in a very concentrated form.

In fact, we are so used to extremes today that we've become immune to the subtleties of taste and smell. We eat foods that are so off-the-charts sweet that we can no longer appreciate the incredible real sweetness of a piece of fruit. We are so bombarded with crazily strong, synthetic fragrances every day that we can no longer appreciate the subtle and exquisite scents around us.

To counteract this immunity, we have to give up our addiction to overly strong scents and tastes, which basically means getting them out of our homes. Ditch the artificial sweeteners and fragrances for a while, and you'll get your subtle taste and smell back again quite quickly.

This is why I always recommend that you use natural perfumes. Luckily, artisan perfumers are on the rise, so it's much easier to get hand-blended perfumes made from primarily pure essential oils instead of synthetic compounds. Here are the pros and cons of these handcrafted beauties.

Pros:

- You won't expose yourself to chemicals that could make you sick.

- You can enjoy a beautifully subtle scent (which, incidentally, most men prefer because they don't like a strong perfume drowning out your gorgeous, natural scent).

- You won't be offending anyone around you. Trust me, most people can't stand the strong smell of a perfume they didn't pick invading their personal space.

Cons:

- Natural perfumes may be more expensive because pure essential oils are pricier than the cheap synthetics used in drugstore and designer perfumes.

- The scent won't last as long, so you may need to pop a bottle in your purse for repeated applications.

The other option for natural perfumes is to make your own, which can be a sensuous and deeply satisfying project. You get to customize the scent exactly the way you want it, and once you get good at this, you can give or sell your signature blends to friends. To learn how to make your own perfume, go to page 389.

Chapter 4

Gorgeously Green Skin from the Décolleté Up

Primping with makeup and hair care is one thing, but if you really want to glow, you need to go deeper. The next step: caring for the health of your skin.

The condition of our facial skin is a reflection of our general health and wellness, inside and out. When I'm stressed out, traveling, and subsisting on airport food, my skin takes a turn for the worse. Conversely, if I take care of myself with meditation, exercise, and tons of gorgeous greens, my skin glows. Before I understood all the ins and outs of skin care formulations, and the fact that beautiful skin begins on the inside—I have to admit that I wasted way too much money on completely useless products with empty promises. It's so hard not to fall for the quick fix thing. When an adorable YouTuber or model tells us that a quick slick of a particular eye cream will banish dark circles for good, we just want so badly to believe it's true. But, unfortunately, there are no shortcuts to lasting beauty and skin that looks gorgeous with or without makeup.

We've discussed how skin care is best done holistically, which means that the skin is no longer treated as a separate entity from the rest of the body. Your skin's health and beauty, or lack of them, is always determined by your overall health. If your liver and kidneys are congested, you'll be more likely to have dark circles under your eyes, and if your hormones are out of balance, you'll be more likely to suffer from breakouts, and so on. Moreover, if your digestion is out of whack, your skin will be so lackluster that no cream or potion can bring the bloom back to your cheeks. So the first step in taking care of your skin is to consider what might be causing certain skin conditions that you don't like. Your diet is almost always the first area to look at if your skin isn't looking as gorgeous as you'd like it to.

Look and Listen

You can learn a lot by slowing down and listening to what your body is telling you. Any imbalances in your life will likely be reflected in your appearance. If you know that your digestion is sluggish or that your hormones are out of balance (you might be motoring to, through, or past menopause), you need to address the issue before you even consider how to deal with your skin.

Moreover, if you lead an incredibly stressful life, it will be reflected in your skin because when you're stressed, your body releases a steroid called *cortisol*, a stress hormone that causes a whole cascade of biochemical reactions that throw your entire system out of balance. This is probably the main reason for the apparent increase in women who suffer from rosacea, eczema, and psoriasis—conditions that are now being associated with inflammation caused by stress.

We need to learn to balance our entire physiologies to have the most beautiful skin possible. Don't worry—we'll go much more deeply into how to do this in the next section of the book. For now, I just want to open your eyes to some of the clues that your appearance can give you about your health:

- **Dark under-eye circles:** Can be caused by adrenal burnout (too much stress), not enough sleep, allergies, vitamin K deficiency, and liver or kidney issues

- **Thin and very dry skin:** Can be caused by low estrogen levels

- **Eczema:** Can be due to allergies to certain foods including wheat, dairy, and soy

- **Psoriasis:** Can be due to a malfunctioning immune system and inflammation

- **Coarse, thick, and scaly skin:** Can be a symptom of hypothyroidism

- **Rosacea/inflamed skin:** Can be a symptom of an inflamed gut

- **Hair loss:** Can be due to hyper- or hypothyroidism

- **Dull, lackluster skin:** Can be caused by digestive issues and stress

Most of us know in our gut if something needs to be addressed. If we stand still for long enough and take a good, honest look in the mirror, it takes just a few seconds to assess our situations. A few years ago, when I was traveling every week, not eating as well as I usually do, and under tremendous pressure, I developed little patches of psoriasis on my legs, chest, and face. One morning, I stood still in front of the mirror, looked into my eyes, and saw an exhausted and depleted Sophie. I knew that there was absolutely nothing that I could apply to my skin to fix all these problems. I also knew if I went to the dermatologist, she would prescribe steroids for the psoriasis and likely some other cream that a large pharmaceutical company had hawked to her. I knew in my heart that the only thing that would make my skin better would be for me to get my diet back on track and hit the meditation mat.

What's Up with Your Thyroid?

In my mid-40s, I discovered that I had hypothyroidism and that this condition is extremely common in women 45 and older. Who knew that my perpetually cold feet, cracked heels, and low energy were symptoms of my thyroid firing improperly? I learned about specific nutrients to include in my diet and specific supplements, which my doctor prescribed, and all my symptoms disappeared. But in the meantime, I did a great deal of research on hypothyroidism and discovered that it also creates visible signs of aging. Yikes! Some of these symptoms include rough or scaly skin, thinning skin and hair, paler-than-usual complexion, and dry, cracked skin on the palms of your hands and soles of your feet. If you experience any of these symptoms, you might want to get your thyroid checked out. You can either go to the doc to get a simple blood test, or try the "Barnes Basal Temperature Test": Place a thermometer in your armpit for ten minutes immediately after waking up. A reading of 97.8° F or below may indicate hypothyroidism.

"Inflammaging"

Another issue that greatly affects the look of your skin is inflammation. In fact, inflammation has been found to be one of the prime causes of prematurely aging skin—not to mention disease. We tend to think of inflamed skin as bright red or irritated; conditions such as rosacea and eczema come to mind. Although these conditions are absolutely caused by inflammation, another kind of chronic inflammation affects many of us as we age—and that is not so obvious to the naked eye. According to holistic aesthetician Emily Fritchey, this is known as low-level inflammation, and, over time, its effects show in our skin.

When you injure yourself, your body sends inflammatory substances to deal with bacteria, and as a result, you see swelling and redness (inflammation). This is nature's way of protecting our bodies from foreign invaders, but the problem is that we now face a plethora of environmental invaders, which is overkill for our bodies to deal with—hence, low-level and continuous inflammation.

What are these invaders?

- **Digestion problems:** If you suffer from bloating, gas, bouts of diarrhea, constipation, or heartburn (acid reflux), you may have an inflamed digestive tract. This is why it's imperative that you follow an anti-inflammation diet, which I address in Chapter 7. In addition, all of my recipes in Chapter 12 are made up of anti-inflammatory foods.

- **Hormonal imbalance:** As we age, particularly during and after menopause, symptoms of chronic inflammation that might be seen as skin irritation and extra sensitivity may worsen. Hormonal changes leading up to menopause may also pack on extra pounds around the midsection. We know these extra fat cells add to systemic inflammation because they produce inflammation markers such as cytokines and C-reactive protein.

- **Environmental stress:** This is a huge inflammation trigger. We really weren't designed to deal with the onslaught of toxic chemicals that are pretty much everywhere today. Just walk into an office building, and your body might have to deal with toxins emitted from synthetic flooring, particleboard furniture, latex glue, air "fresheners," and toxic cleaning supplies. Add pesticides, heavy metals, and hormone-mimicking chemicals to this cocktail, and it's no wonder that our immune responses are in overdrive, causing a full-on inflammatory response.

- **Stress in general:** The reason we look awful when we've been through periods of high stress is because our body releases cortisol, which sets a skin-damaging process into motion. As if that weren't enough, the release of adrenaline causes a massive decrease in blood flow to the skin, and we all know that the nutrients and oxygen that our skin needs come via the blood.

How to Minimize Skin Inflammation

1. Use skin care products that contain soothing anti-inflammatory and antioxidant ingredients (see box)

2. Follow an anti-inflammatory diet (see Chapter 7)

3. Check your hormone levels and perhaps get help with balancing them

4. Meditate

Inflammation Facial Soothers

- Allantoin
- Aloe vera
- Boswellia serrata
- Calendula
- Chamomile
- Coffeeberry
- Colloidal oatmeal
- Colloidal silver
- Ginkgo biloba
- Glucosamine
- Grape seed extract
- Licorice extract

- Mangosteen
- Niacinamide
- Noni
- Pine bark
- Plant peptides
- Pomegranate
- Quercetin
- Resveratrol
- Sea kelp
- Silymarin
- Soy isoflavones
- Turmeric

Hormone Heaven (or Hell!)

Before we move into a more general discussion of skin care, I'd like to go a bit deeper into the subject of shifting hormones and hormonal imbalance. You probably first experienced hormonal issues when you were an adolescent, right? You moved from having the pristine skin of a child to being an oily, confused mess of a near-adult. And once you got a routine worked out to deal with this, something changed again. Argh!

That's just one of the things we've all had to deal with. Hormones change throughout adulthood, but if you are in perimenopause, menopause, or postmenopause, it's likely that you've experienced some major changes in your body that go well beyond general fluctuations. One of those is probably a huge change in the texture of your skin. If this is something you've faced, don't worry. It happens to nearly everyone—and there is definitely something you can do about it.

I'm a big fan of finding a good endocrinologist who can help you get your hormone levels back on track. Although there's a ton of controversy about hormone replacement therapy, I like to take as natural an approach as possible when tweaking my hormone levels back into balance, by using topical bioidentical hormones that come from a plant source. However, I believe that diet and exercise also play huge roles in hormone balance, which is why I've included both in your 30-day program. If I am not exercising regularly, eating poorly, and *not* managing my stress levels, I can almost feel my hormones going crazy, because they crave balance.

When I asked the wonderful Dr. Christiane Northrup about hormone balance and the use of bioidentical hormones, she said, "At the end of the day, it's the excess stress hormones (cortisol and epinephrine) and too much sugar that really wreak havoc with hormones. Once you clean up your diet, the hormones tend to take care of themselves . . . with a little help from progesterone."

I like to get my hormones checked once a year, but Dr. Northrup says we need to be smart about *how* we get them checked. "You need to get the right test," she emphasized. "After years and years in this field, I have found that urine testing, using strips, is the most accurate." And it's also easy. If you are interested in trying out this kind of testing with strips, Dr. Northrup recommends Precision Analytical (www.precisionhormones.com).

Now that you understand a few of the things that can affect your skin, let's move into a discussion of the magic that exists once your health and your life are in balance. And you can start doing some helpful things right away. Even without working on diet, exercise, and self-care, they will help you look more beautiful.

Skin Basics

Most of us really don't understand how to take care of our skin. We kind of know the broad strokes, and then as we get older and start to see things that we don't like, we grab for straws. We throw ingredients into our regimens that we've heard might turn us into glowing Gwyneth Paltrows or Cate Blanchetts overnight— after all, if *she* uses it, it must be good, right? We also tend to think that more is better: *If I throw as many fruit acids and glycolic peels at my skin as I can, I'll look brighter and younger.* But it isn't necessarily the case. Unless we know how to create a core regimen that supports the natural functions of our skin first, these other great ingredients can do more harm than good.

I've had all kinds of products and skin care lines recommended to me by different dermatologists over the years that actually created inflammation in my skin that wasn't there to begin with. Through trial and error and working with a handful of brilliant professionals, I've come to understand that a daily routine that supports the integrity of my skin is the most important thing to put in place. Having established a healthy foundation where inflammation and oxidation are minimized, I can then add "booster" ingredients bit by bit.

In this chapter and in your 30-day program, I teach you how to create a basic daily regimen that will restore your skin's natural, healthy glow, refine its texture, brighten it, and dramatically improve its elasticity. My aim is to get you to the point where you would be okay *not* wearing foundation because your skin looks so great. But, for now, let's look at the physiology of the skin so that we can get a better understanding of what we are dealing with.

Your Largest Organ (Yes, *Really*)

Your skin really is your largest organ. It lives and breathes, which means that it needs to be taken care of, not simply looked at as a protective layer against the elements. In fact, it needs to be protected against the elements itself—just like the parts of your body that *it* protects. To do this, it's important to understand a bit of its structure, which is composed of three layers.

Subcutaneous (bottom layer): This is the deepest layer, where all the action takes place. It's full of connective tissue, fat cells, and nerves. It contains all the blood vessels that nourish your skin. This layer contains almost 50 percent of your body fat and thus keeps you warm, cozy, and protected. This is the layer of skin that regulates the temperature of your skin and your body. As we get on in life, this layer of fat thins out, so you could start looking a bit gaunt, especially if you're purposely trying to lose weight. This is why maintaining a healthy weight is imperative if you don't wish to look older than you are.

Dermis (middle layer): This layer contains blood vessels, lymph vessels, sweat glands, and hair follicles, but the main component is a bundle of fibrous proteins called *collagen*, which are held together by another protein called *elastin*. Collagen gives your face its structure, and elastin gives it its suppleness and bounce. If you've still got loads of elastin in your skin, when you pinch it, it'll spring back flat as soon as you let go. As you get older, it won't spring back quite so speedily. The breakdown of collagen and elastin as we age makes our skin appear wrinkled and saggy.

The dermis also contains cells called *fibroblasts*, which are mini-factories that produce:

- Collagen
- Elastin
- Hyaluronic acid (HA)

Hyaluronic acid affects the texture and fullness of your skin. Up until the age of around 30, your HA is like Jell-O that's been chilled in your fridge. After 30, it begins to get softer and more like Jell-O that's been left out at room temperature. Eventually, your body stops making it altogether. This is why hyaluronic injectable fillers have become so popular; they serve to replace this lost HA and thus the texture you had when you were a spring chicken.

Epidermis (top layer): The epidermis is stuck to the dermis with a porous membrane that regulates cell migration from the bottom layer up to the top. The epidermis has five layers, but in the name of glowing skin, you really only need to understand two of them:

1. Basal layer (bottom layer of the epidermis): It produces melanin, a brown pigment that creates your skin color. The important thing about this layer is that the basal cells continually divide to form shiny new cells that replace the old ones shed from the skin's surface.

2. Cornified layer (very top layer of the epidermis): This layer is responsible for maintaining healthy skin. It acts as a barrier that prevents moisture loss and damage from outside oxidants, much like the shingles on the roof of a house. Most important, it contains hormone receptors and little signal stations that can mobilize a full-on immune response to invading allergens and microbes. This layer used to be thought of as only dead skin cells, but it's now understood to have an intelligence all its own.

Now let's jump into some of the ingredients and techniques that will help you get gorgeous for good. These recommendations are great to keep skin of every age as healthy as possible, but they are invaluable if you are trying to minimize or reverse the effects of aging.

Skin Care Ingredients

It's important to know that skin care products generally contain two types of ingredients: functional and active.

Functional ingredients bind the formulation together and ensure that it stays fresh. They deliver specific ingredients where they need to go and keep everything stable. Examples of functional ingredients are emulsifiers (xanthan gum, glycerin, lecithin), thickeners (xantham gum, carbomer), chelating agents to remove metallic impurities (phytic, citric, or glucuronic acid), humectants, preservatives, and pH adjusters.

Functional ingredients that I like to look for are:

- Hyaluronic acid
- Aloe vera
- Cold-pressed plant oils
- Plant butters
- Glycerin
- Squalane*

Active ingredients, on the other hand, are things that actually change your skin and go deep into the dermis to perform their work. These are what deliver on the promises of the product. In essence, they do the work of any product you buy. If the product claims to tighten your skin, the active ingredients are what do it. If the product claims to get rid of wrinkles, again—that's the job of an active ingredient.

We'll go much deeper into which active ingredients to look for as we work our way through this chapter. But one general rule about choosing a skin care product is this: you get what you pay for. Inexpensive, mass-produced skin care products are unlikely to

---

*Squalane is a hydrogenated form of squalene. In this case, hydrogenation is actually a good thing because it extends shelf life and stops the ingredient from becoming rancid. But my big caveat about squalene is that it must be 100 percent plant derived. Many skin care products use squalene that comes from sharks, and the particular sharks from which the squalene is harvested are on the brink of extinction. If the label doesn't say it's plant derived, e-mail the company to ask what kind of squalene it uses.

carry out the lofty promises of their active ingredients. They are more than likely filled with preservatives and cheap ingredients to make their profit margins work. The most inexpensive ingredients are often petroleum derived. Propylene glycol, which is a great moisturizer that also helps deliver other ingredients into the skin, is just one example. It's in a great number of skin care products even though there are possible health issues with it. Just remember, there are way better alternatives. Even if you don't care about the petroleum-derived aspect, moisturizing ingredients such as hyaluronic acid come without the potential toxicity of propylene glycol and work better.

There are literally hundreds of incredibly effective, potent ingredients that you could be applying to your skin, and there are now hundreds, if not thousands, of companies that are using these ingredients in stellar formulations. I urge you to visit my website, www.sophieuliano.com, where you'll find a plethora of product recommendations. I've tried to include products for every budget, but if they all seem out of your price range, consider making some of your own (see Chapter 13). Plus, they'll be even more active and nourishing than anything you can buy in a store.

Ingredients My Skin *Loves*

My skin is so happy when I nourish it with any of the following ingredients. I feel as if I am feeding the living, breathing organ that is my skin with the best that nature has to offer. I like to think of these ingredients as real food for my skin.

- **Pure plant oils:** Sweet almond, rose hip seed, coconut, avocado, apricot, grape seed, olive, argan, and sesame oils are wonderful, natural moisturizers.
- **Plant butters**: Shea, mango, and cocoa butters are great moisturizers.
- **Plant waxes:** Jojoba oil (which is technically a wax) is a great moisturizer for those who tend to break out.

- **Pure essential oils**: There's a plethora of pure essential oils that provide such amazing skin care benefits that I include them in almost all my skin care recipes. Blends of essential oils such as rosemary, thyme, lemon, oregano, clove, and cinnamon are also great preservatives.
- **Natural astringents:** Aloe vera juice or gel and apple cider vinegar are wonderful toners.

Five Things to Consider When Purchasing New Skin Care Products

1. **Is the "active" ingredient stable?** This is really important, because many of the most powerful ingredients are highly unstable, especially when exposed to light. Make sure that the product uses a stable form of that ingredient—the company will be happy to elaborate if so. It's also a good sign if the product is packaged in an opaque container, because most active ingredients begin to degrade when exposed to light, and some, such as vitamin C, oxidize when exposed to light. Oxidation means that something loses its efficacy and can form free radicals.

2. **Is the active ingredient fresh?** This question bleeds into the stability question, but I add it as a separate point because I always try to buy from companies that make products in small batches or microbrew their formulations. This obviously means that a widely available drugstore brand may not be able to offer the proactive efficacy of a smaller, "boutique" brand. Make sure there is a clear expiration date on every product you buy.

3. **What is the concentration of the active ingredient?** You need to make sure that there's *enough* of the active ingredient in your skin care product to

make a difference. This is hard to find out. The only ingredients for which an actual percentage is mentioned are retinol, AHAs, and vitamin C. For other ingredients that you are interested in, at least check how far up the ingredient list they are. If they are near the end, as we've noted, the product only contains minimal amounts. Don't get hung up on given percentage numbers, because they are often only marketing tools rather than exact measurements.

4. **Is the formulation chirally correct?** You will soon hear more and more about "chirally correct" ingredients. Although the phrase is often used to market a product, there is valid science behind such claims. It means that an ingredient's molecule must be able to fit into its target receptor in your skin to be effective and for its side effects to be minimized. It's very hard to figure out whether or not an ingredient is chirally correct from an ingredient label, but many forward-thinking companies can offer you a lot of information on their websites about how they formulate in this way.

5. **Is the product from a "good" company or brand?** You need to do your research here. I like to buy from companies that have good sustainable, ethical, and scientific practices. I like to purchase from companies who put my health first.

Divine Dozen

These are my favorite plant oils for using on my skin because they are all loaded with antioxidants and vitamins, especially when fresh and cold pressed. You can either use them alone or look for them blended together in specific, synergistic formulations:

1.	Argan	7.	Meadowfoam seed
2.	Avocado	8.	Monoi
3.	Black cumin seed	9.	Moringa
4.	Borage	10.	Rose hip seed
5.	Evening primrose	11.	Sea buckthorn
6.	Grape seed	12.	Tamanu

Damage Control: The Magical Four Ingredients

When I reached my 40s, I decided I wanted to get a little more proactive about my skin. I began to notice quite a bit of sun damage (brown spots suddenly appeared) and a coarser texture, not to mention an almost overnight appearance of fine wrinkles (which I actually don't mind, because I'd look weird if I didn't have any). Fortunately, there is so much we can now do to smooth skin texture and even out the tone—and to protect from these things if we haven't yet started to experience them.

There are only a handful of active ingredients that have proven effective in this respect. The important thing to realize is that no one ingredient on its own is a miracle worker. I look for products that contain a carefully formulated blend of specific ingredients.

I only recommend active ingredients that have published, peer-reviewed, double-blind, placebo-controlled studies backing them up. I'm a stickler for this kind of scientific research because there are so many bogus marketing claims out there, and I don't want you to waste your hard-earned money on something that doesn't really work.

There's a big distinction between active ingredients that can actually reverse damage and signs of aging and active ingredients that can help minimize any further damage. Let's take a peek at the hard-hitters first:

- Retinol

- Vitamin C

- AHAs/BHAs/LHAs
- Peptides

Retinol: Do I Really Need It?

Retinoids are vitamin A derivatives, which have become one of the most researched antiaging ingredients on the market. For women who are already concerned about aging skin, these are must-have proactive ingredients because they have been proven to stimulate collagen production, unclog pores, and stimulate cell turnover, which makes your skin softer, smoother, and less wrinkled—love it, right? If you're not worried about your aging skin, you technically don't need to use this; however, it won't hurt, so I suggest you begin this powerful proactive regimen now.

The first retinoid to be approved for use was a prescription retinoic acid called *tretinoin*. Dermatologists found that not only did the retinoic acid in tretinoin treat acne, but it also significantly helped to thicken skin and restore its youthful luminosity. However, it came with side effects such as dryness, peeling, and scaly patches.

Retinol (vitamin A alcohol) is a precursor for the synthesis of retinoic acid, and it was discovered that retinol provided the same benefits as tretinoin without the annoying side effects. Thus, it became popular as a potent ingredient in antiaging beauty products. But retinol is not very stable; it loses efficacy when exposed to light. It can also still cause skin irritation and dryness until you get used to it. To deal with these issues, retinol derivatives such as retinyl acetate, retinyl palmitate, and retinaldehyde were created.

So, to sum it all up, the mother (and most potent) retinoid is tretinoin, which is typically administered to patients with severe acne, and it is prescription only. Next up in the potency department is retinol, which you will find in hundreds of OTC products in varying concentrations. The least potent are the derivatives, but if you want to dramatically minimize side effects, these would be a good choice.

It's important to understand that retinol and its derivatives have to be converted to retinoic acid to be absorbed by the body. This means that though retinol has only one step to get converted into something that the body can use, the derivatives have two steps. Phew! This may seem complicated, but it's important to understand when choosing which retinoid might be the best for you.

Here are some considerations that will help you choose the best retinol product for you:

- **Severe acne:** A dermatologist can tell you if tretinoin or one of the next-generation retinoic acids is a good call for you.

- **Sun-damaged, normal-to-dry skin:** If your skin is mature or dry (and not sensitive) and you have quite a lot of sun damage, you might want to consider retinol. Instead of getting caught up in deciding which concentration you need, it's more important to buy a product that contains nontoxic, nourishing functional ingredients alongside the retinol.

- **Sensitive skin:** If your skin is very sensitive, you may be better off using one of the retinol derivatives.

When you are shopping for a retinol product, keep the following points in the forefront of your mind:

- Retinol is very unstable, especially when exposed to light. Make sure that your product is packaged in an opaque tube or jar.

- Because of its instability, pay particular attention to the shelf life. This is one of the main reasons that I purchase products manufactured in the U.S. in small batches that won't sit on a store shelf for years.

- Look for companies that speak to both the stability and the efficacy of the retinol they use. There are a few new ingredients on the market, such as IconicA, that show great promise because they remain stable while delivering a nice, hefty dose of retinoic acid minus the extreme side effects.

- Look for progressive, "clean" companies that now use encapsulated forms of retinol, which again minimize side effects.

How do I use retinoids? You always use retinoids at night, because they make your skin photosensitive. After cleansing, apply your retinol product next (before your serums and/or moisturizers). You need a thin layer over your face, neck, and chest. If you are a newbie to retinol, it may take a few days for your skin to get used to it. This means that you may experience redness or dry, flaky skin for a couple of days.

You should use your retinol every three days to start with; then, once your skin acclimates, move to every two days, then every day. Any symptoms should subside after a few days, but if they persist or get worse, the product may be too strong for you. It's also super important that you use your sunscreen religiously once you start using retinol, because your skin will become more sensitive to the sun.

Is there anyone who shouldn't use it? I would steer well away if you have rosacea or eczema and also if your skin is super sensitive.

Are there more "natural" alternatives? Absolutely! A handful of innovative companies have figured out that certain plant compounds may be able to mimic the effect of retinol and are kinder to the skin. Some of these compounds come from roots and seeds such as rose hips and chicory. However, I haven't found any convincing trials or studies proving their antiaging efficacy thus far, so I will be watching this space, as I'm quite convinced that these bioretinoids hold great future promise.

Vitamin C: What's the Big Deal?

The big deal on vitamin C is that it's one of the few skin care ingredients that has substantiated evidence proving that it significantly helps improve the look and texture of your skin. A groundbreaking study found that L-ascorbic acid (a synthesized form of vitamin C) considerably reduced the visible signs of sun damage on the backs of hairless pigs! If it can do that for a little piggy, it can do it for you, too. Needless to say, I'm obsessed with the stuff because I slathered myself in zero-SPF oil and roasted myself within an inch of my life up until my mid-30s, when the brown spots began to appear. Aside from helping with sunspots, this is what else vitamin C can do for you:

- Protect your skin from UV damage
- Strengthen your skin's barrier response
- Reduce inflammation
- Build collagen
- Lessen hyperpigmentation
- Boost efficacy of sunscreen actives

The most stable and effective forms of vitamin C are: L-ascorbic acid (in powder form), ascorbyl palmitate, sodium ascorbyl phosphate, retinyl ascorbate, tetrahexyldecyl ascorbate, and magnesium ascorbyl phosphate.

How do I use vitamin C? Use it every morning to help protect your skin for the day. I prefer to use it in powdered form because it is at its most active before you add it to a liquid. I mix micronized, water-soluble crystals into my serum, moisturizer, or a simple aloe gel. I then apply directly to my face, neck, and back of hands after cleansing and exfoliating. If you don't wish to use the powder, choose a serum that contains a proven-stable form of vitamin C.

Is there anyone who shouldn't use it? If your skin is broken and/or super sensitive, you need to be cautious. L-ascorbic acid is a hard-hitter (great for tough, coarse, wrinkled skin), but if you are very sensitive, you might want to consider one of these more gentle forms of vitamin C: ascorbyl palmitate, sodium ascorbyl phosphate, retinyl ascorbate, tetrahexyldecyl ascorbate, or magnesium ascorbyl phosphate.

Is there a more "natural" alternative? We tend to think of vitamin C as natural (with a pretty visual of an orange in our minds), but L-ascorbic acid and all the forms mentioned above are synthetic. There are plenty of plant oils and super foods that have really high concentrations of natural vitamin C; however, the oil must be absolutely fresh for the vitamin C to be active. Unfortunately, it's really tough to find out how many weeks old the serum or moisturizer might be. As much as I love to use vitamin C–packed oils such as rose hip and pumpkin seed oils, if I want outstanding results, my best bet is to stick with L-ascorbic acid.

Vitamin C 101

Vitamin C in all of its forms is very unstable. This means that it oxidizes and begins to lose its efficacy the moment it's exposed to light or to a liquid. Even if your vitamin C product is in its stable form and packaged in opaque packaging (which it always should be), it should be discarded after six months. However, it's tough to know how long a product has been sitting on a shelf, so even this guideline isn't perfect. This is why I use L-ascorbic acid in its dry (completely stable) form—with this, I know I'm getting maximum potency.

AHAs/BHAs/LHAs: Are These Part of the Package?

Most definitely! Alpha hydroxy acids (AHAs), beta hydroxy acids (BHAs), and β-lipohydroxy acids (LHAs) work to dissolve the protein bonds that hold dead skin cells in the epidermis together and thus hugely assist in exfoliation, which gets rid of old, lackluster skin and brings new skin cells to the surface.

AHAs are typically found in the form of glycolic acid from sugar cane, lactic acid from dairy products, tartaric acid from grapes, malic acid from fruit, citric acid from citrus fruits, and antioxidant ellagic acid from raspberries, cranberries, and pomegranates.

BHAs, which are also known as salicylic acids, occur naturally in plants such as willow bark, wintergreen, licorice, marigold, and sweet birch. LHAs are a little newer to the scene in terms of skin care, but they hold a lot of promise, especially for those with acne or persistent breakouts, because they decrease bacteria within a pore, and they're an excellent exfoliator, even at low concentrations. LHAs also stimulate the renewal of epidermal cells in a similar manner to retinoids.

While AHAs, BHAs, and LHAs assist in exfoliation, BHAs and LHAs are best for people with oily skin and blackheads because, unlike AHAs, they are fat soluble. This means that they can cut through the oil and get right into clogged pores. AHAs are great for normal skin. If you have combination skin, you might want to look for a product that contains all three.

How do I use hydroxy acids? I've found that cleansers containing AHAs, BHAs, and/or LHAs generally give great results, as they slowly exfoliate over time. However, there are other options available, which I cover much more fully on page 113. If you have acne, you may want to consider a serum that contains BHAs and AHAs, because when left on the skin (as opposed to being rinsed off), the acids will be more potent.

Is there anyone who shouldn't use them? If you have rosacea, broken skin, severe acne, or really sensitive skin, you might want to skip AHAs and BHAs in your products because they might be a little too harsh for you. For exfoliation, you can lean toward fruit enzymes such as papaya and pumpkin as the key ingredient in an enzyme peel (rather than an acid peel). These can be just as effective at dissolving dead skin cells, but they don't cause any inflammation and can be used in perpetuity with zero side effects.

Is there a more "natural" alternative? These acids *are* natural.

Peptides: Are They for Real?

Peptides are short chains of amino acids, which are the basic building blocks of proteins and many other different types of organic molecules. Cosmetic peptides are not just a marketing ploy, and the science behind many of the new ones being added to formulations is very promising. Studies have found that peptides, especially when used with niacinamide, can be as effective as retinoids (if not more so). These peptides are synthesized; however, they are safe and can be a powerful wake-up call for the complexion. Many of them are considered to contain moisture-binding and cell-communicating properties. Since the molecules are large, they need to be synthesized in a lab so that they can be structured to penetrate the skin.

As was true of most of the effective antiaging ingredients, peptides were not discovered in a search for glamour. They were originally used to heal wounds and prevent scar tissue from forming because they can speed up skin cell turnover and help with inflammatory conditions. Peptides that are synthesized from plants are nontoxic, safe, and really effective in helping the skin to build more collagen.

How do I use them? Look for them in ingredient lists on serums and moisturizers. It's really hard to tell the efficacy of the peptide being used, but as is the case with almost all active ingredients, if the product's company has a great reputation, it's likely that it will use effective peptides with a good delivery system.

Is there anyone who shouldn't use them? Peptides are pretty much safe for everyone to use and have few side effects.

Are there any "natural" alternatives? No, because these have to be synthesized in order to be able to penetrate the skin.

Natural Damage Control

Ingredients scientifically proven to work aren't your only options for keeping your skin looking fresh and healthy. Some natural ingredients can work toward this as well. Antioxidants are the rock stars of natural damage control and help with one of the most aging processes in the skin: inflammation. Here are some of the antioxidants that I look for in a skin care product:

- Alpha lipoic acid
- Coffeeberry
- Ferulic acid
- Genistein
- Grape seed
- Green tea

- Lycopene
- Niacinamide*
- Resveratrol
- Vitamin C
- Vitamin E

*Niacinamide is sometimes known as vitamin B3, and it's absolutely an ingredient to look for in your skin care products. It has a plethora of proactive benefits, including improving your skin's elasticity, barrier function, discoloration, texture, and tone.

Other ingredients that are showing a lot of promise in terms of helping to keep your skin even and toned are:

- Dimethylaminoethanol (DMAE), an anti-inflammatory that may cause muscles to contract and tighten
- Methylsulfonylmethane (MSM)
- Oat beta glucan (stimulates collagen production)

Certain ingredients work synergistically with others to either enhance or stabilize formulations. A great example is the winning combination of vitamin C, ferulic acid, and vitamin E. A study performed by scientists at Duke University found that the antioxidant ferulic acid not only stabilizes these vitamins but also makes them more potent.

Skin Care Techniques

While using the right ingredients is a must, it's also essential that you bring them into a skin care process that uses techniques that help create a fresh, beautiful glow. The three things that need to be in every skin care regimen are exfoliation, cleansing, and hydrating/nourishing. If you are doing all of these processes daily, using products that include the ingredients we've already talked about, you'll see amazing results.

Exfoliation: Your New BFF

Before you can fully understand how exfoliation will help you, you have to understand the journey of a skin cell.

A skin cell (basal cell) is created in the bottom layer of the epidermis. It travels up through the various layers of the epidermis, flattening out as it goes, until it reaches the top cornified layer. It's still active and connected to other cells until it eventually reaches the final sloughing point, where it flakes off. This entire journey takes about 28 days in a 20-year-old, and at least double that time in someone over 50.

So, if you take anything from my mini science lesson, take this: as we get older, if we want fresh, shiny new skin, we need to try to *speed up* this journey, and the fantastic news is that we can do this, in part, with the right kind of exfoliation.

Exfoliating your skin is the process of not only removing all those dead skin cells, which instantly freshens and brightens your skin, but also stimulating the messengers (cytokines and hormones) in the cornified layer to get on with their job of nudging the epidermis to make new skin cells. Alarm bells go off when the skin is deeply exfoliated, because these messengers can't really tell the difference between an injury and exfoliation. They only know that something is off and that they must signal for new cells to be delivered up to the top floor ASAP.

There are two different ways you can exfoliate your skin:

1. **Natural acid exfoliators:** For the most part, this means AHAs, BHAs, and LHAs. L-ascorbic acid is also an exfoliating agent; however, I recommend the use of products with AHAs, BHAs, and LHAs for the best exfoliation. AHAs, BHAs, and LHAs should be used with caution if you have sensitive skin—especially if you have inflammatory conditions such as rosacea. The other thing about these acids is that they can prompt the fibroblast cells in your dermis to produce more collagen.

2. **Mechanical polishing:** Much like polishing tarnish off a beautiful piece of silver jewelry, a mechanical skin polish involves the use of something mildly abrasive such as a brush, rice bran, oatmeal, or jojoba beads. I am very careful with this kind of "polishing" because, depending on the method or ingredient used, the skin can easily be damaged.

Avoid Plastic Micro Beads!

Many exfoliating cleansers contain "micro beads" as their exfoliating agent. These beads are made from plastic and are horrible for the environment because they flush straight into our water supply and don't biodegrade for hundreds—if not thousands—of years!

Choosing an AHA, BHA, or LHA Exfoliator

Products containing AHAs/BHAs/LHAs include cleansers, masks and peels, toners, gels, and serums. The main difference between these acids is that AHAs are water soluble, and BHAs/LHAs are fat soluble. If your skin is normal, AHAs are the way to go. If your skin is oily/acne prone, BHAs/LHAs are the way to go.

AHAs, BHAs, and LHAs come in many different forms, so you just need to find the one that works best for you.

- **Cleanser/exfoliating cleanser:** If you have normal skin, a cleanser and/or exfoliator that contains AHAs and/or BHAs is a potent daily tool. Some of these products also contain mechanical exfoliants such as jojoba beads, but for everyday use, I prefer one without because I only like to use the mechanical exfoliating agents a couple of times a week. If your cleanser contains hydroxy acids, it's best to leave it on for a couple of minutes before rinsing it off, because the acids need a little time to dissolve the dead skin cells.

- **Toner:** I've found some excellent toners that contain AHAs and BHAs. You don't need your cleanser *and* your toner to contain these exfoliating acids, so choose whichever you prefer.

- **Serum:** There are some excellent AHA/BHA and enzyme serums on the market. These tend to be pretty strong because they're designed to "resurface" your skin overnight. If you choose a serum like this, make sure you use it on a night when you are not using your retinol. An AHA/BHA/LHA serum might be a good choice if you have acne, but be cautious if your skin is inflamed or very dry.

- **Gel:** If you suffer from breakouts or have very oily skin, you might want to consider a soothing gel that contains BHAs, because you can dot the gel over your blemishes and oily areas.

- **Mask:** You'll be able to find some beautiful masks containing AHAs, BHAs, and LHAs. The concentrations tend to be strong, as they are designed to sit on the skin for a few minutes before being rinsed off. These masks serve as a good option for a once-a-week (or once-a-month) deep cleanse.

- **Cleansing pads:** A couple of companies I love offer pads saturated with deep-cleansing acids. They are super strong, so use them only if your skin is normal.

Once you figure out if AHAs, BHAs, and LHAs—or a combination of two or three of them—are best for your skin and how you want to apply them, the next thing to look at is the concentrations of these ingredients.

If you are relatively new to using AHAs on your face, I recommend a cleanser, mask/peel, toner, or serum with a 5 percent concentration. If you have been using AHAs for a while as I have, you might want to try dialing it up to 10 to 15 percent. Your skin will tell you how much is acid is enough! Most OTC products contain concentrations of 1 to 30 percent, so you want to aim for somewhere in the middle. Interestingly, dermatologists and some aestheticians can use concentrations of 30 to 70 percent, but this strength of product shouldn't be used on a daily basis.

For BHAs, newbies will want to start with a 1 percent concentration, and when your skin gets used to it, move up to 2 percent.

The most important thing to remember when choosing a product is to purchase from a company that works with quality ingredients. Concentrations are secondary when it comes to quality, so don't fret too much about finding the perfect one. Remember that measuring the concentration of any ingredient in a product isn't an exact science. The concentration of a specific ingredient listed on a product label is an approximation.

Using an AHA, BHA, or LHA Exfoliator

If you have completely normal skin with no sensitivity issues, I recommend using an AHA, BHA, or LHA product in a cleanser every day. However, if your skin feels like it's becoming too dry, dial it back to every other day and use an acid-free cleanser in the interim.

If you are a newbie with these ingredients, go slowly to begin with. This means that if you experience any kind of irritation, you may want to eschew your mask or cleanser for a few days to allow your skin time to calm down.

Choosing a Mechanical Exfoliator

A "mechanical" exfoliating product has an abrasive agent such as jojoba beads, aluminum oxide crystals, or oatmeal. Some of the companies I love have become extremely creative in finding exfoliating agents such as volcanic sand and fruit seed powder. Some of the companies that I don't love use plastic exfoliating micro beads, which, as I've said, are terrible for the environment. Whatever the agent used, the rest of the formulation should be a creamy, soothing mix of plant waxes, oils, butters, and gels.

Love . . . the Brush!

I love an electronic exfoliating brush because it enables me to perform a much deeper cleanse that I would ever be able to do with my fingers or a cloth. What I love about some of the electronic exfoliating brushes is that I can choose my level of exfoliation by the firmness of the bristle. The science behind many of these brush devices is in their movement, which allows them to dig deep and in some cases actually penetrate dirty pores, thus removing wax and built-up debris. If, however, you are battling enlarged pores or stubborn blackheads, the brush alone won't do the trick. You need to use it in conjunction with your AHA/BHA/LHA cleanser. Apply your cleanser to your face or to your brush, and let the bristles assist in driving the product into your pores.

There are now a few brushes on the market—many of which do a decent job. When choosing a brush, consider:

- Do you want oscillating bristles? They have the effect of micro-massaging your skin in addition to exfoliating.
- Do you want a rotating brush? Some of the less expensive models have a rotating rather than an oscillating brush.
- Do you want a brush that offers interchangeable heads?
- Do you want a brush that charges directly or uses batteries?
- What other options do you want? Variable speeds? A timed shutoff? Signals for you to move it to another area?

Using a Mechanical Exfoliator

If you choose to use a brush or an exfoliating cleanser containing an abrasive, you need to decide how often you should use it. It all depends on your level of sensitivity. While some may feel great using it every day, for others this is way too much. I use my brush about every other day, and I'll occasionally throw an abrasive exfoliating cleanser into the mix, but for the most part, I prefer to use acids and natural enzymes for deep and consistent exfoliation.

Cleansing: Getting Squeaky Clean

Most women don't cleanse thoroughly enough at night. If you wear makeup—even if only a smear of tinted moisturizer or sunscreen—your skin picks up all kinds of grime and debris throughout the day. Combine all this with the sebum that your skin secretes, and you get a film of goop that can't be removed with a quick, 15-second cleanse.

You need to perform a two-step cleanse every single night to keep your skin looking its best. This might seem like hard work, but once you get the hang of it, it can be really quick. And don't worry— I'll walk you through exactly how to do this in the 30-day program. For now, here's a quick overview:

- **Step 1:** Melting the makeup and layer of oily grime off your skin with a really good, emollient cleanser. You want to look for a creamy cleanser that might contain aloe vera gel and plant oils or butters. Or, you can even try using a light fruit oil such as grape seed oil. A cleanser that can help melt off your makeup will typically be called a "cleansing milk," "cleansing lotion," or a "hot cloth" cleanser. Massage it into your face, neck, and chest in circular motions. Do not mix it with water unless your face feels really dry. Massage for a good 30 seconds, and then remove with a hot washcloth.

- **Step 2:** Using a lighter "brightening" cleanser. This step digs down deeper to refine the skin's texture, lighten skin discoloration, clear breakouts, and balance blotchy skin. This refreshing step will leave your skin feeling squeaky clean but not tight and dry. I recommend finding a cleanser that contains "next-generation" flower acids such as mandelic, hibiscus, azaleic, betulinic, malic, and lactic acids along with antioxidants and minerals to help brighten, soften, and "jump-start" your program's results and speed you on your way to clear, healthy skin. If you are using a daily cleanser with acids, it should be in this step. A cleanser that will work here will typically be called a "gel cleanser," "purifying cleanser," "foaming cleanser," or "exfoliating cleanser." For a foaming cleanser, make sure that the foaming agent is not SLS, because that will dry out your skin.

Oil and Butter Cleansing

Many wonderful aestheticians and skin care brands love the plant oil or butter cleansing method. An oil cleanser by Eve Lom, a French aesthetician, garnered a cult following in Europe and has now reached an almost iconic status. The technique is to massage a greasy, balm-like goop into your face and then remove it with a hot muslin cloth. The concept is that the oil adheres to the oil and dirt in your skin, thus making it easier to remove. The bonus is that your skin gets massaged and hydrated at the same time. I love the idea, but only if it's done with products that use organic nut butters and plant oils. There are many women with oily skin who love this technique because they believe that the oil mimics the sebum in their skin, so less oil is produced. I'm on the fence about this and honestly think that if you are prone to breakouts and acne, you're better off with a less oily product.

Hydrating and Nourishing: Feeding Your Skin

Good hydration is another essential element in maintaining healthy skin. Remember, hydration comes from both the inside and the outside, which is why some skin care ingredients (humectants) are designed to draw moisture up to the top layer of skin from the epidermis, while others (emollients) provide a protective barrier to the top layer to avoid moisture loss. We also moisturize this top layer of skin by way of natural oil and water secretions and external moisturizers. And all of this is important.

As the expert holistic aesthetician Emily Fritchey (aka "the Skin Whisperer") explained to me:

> Maintaining the health and integrity of the skin's protective barrier function (the acid mantle) is vital for smooth, healthy skin so it can ward off the growth of bacteria and fungi that can lead to chronic inflammation and sensitive, problem skin conditions. The mantle is maintained by the skin's natural sebum (body oils) and water produced from the deepest layers of the skin. Skin that has lost the slightly acidic coat is not only prone to dryness, itchiness, and premature wrinkling, but also very vulnerable to infection. Anyone who has ever suffered the tight, dry feeling of their skin when they wash with a strong soap knows what it feels like to strip away the natural oils that protect its protective acid mantle.
>
> Careful attention to topical skin care ingredients, especially when it comes to skin cleansing and correction, is a must to avoid the unintentional destruction of this protective skin film. Maintaining the skin's delicate pH (your beauty ecosystem!) is super important. Harsh, acid-based products, topical acne meds, ablative antiaging procedures, and many strong wrinkle treatments can all too often be more destructive than helpful. Interestingly, products that are too alkaline can be even worse and create major redness and skin issues. Common OTC cleansing soaps marketed as mild and gentle can be highly alkaline and create a cascade of skin imbalances. Know your ingredients, and remember—balance is the key!

These are some of the factors that can lead to overly dry and irritated skin:

- Harsh, acidic skin care products
- Soap containing SLS
- Soaps and facial washes marketed as "gentle"
- Retinol used too frequently when skin hasn't adjusted
- Sun damage
- Environmental pollutants

Choosing and Using a Moisturizer

Selecting a moisturizer that works with your skin type is important, but here again, it's all about the quality of the ingredients. In any good moisturizer, there should be both humectants and emollients.

Humectants draw moisture from the dermis to the epidermis and prevent skin from losing moisture. Typical healthy and nourishing humectants might be hyaluronic acid, vegetable glycerin, and even honey.

Emollients lubricate the surface of the skin to make it feel softer. Most plant oils are emollients (see the box below for more information). They also form a protective layer that may prevent further moisture loss. Cheaper emollients include mineral oil derivatives such as propylene or butylene glycol and silicones.

Emollient Heroes

I love exotic, cold-pressed plant oils for hydrating my skin. The top layer of skin is held together by lipids, and as we get older, our lipids deteriorate, which means that we need to supplement them to keep this protective barrier intact. The fatty acids in these wonderful oils help to keep everything in tip-top condition. Some of my favorite oils include avocado, rose hip seed, pomegranate seed, tamanu, baobab, borage seed, argan, and bassu.

The other thing to decide on is the form of your moisturizer:

- **Water-based ("oil-free")**: A lot of women with oily or problem skin opt for water-based moisturizers because they are afraid of adding more oil to their skin. However, it's important to understand that a "cream" has to contain some kind of oil (or oil substitute) to create its texture. In a "water-based" cream, the ratio of water to oil is simply higher, and the "oil" in it may well be a synthetic oil derivative such as propylene glycol. It will also likely be loaded with glycerin and silicones to give it a rich and creamy texture.

- **Oil-based**: Good oil-based moisturizers are formulated with the cold-pressed plant oils I mentioned above, along with all kinds of other nourishing ingredients. Depending on the ratio of water to oil (and to the other ingredients), the moisturizer may be a gel, a lotion, a cream, or a balm. If you choose an oil-based moisturizer, you are better off using gel or lotion forms for oily or problem skin and a cream or balm for dry skin.

- **Oil**: Many fantastic moisturizers are just simple plant oils such as rose hip seed, argan, sweet almond, and so on, without any water added. The advantage of these formulations is that they are very stable, so preservatives don't need to be added. Also, many of these plant oils, if fresh, can be pretty potent. If you tend to break out or have acne or rosacea, I recommend steering away from using pure plant oils.

The most important thing to look for in a moisturizer is a formulation that contains ingredients that serve the greater good of your skin. Many skin care ingredients are thrown into big brand formulations because they make the product feel or look better—and because they are cheap. This is where I want you to be cautious. There is no point in spending your hard-earned money on a cream that does your skin little good in the long run. You do get what you pay for here, so if you splurge on any item, it should be your serum or moisturizer.

Do I Really Need . . . ?

When it comes to moisturizing and nourishing our skin, many women wonder if it's absolutely necessary to get a separate eye cream, night cream, or even neck cream. The truth is that it's not vital, and in some cases, you are better off with just one cream. However, many of us want special potions and ingredients to target different areas of our skin, so let's take a closer look at some of the options.

Eye Cream: Eye creams are usually touted as necessary for treating the delicate area of the skin around your eyes. I can see the logic in this because the skin is thinner there, but I've found my regular moisturizer to be just as effective in keeping the area under my eyes well moisturized. The advantage of some eye creams is that they can be thinner than your moisturizer or may come in a gel form. This is important because you don't want to weigh down your under-eye skin with a thick, rich cream that might sit in your wrinkles. But watch out for a lot of marketing hype, such as the promise of removing dark circles or puffy eyes, and even of "lifting" the eye area. There are no miraculous ingredients that can do any of the above, especially as the causes of dark circles, puffy eyes, and saggy skin are certainly more than skin deep.

Eye creams are also way more expensive per ounce than facial moisturizers because they supposedly contain special ingredients; however, I mostly choose to save my money. This is not to say that I am against eye creams—if you have the budget and enjoy a lot of moving parts in your beauty regimen, there is nothing wrong with a cute tube of gel or cream that contains specialized ingredients . . . just don't expect it to work miracles.

Night Creams: Contrary to what marketers would have us believe, our skin doesn't behave differently when we go to sleep. I've been told many a story about what happens to my skin when I sleep, but honestly, aside from the fact that my cheeks might be scrunching against my pillow, it behaves the same way as it does in the day. Sure, at night my skin isn't as exposed to the elements, but does this mean that I need a separate night cream? No. You don't *need* one—absolutely not. But some people like to use different kinds of products in the day and in the evening. For example, I sometimes like to use a replenishing facial oil at night, whereas I don't like using facial oils in the morning because they feel too greasy under makeup. There are also a few ingredients that will make your skin more susceptible to UV damage and thus should never be applied in the daytime—for example, retinol and citrus essential oils.

Serums: I am a huge fan of serums. The other day, my mother, who would like to believe that a jar of cold cream or petroleum jelly does just as good a job as any newfangled concoction, asked me about serums. "What is a *serum*?" she asked with a suspicious lift of her eyebrows (and a slight smirk on her face). I think she was convinced that I was either going to fumble my answer or cop to the concept of a "serum" being indeed another load of marketing hogwash. But *no*, dear Mother—a serum is a very good invention, and here's why: it's a concentrated boost of a particular active ingredient in a highly absorbable base.

Unlike a cream, which contains loads of functional ingredients to moisturize the skin, a serum has one job only: to infuse the skin with ingredients that help mitigate past damage or prevent any further damage—or both. A serum is truly the workhorse of any good brand and contains the most potent dose of active ingredients. Most serums are water based and absorb so quickly that within a couple of minutes of application, skin will feel quite dry. This is why the serums of most good skin care lines need to be used before the moisturizers are applied.

Another great thing about serums is that different ones can be used at different times of the day. For example, I highly recommend a vitamin C serum in the morning, whereas I'd recommend an alpha hydroxy serum at night.

When shopping for a serum, you need to be very clear on what you are looking for: brightening, resurfacing, and antioxidation are just some of the functions that you might want to target. Serums tend to be more expensive because of the concentration of active ingredients involved. However, a small, one-to two-ounce bottle should last you a long time because you'll only need a few drops per use.

Neck and Décolleté Cream: Our neck and décolleté (love that word!) are often seriously neglected. Ever heard of "freeway chest"? It apparently refers to the chest of a woman who has spent many a year cruising around without a mega SPF on the area. Gosh—if only I had known that UVA rays actually penetrate glass. I have been dealing with a minor case of "freeway chest" for the past couple of years and have seen massive improvements, so this problem will be addressed in your 30-day program.

Do you *need* different products for these less-taken-care-of areas? Not really. I just take the products I use on my face all the way down to my cleavage. This can get a little pricey, because you do use a lot more product. But to mitigate this, you can do one day on and one day off. The key going forward is obviously bucketloads of sunscreen daily.

Oh, and a note about neck creams: marketers always try to hit our vulnerable spots, and they know that women over a certain age start freaking out about their turkey gobblers and saggy neck skin; however, there is currently no formulation that will even slightly "lift" the skin on your neck, so don't shell out hard-earned dollars for a load of snake oil. That being said, the skin on your neck is super thin, so your facial serums containing retinol (which thickens skin), vitamins, and peptides should always be taken down onto your neck and chest, too.

Masks: I love masks because they stay on your face for an extended period, and with the right active ingredients, they can work wonders. I try to save money by making a lot of masks myself (see Chapter 13) because then I can invest more in the kinds of serums that are harder to make.

The ingredients that I like to see or use in masks are:

- Clay (draws out impurities)
- Glycolic acid or natural fruit acids (help resurface the skin)
- Omega-3 fatty acids such as avocado and flaxseed oil ("feed" the skin with vital nutrients)
- Yogurt or powdered milk (contain exfoliating lactic acid)

- Antibacterial ingredients such as honey and cinnamon (help keep acne-causing bacteria at bay)

Must haves

Stash Away

I highly recommend that you always have the following three ingredients stashed away in your kitchen cabinets, because I can promise you that you'll be sneaking them into your bathroom to use on your skin for all kinds of beauty fixes.

- **100% organic, whole-leaf aloe vera juice and gel:** You can use the juice in place of a toner and the gel as a serum base for your vitamin C powder.
- **Raw, virgin coconut oil:** You can use this as an all-body moisturizer, a facial cleanser and moisturizer, a deodorant, and a hair mask.
- **Organic apple cider vinegar:** You can use this to remove excess oil and bacteria from acne-prone skin.

Putting It All Together

I know I've given you a lot of information here, so now I'd like to do a quick sum-up so you can see how all of this fits into daily routines. Here is what I recommend:

Morning Routine:

1. **Cleanse** with a brightening, purifying cleanser containing natural acids and enzymes*

2. **Feed** with an antioxidant and vitamin serum

3. **Boost** with collagen-building, protective vitamins, antioxidants, and peptides

4. **Hydrate** with a moisturizer that contains hyaluronic acid along with other proactive ingredients

5. **Protect** with a mineral sunscreen (SPF 30–40)

*If you have sensitive or inflamed skin, forgo acids and enzymes in your daily brightening cleanser and opt for a soothing gel cleanser instead.

Order of Application

After cleansing, it's important that you apply the rest of your products in the right order. The most active ingredient goes on first. Here is a list of the most active ingredients in descending order:

1. Vitamin C product (in the morning) or retinol product (at night)
2. Peptide firming/lightening product (morning and night)
3. Antioxidant and other botanic actives (morning and night)
4. Protect with your moisturizer and sunscreen

Evening Routine

1. **Two-step cleanse** with an emulsifying, makeup-melting cleanser followed by your brightening cleanser

2. **Boost** collagen production with your retinol products applied straight onto cleansed skin

3. **Feed** your skin with your antioxidant- and/or peptide-packed serum

4. **Hydrate** with your moisturizer

Twice each week: Exfoliate with a brush and/or a mechanical exfoliating agent.

Once each week: Do a mask or peel for extra exfoliation and nourishment.

In the Gorgeous for Good 30-day program, I'm going to walk you through the process of incorporating each of these steps into your daily life one by one, but if you'd rather follow a process of your own, the above summary can help you get started.

Going Further

While taking care of your skin by following the information in this chapter regularly will make a world of difference in how you look, people often turn to more dramatic procedures to combat damage that's already been done. Here's the thing: many consider these cosmetic treatments, such as fillers and lasers, to be preventative—in the sense that they may prevent a woman freaking out about seriously sagging skin and feeling like she needs a face-lift by the age of 60 or 70. A full-on face-lift is not for the faint of heart—it comes with surgical risks and oodles of downtime, not to mention remortgaging your home to pay for it.

I consider some of the following treatments proactive because they promote new collagen growth while giving an instant lift and bloom to a tired-looking face. For me, it's all about looking *refreshed* instead of "done." There is such a fine line between the two, and this lies in the hands of the person wielding the needle or laser gun—so choose wisely.

Fillers: What's the Deal?

Fillers are one of those things that you obviously don't *need*. Plenty of women look absolutely stunning in their 70s and 80s without going near a needle; however, there's nothing wrong with wanting a little juice-up here and there. But less is more when it comes to fillers, because overly pumped-up cheeks and blown-out nasolabial folds look completely unnatural. Getting too needle happy can actually have the opposite effect than what you want and can make you look older than you actually are because something in your face just seems off. We only need open a gossip magazine to see plenty of examples of horrendously overfilled faces.

When fillers are administered by a really great dermatologist or other doctor, they can plump up areas of your face where you notice volume loss. Fillers can be pretty awesome when administered by the right dermatologist properly, but if they're not, you can get some scary results. Filling a woman's face with a hyaluronic gel is something of an art, and it's imperative that you see testimonials and get at least three personal recommendations for the doctor you are considering.

Everyone loses a bit of facial volume as they age. However, if you have been a yo-yo dieter or seriously stressed or sick, the volume loss may be worse, especially in your cheeks. It's great that we can now add some fullness to an area that might look a little like a cake that's been taken out of the oven too early. The area around our temples can also lose a lot of volume, especially during and after menopause. When this happens, our faces can take on a kind of peanut shape. So, a little filler in specific areas can help to round out and soften our features.

Rebecca Fitzgerald, M.D., is one of the top aesthetic dermatologists in Los Angeles, and she is known for her outstanding research and work in helping to build back volume and shape in patients with HIV. I asked Dr. Fitzgerald which fillers she thinks are best for most people. Unlike many aesthetic dermatologists I've consulted, Dr. Fitzgerald takes a "global" approach to how she treats a face. Instead of filling up areas that most women think need help (nasolabial folds and lips), she considers the age of her patient and the overall look that she is probably after, which for most women is a very natural one. "You can't put thirty-year-old lips on a fifty-year-old woman," she explain. "And you can't puff up nasolabial folds on a face that otherwise doesn't have plumpness because it immediately screams that you've had work done." Dr. Fitzgerald insists that placement of the product is way more important than the kind of product used. "You need to work with an experienced aesthetic dermatologist who understands that injecting filler in one area of the face will affect every other area of the face." I asked her if she considered fillers to be "natural" (and I expected her to laugh, as most people do). She explained that most of the fillers she uses are made from a stabilized form of hyaluronic acid that actually helps to stimulate the natural production of collagen. So yes, of course the ingredients are synthetic, but they can stimulate natural processes that can help you look better.

There are three types of popular fillers that most people use:

Hyaluronic Acid Fillers: Most of the fillers that you may have heard about—Juvéderm, Perlane, Restylane, and Belotero, to name a few—are made with hyaluronic gel in some form or another. As you

2 YR. lasting filler Voluma

now know, hyaluronic acid is actually made in our own bodies, but the version used in these kinds of fillers is cultivated in a lab from a bacteria. It is extremely safe and requires no prior allergy testing because it has negligible allergenic side effects. An anesthetic called *lidocaine* is added to the mixture to help you deal with a rather long needle. The results are immediate, and if you don't like the result, the gel can be dissolved with a quick shot of the enzyme hyaluronidase. These fillers generally last for six to nine months; however, Voluma, the latest incarnation of this type of product, can last for up to two years.

Collagen-Boosting Fillers: Currently, two fillers have been found to actually stimulate collagen growth from deep within, which is very promising. Radiesse is a filler made from calcium hydroxylapatite, which aims to stimulate collagen production in addition to creating an instant fill. The advantage of this kind of filler is that you get the immediate plumping effect, knowing that it helps your skin from within, too. It lasts for about one year; however, note that it is not reversible should you not like the results.

Sculptra is another collagen-boosting filler, but this is made from the naturally occurring substance called poly-L-lactic acid. It was originally used to help fill in the gaunt faces of HIV patients and was subsequently approved for cosmetic use. The results grow slowly over time and are way more natural looking than those of the other fillers, because instead of a gel pumping up your face, Sculptra *only* works by depositing tiny particles of Sculptra, which act as irritants that force your body into creating more and more collagen. That said, it's also the most expensive filler of them all, and it requires follow-up visits to get the volume right. A great deal of patience is also required with Sculptra because it can take four to eight weeks for the new collagen to be produced. The other downside is that it is also not reversible. But if you want a way more natural look, it's the way to go. Dr. Fitzgerald teaches doctors and dermatologists all over the world how to inject Sculptra. After chatting with her about it, I realized that it requires exceptional skill, experience, and a little artistry to get it right.

Dr. Fitzgerald recommends that you get personal referrals if you are considering investing in this procedure.

Botox: Ahhhh, Botox. We've all heard horror stories about Botox—someone used too much, and now her face looks weirdly masklike. Or something's a bit off about someone because he looks perpetually surprised. But Botox isn't just used to keep foreheads wrinkle free. Interestingly, at least 50 percent of Botox treatment in the U.S. is used for medical conditions such as severe neck pain, migraines, voice or swallowing problems, drooling, crossed eyes, muscle spasms, and even an overactive bladder.

As far as cosmetic use is concerned, all of our faces frown and crease quite differently. I've seen women who've never had Botox and who barely have a line on their foreheads. On the other hand, I've seen plenty of women who have deep lines etched between their eyebrows, making them look perpetually tired and angry when they're really not. Botox is one of the only procedures to date that is effective at stopping your frowning so that those wrinkles disappear.

Although Botox is obviously a toxin, it's interestingly one of the drugs that is most studied for safety, and it has been found to be way safer than many OTC drugs—even aspirin. The rare cases where the drug has spread from the injection site and caused serious problems or death have, for the most part, been in children with cerebral palsy who were injected with huge amounts. That being said, if you use Botox to keep wrinkles at bay, you *are* having tiny, poisoned arrows injected into your muscles to cause paralysis. If people came down from Mars and saw that women on Earth were willing to put themselves through this and pay a handsome fee for it, they would think that we'd taken leave of our senses—and maybe we have! I have to remind myself here that almost every older woman who I think is stunningly beautiful has a few well-earned wrinkles on her face.

Because Botox is a drug, you must speak to a highly qualified dermatologist or doctor to assess its safety for you. My feeling is that, as with most cosmetic procedures, if you insist on injecting something into your face, less is more. Don't completely freeze your entire face (some women have it put around their eyes, in their cheeks, and even around their mouths). Don't be one of those horror stories. Remember, it's all about who does it for you, and if someone's coming near your face with a needle, triple-check their credentials and get some personal references.

There are a couple of very similar but slightly different incarnations of Botox as well. One is Dysport, which is essentially the same except for the dosages and the way it spreads; some patients think that it is more effective in the way it spreads to other muscles. Xeomin is a "tox" from which the proteins have been taken out, leaving it a "naked tox." This is thought to lessen the very rare chance of a patient developing an antibody to the tox, which renders it less effective. Either way, though, a tox is a tox!

Picking the Right Filler

In an ideal world, I recommend going without any fillers or injectables, period. They are expensive, they can hurt, and they can leave huge bruises. And let's be honest—injecting our faces with even the most "natural" substance is still not exactly allowing nature to take its course. But, if you feel for one reason or another that you just need a little plumping here and there, be sure to choose the right filler.

According to all the plastic surgeons and dermatologists I spoke to, these are the right injectables for each issue:

- **Forehead frown lines and/or crow's feet:** Botox, Dysport, or Xeomin

- **Loss of volume in cheeks and around temples:** Sculptra, Juvéderm, Voluma, or Radiesse. Sculptra is the most subtle (it won't look like you've had filler) and lasts the longest.

- **Marionette lines and deep folds:** Radiesse

- **Nasolabial folds, smile lines, and lips:** Restylane

- **Instant cheek plumping (baby cheeks):** Juvéderm or Voluma

- **Deep furrows, glabellar lines:** Belotero

Serum [handwritten margin note]

Factor This In . . .

Emily Fritchey, "the Skin Whisperer," explained to me that if her clients have been using fillers and Botox for years, she notices a laxity in their skin, which she believes is partly due to lack of muscular action: the muscles seem to get "flabby" after extended periods of inactivity and lack of daily use. This makes sense, particularly with Botox, with which the muscles are rendered pretty much immobile. If the muscles in your arms and legs cannot contract anymore, they get soft and flabby, so it stands to reason that the muscles in your face will do the same. Emily's advice to her needle-happy clients is to make sure to use a daily serum that contains muscle-tightening peptides such as copper, matrixyl (pentapeptide), argireline (hexapeptide-3), palmitoyl oligopeptide, or palmitoyl tetrapeptide-7—to name just a few.

Lasers: Are They as Miraculous as They Sound?

Laser treatments are on every plastic surgeon and dermatologist's menu of services. But are they safe? And can they deliver on their promises? I turned to Julia Tatum Hunter, M.D., to help me make sense of this rather complicated topic. I love Dr. Hunter because her philosophy embraces the latest scientific advances coupled with a smart, holistic approach.

So the question is, "If I want a laser treatment, what should I look for?" Dr. Hunter believes that skin laxity and loss of subcutaneous fat can be really helped with lasers; however, she advises women to be very selective in their choice of treatment. She told me that good lasers can visibly volumize, lift, and tighten the skin, which means that new collagen is being produced. She added that hyperpigmentation, scarring, and abnormal veins can also be treated with lasers and reduced. Not only did she stress that you need to choose the right laser treatment—choosing the right doctor is even more important. A good laser in inexperienced hands can lead to really bad results, as can a poor machine in good hands. She says that laser treatments are both an art and a science.

According to Dr. Hunter, even the best lasers are only as good as the knowledge and meticulousness of the person using them. Practitioners or salons may buy lasers without understanding the limitations or side effects of the technology, and they often try to overreach the technology's limits. This is when problems and side effects occur. The practitioner *has* to know his or her technology. He or she must continually observe and improve delivery methods for best results and choose the right laser to address each individual patient's challenges and goals.

Lasers work on collagen, so it makes sense that you *first* want to improve the amount of collagen you have by optimizing your diet and exercise and using therapeutic skin care products that give you visible results. Then, when you spend the time and money on a laser procedure, you get the best use of that time and money. Remember that to get the full results of any laser procedure takes 6 to 12 weeks, because this is how long the collagen production cycle takes.

What about downtime and sun photosensitivity? Dr. Hunter says that yes, there is a compromise with any procedure that penetrates the deeper layers of the skin. With an "ablative" laser, which removes the top layer of skin, there will be at least five days' downtime during which you cannot put anything on your skin—which will look a little . . . let's say . . . interesting! Moreover, as Dr. Hunter pointed out, the deep, ablative lasers will bring old sun damage right up to the surface, so your skin may look even more sun damaged than before. This, however, is a good thing, because nontoxic peels (when the skin is ready for them) can slough off the newly surfaced damage.

Which Laser Might Be Best for Me?

The biggest difference in skin-resurfacing lasers is between the ablative and nonablative types. In short, the former whips off a whole layer of your skin, and the latter doesn't. But here's a bit more technical detail:

- **Ablative:** An ablative laser "ablates" or removes the top layer of skin and part of the sublayer. It is invasive, requires a couple of weeks of downtime, and carries a risk of infection. It also requires anesthesia. It will, however, deliver the most dramatic results in terms of wrinkle and sun damage removal. A single procedure lasts for up to five years, but this depends on how well you take care of your skin going forward (and especially how religious you are about applying your sunscreen).

- **Nonablative:** A nonablative laser delivers energy (heat or laser) into the dermis but does not remove the skin. Nonablative laser treatments are typically done in a series of three or four sessions, where little or no downtime is required. There are lots of different kinds of nonablative lasers, and I'm sure there'll be many more to come.

- **Fractionated:** A fractionated laser can come in both ablative and nonablative forms. The advantage of an ablative fractionated laser is that it reduces the amount of downtime because the laser beam is broken up into separate beams (as opposed to one giant beam), each sending microscopic columns of energy into the skin to destroy the tissue. Only specific areas of targeted skin are wounded, which means that the surrounding healthy tissue can help speed the healing process. The beams that penetrate down into the dermis stimulate the growth of new collagen.

Go chat with a dermatologist or plastic surgeon about which procedure they think is best for you, but remember that they are going to push the laser machine in which they have just invested a huge amount of money. However, they obviously purchased it because they believe that it will deliver the best results. Still, I think that if you are about to spend a lot of your own hard-earned money, you should consult a couple of different dermatologists—after all, it's your precious face that's at stake, and some of these procedures are heavy-duty. I would also double the downtime and pain factors they estimate. I've watched many videos of bloggers and YouTubers who have cataloged their day-to-day recoveries, and their experiences are often way worse than the docs told them they would be!

I haven't yet tried a laser (I'm a bit of a baby when it comes to that kind of pain, because I don't want to be reminded of a terrible facial burn that I suffered a decade ago), but I am open to giving one of the gentler ones a try. Like most people, I have a degree of sun damage that I'd like to see reduced. That's not to say that I want to walk around with a strange, white, shiny face (yes, I see many of these in Beverly Hills). I like my freckles and a certain amount of wear and tear!

Just like fillers, certain lasers are better for certain concerns:

- **Deep wrinkles, sagging skin, and extreme sun damage:** a fractionated, ablative procedure

- **Fine lines, sun damage, and coarse texture:** a nonablative, fractionated laser

- **Rosacea, broken facial veins:** a V-beam laser, which delivers an intense pulse of light into the skin, destroying blood vessels and allowing them to be reabsorbed into the body

- **Brown spots and broken capillaries:** an intense pulsed light (IPL) photofacial, in which computer-controlled pulses of light heat the subsurface layers of your skin

Before I finished my discussion with Dr. Hunter, I asked her for some tips to help people get the best results from any procedure they decide to try.

Here's what she told me:

- Before you even think about any procedure, make sure that your skin is healthy by way of diet and nontoxic, therapeutic skin care products.

- Don't trust what you read on the Internet, because most of it is marketing.

- Do thorough research to find a highly skilled doctor with an excellent track record and pristine credentials. Make sure that the doctor takes your particular skin concerns and goals into account when recommending a procedure.

- Personal referrals are great, because you can actually see someone's skin three to six months postprocedure, which is important.

Radiofrequency Procedures

While discussing laser treatments, you may also hear mention of radiofrequency procedures. But don't be fooled—these are very different from lasers. A radiofrequency device uses heat to tighten the underlying tissues of your face to "lift" it. These procedures do not work on the surface layers of the skin, so they won't affect sun damage or skin texture, meaning the results are generally less dramatic than you get from a laser. The good news is that there is no downtime.

Chapter 5

Nourishing and Protecting Your Temple

Taking care of your body is as important as taking care of your face. There is no point in having a glowing face and lackluster, dry arms and legs. Let's get the whole of you looking gorgeous!

Protecting Yourself

I'd like to start this chapter off with something about health and beauty—something that is essential to looking good and feeling well: sun protection.

It's now common knowledge that UV (ultraviolet) rays damage our skin and accelerate aging. UVA rays can pass through clouds and glass. They penetrate deep into our skin, damaging the collagen and elastin, causing uneven pigmentation and brown spots, damaging DNA, and potentially causing the deadly skin cancer malignant melanoma. The other UV rays are UVBs, which are the ones we commonly think of when we think of sunblock because they are stronger, and they're the ones that cause our skin to burn. UVB rays can also cause cancer. It's important to note here that we do need a little sun in order to make vitamin D (many of us are deficient in this vital vitamin). Sun exposure, however, should be moderate and controlled (see page 143), and it's best to avoid sun exposure on the face, neck, and chest, where the skin is thinner.

It's interesting that despite the fact that everyone knows that we should plaster ourselves with the highest-SPF (sun-protection factor) sunblock we can find, rates of deadly skin cancer are increasing by 1.9 percent per year. This might have something to do with high SPF factors fooling us into thinking we can spend hours frolicking around in full-on sun, and/or the chemicals in some sunscreens that are thought to damage DNA. SPF measures a product's ability to screen skin-burning rays, primarily UVBs. However, SPF does not reflect a product's ability to screen out UVA rays, which are the ones most responsible for cell damage, aging, and possibly melanoma—this holds true even if the sun product is labeled "broad spectrum." Another problem with our current sunscreens is that the SPF claims are often quite inaccurate. Many sunscreens, no matter what their stated SPF, fall well short of an adequate level of protection. And many health professionals believe that any claims of SPFs over 30 are just marketing. All this means that finding the best sunscreen for you can take some work.

Choosing a Sunscreen

Sun protection products have become a hot-button issue of late because it's been discovered that chemical sunscreens may not be good for your health. While the FDA has approved 17 ingredients for sun protection, 15 of them are chemical compounds, and 2 are physical minerals. The chemicals (such as oxybenzone and avobenzone) work by absorbing and scattering the UV light, whereas the minerals reflect it physically.

I personally don't love chemical sunscreens. Because they work by absorbing the sun's rays, you need to apply them at least 30 minutes before heading into the sun, which many people forget. And some of the chemicals, such as oxybenzone, have been found to be endocrine disruptors, so the fact that they are absorbed by the skin worries me. A vitamin A derivative, retinyl palmitate, is often added to sunscreens, too, and this ingredient has been found to possibly promote tumor growth. Moreover, the chemical sunscreens typically contain a bunch of other worrying ingredients, including preservatives and artificial fragrances.

Chemicals to Avoid in Sunscreen

The following ingredients have been linked to cancer, DNA damage, or allergic reactions:

- Benzophenones (dioxybenzone, oxybenzone)
- PABA and PABA esters (ethyl dihydroxypropyl PABA, glyceryl PABA, p-aminobenzoic acid, padimate O, or octyl dimethyl PABA)
- Cinnamates (cinoxate, isobutyl salicyl cinnamate, octyl methoxycinnamate, octinoxate, octocrylene (2-ethylhexyl-2-ciano-3, 3-diphenyl acrylate)
- Salicylates (ethylhexyl salicylate, homosalate, octyl salicylate)*
- Avobenzone (butyl methyoxydibenzoylmethane, parsol 1789)
- Digalloyl trioleate
- Methyl anthranilate

*These are derivatives of the natural plant-based salicylic acid that is used in skin care products for oily skin.

Although not perfect, mineral sunblock is a great option. Because it provides an immediate block, you can go out in the sun directly after application. The two minerals used are zinc oxide and titanium dioxide. Zinc oxide in particular is very good at reflecting UV rays. One of the downsides of these minerals, though, is that unless they are crushed so fine that they become nanoparticles, they look like white, opaque grease sitting on your skin—not so pretty. Therefore, manufacturers choose to use nanoparticles to create a more transparent sunscreen. Is this an issue? The jury is still out on whether or not engineered nanoparticles in a cream formulation can penetrate the skin and enter the bloodstream, where they could cause cell damage. There has been a lot of concern about engineered nanoparticles of zinc oxide, and although most health experts deem it to be safe because it's unlikely to get beyond the dermis, I choose to steer clear until long-term safety studies have been conducted. I always ask companies whether or not they use nanoparticles.

In the case of a sunscreen spray or mineral powder, however, it seems very likely that nanoparticles could be a problem because inhaling tiny particles of any mineral could cause severe lung issues.

When looking for a mineral sunscreen, also make sure that the rest of the ingredients in the formulation are good, and avoid sunscreens that contain synthetic fragrance.

The Great Vitamin D Debate

There is also an interesting debate about whether or not giving our skin a dose of daily sunlight is good for building our reserves of vitamin D. The dermatologists I've spoken to don't advise that you *ever* allow your unprotected skin to be blasted by the sun's rays; however, many natural health advocates disagree because they believe the most effective way to get your vitamin D is through direct sunlight.

Dr. John Douillard, author of six books on Ayurvedic health care, explains that vitamin D is actually a hormone responsible for promoting many vital, healthy processes in the body, especially regulating calcium and protecting our bones. Dr. Douillard is an advocate of getting your daily dose of sun because its UVB rays convert cholesterol in the skin to vitamin D3 (which he prefers to the more popular D2 because its absorptive affinity is better, and it's less toxic). He recommends lying out in the sun for 15 minutes (baring as much of your flesh as possible), or until your skin starts to turn pink. Dr. Douillard also recommends that you don't shower off until at least an hour later because it takes that amount of time for the cholesterol in your skin to convert and the vitamin D to be absorbed into your body. However, the UV index of where you live must be 3 or above when you go out, or it won't be strong enough. To find out the UV index in your area, you can visit www.uvawareness.com and type in your ZIP code—it will tell you what your UV index is for every hour of the day. When your UV index falls below 3, which in many places it does in the winter months, Dr. Douillard suggests that you supplement with 4,000 IU of vitamin D per day.

To find out if you're deficient in vitamin D, a simple blood test will tell you your levels, and your doctor will recommend the right supplemental dosage for you.

In my own life, I try to get a bit of natural vitamin D each day—more along the lines of what Dr. Douillard suggests. It seems natural and healthy, and it makes me feel better, which is generally a good thing. That being said, I always protect the skin on my face and neck because the skin is thinner on these areas and thus way more susceptible to sun damage.

Unfortunately, there doesn't seem to be a definitive answer on whether or not a little sun will hurt you, so you'll have to decide this one on your own. For me, it falls into that "everything in moderation" category. I go with the fact that the superior way for making sure my vitamin D levels are good is to allow the sun to manufacture it in my skin. I am, however, careful not to overdo it, and I always keep my face and chest well covered because my skin is thinner in these areas and thus more prone to sun damage.

Sophie's Top Sun Protection Tips

- Stay out of the sun between noon and 2 P.M.
- Wear SPF-protective hats and clothing if you will get prolonged sun exposure.
- Reapply mineral sunscreen every two hours.
- Make sure you thoroughly cover your face, neck, and chest with sunscreen each day.
- Layer your mineral sunscreen, especially over areas like your neck and chest, where your skin is thinner.

- If you are going to be in direct sunlight for more than a couple of minutes, don't rely on mineral powder sunscreen for your face.
- Wear protective SPF gloves for driving. (According to my daughter, these are the zenith of "creepiness," but I'd rather suffer her derision than have lizardy, spotted hands!)

Faking It

With all of the controversy over whether or not the sun will make you sick, many people have turned to fake tans as a healthier alternative to geting that sun-kissed glow. Almost all sunless tanners use an ingredient called DHA (dihydroxyacetone), which is either made synthetically or derived from sugar. It reacts with the amino acids in the top layer of your skin to produce pigments called melanoidins, which turn your skin brown. DHA has been proven to be nontoxic, and it doesn't migrate beyond the top layer of your skin. It does, however, have a slightly strange odor, but that's cleverly masked in many formulations.

The most important thing to do when shopping for a self-tanner is to look at all the other ingredients in the formula, because there can be some really nasty stuff in there. Fortunately, many sunscreen and skin care companies now create wonderful self-tanners without the toxic ingredients. They vary greatly in texture and scent, so you just have to try them to see which you like. Keep in mind that despite all the claims about the "kind" of tan the product will give you, they all use the same "tanning" ingredient: DHA. The only difference is the intensity of tan, which is dependent on how much DHA they throw into the formula. Products that advertise a soft, buildable tan (e.g., when used as a daily moisturizer) just have a very small concentration of DHA added, so this is often a good place to start.

Some self-tanning products contain a brown coloring agent so that they go on "brown." I quite like this, because it's easier to see if I've applied the product evenly. This brown dye, however, will wash off when you shower. If you don't plan to shower between application and your daily routine, I recommend applying any sunless tanner that has a coloring agent in it in the morning, waiting ten minutes for it to absorb, and then wearing dark colors—because it will get on your clothes and sheets.

Tips for Sunless "Tanning"

- Before applying your tanner, exfoliate really well, because the tan only happens in that uppermost layer of your skin. Those dead skin cells are shed daily, and your tan disappears with them.
- After exfoliation, moisturize areas where the tanning product can get caught in rough patches, such as the toes, heels, elbows, and knees.
- Apply the self-tanner with a mitt to help smooth on the product evenly. It also saves you from having to wash your hands afterward.

Another popular option for faking a tan is spray tanning. The booths for this are a little scary because the airborne particles of DHA can easily be inhaled. If you want a spray tan, be mindful to:

- Have a customized tan where the technician will actually spray you rather than just having the spray come at you at all angles from a machine. It's more expensive, but it means that you can make sure a technician doesn't spray near your face.

- Always wear goggles and nose plugs.

- Always check the ingredients in the products. Compare them against the list in Chapter 1 to avoid anything that's really bad for you.

Cellulite: Our Biggest Foe

Okay. This may not be important to your health, but it is one of the biggest subjects of interest when people ask about having a beautiful body. I seem to be addressing it so often that I've realized that I could become a billionaire very quickly if I came up with a magical cellulite-banishing cream. There is, of course, no such thing, and any lotion or cream that promises to get rid of cellulite is not telling the truth!

But you know what? That's okay. Cellulite is perfectly normal. Ninety percent of women have cellulite, and 10 percent of men. Cellulite doesn't mean you're fat—even very thin women get it. So, what is it? Basically, fat squeezes up between the fibrous connective cords that anchor your skin to your muscle. As more fat accumulates, the fat pushes up against your skin while the tough, old cords pull down. This creates a dimpling on the surface of your skin.

There really isn't anything that will completely get rid of your cellulite forever. There are a number of very expensive treatments that may soften the appearance of your cellulite a little bit (and they require a bunch of ongoing sessions). These treatments include rolling, massaging, and the application of heat via laser. There are also a number of creams that contain methylxanthines, which are a group of chemicals that can break down the fat stores. The problem with these creams is that they cannot deliver anywhere near the concentrations required to make a measurable difference.

So, what options are left? Here's what I recommend:

- Increase your circulation around the areas of cellulite. This can be achieved by daily dry brushing your skin at areas of cellulite (see box on facing page for more information).

- Make sure to take great care of the skin that sits atop your cellulite! I have created a DIY serum that not only helps prevent stretch marks but also contains essential oils to help with detoxification (page 383).

- Give yourself a deep, tissue-manipulating massage with suction cups that are specifically designed for this purpose. I like the ones by Bellabaci (www.bellabaci.com.) You can also give your cellulite a run for its money in terms of deep tissue manipulation with a BelleCore Body Buffer (www.bellecore.com). This is an extraordinary device that not only "moves" your cellulite but also buffs your skin and brings blood to where it needs to circulate.

- It's obvious, I know, but diet and exercise are about the most important part of the equation. Follow my 30-day program, and you'll be on the right track.

My final word on cellulite is this: why focus on it? Granted, it may not be the most attractive thing in the world, but honestly, choose to put your attention on the great things about your body instead: your strength, your soft curves, and how your body serves you so beautifully in getting where you need to go and doing what you need to do. Life is waaaaaay too short to obsess about something that, for the most part, is not even on view for the general public.

Dry Brushing

Dry brushing is essential for healthy-looking skin all over your body. Not only does it exfoliate dry skin, but it also stimulates your lymphatic system, which is your body's natural detoxification system. This is vital when you're trying to minimize cellulite. I recommend that you do this every day and, luckily, it's very simple and quick. Here the skinny on how to do it:

1. Purchase a long-handled, natural-bristle brush.
2. Before you get in the shower, when your skin is dry, use long, firm, upward strokes to brush, starting at your feet and moving up toward your heart. Make sure you brush the fronts and backs of your legs, and don't forget your backside!

3. Next, lift one arm above your head, and starting at your hand, brush down toward your heart. Repeat on the other arm. Brush from the outer edges of your armpits (they have loads of lymph nodes) in toward your breast and heart.
4. Then brush down the back of your neck, from your hairline to your shoulders.
5. Move on to brush your belly in gentle, clockwise circular motions.
6. And, finally, when you are done, jump in the shower and wash as usual.

Deodorant: Another Great Debate

In the green cosmetics world, there has recently been quite a debate about the pros and cons of your standard, store-bought deodorant. There are two super-scary terms that have been linked to ostensibly toxic antiperspirants: breast cancer and Alzheimer's. Now, if you're like me, you don't really need to hear anything more, because even if there's a one percent chance that a family member or I might be struck down with a serious disease from an ingredient, it is not coming into my house.

However, it is important to tease out the Internet rumors here and get to the bottom of the matter. In short, there is currently no reliable evidence that supports a connection between deodorant and cancer or Alzheimer's. That being said, there are a lot of other suspect ingredients lurking in drugstore deodorants. Many underarm products contain aluminum salts, propylene glycol, synthetic fragrance, and parabens—none of which I want in that delicate area extremely close to my lymph nodes, the system that I rely on to expel toxins and keep me healthy.

However, it's hard to find a natural deodorant that really works, and the reason is that the natural formulas don't contain the very substance that blocks your sweat glands: aluminum salts. Although, as previously noted, there is no proven connection between aluminum salts and Alzheimer's, they react with the water

get natural
one w/ essential oil
aloe zinc oxide,
deoderant OK
anti perspir
NO

Nourishing and Protecting Your Temple

in your sweat to create plugs that block your sweat ducts. I think we need to sweat; it's one of the important ways in which our body excretes waste and toxins.

It's important to understand that there are two different kinds of deodorants:

1. **With antiperspirant:** As the name implies, antiperspirants aim to stop you from sweating. They typically contain aluminum compounds because they are some of the few substances that will plug your ducts. Remember, it's not the sweat itself that stinks but the bacteria that breeds when sweat has been sitting in your pits for a while. If you absolutely don't want to sweat at all or have a nerve-wracking meeting or special event where you are going to be wearing a silk blouse, you might want to stash away an antiperspirant to keep you as dry as is possible without having the whole area Botoxed (which I don't advise).

2. **Without antiperspirant:** A plain old deodorant is just as it sounds—it only deals with the odor and won't stop you from sweating, which in my opinion is way healthier. Most truly natural deodorants fall into this category. I look for deodorants that are formulated with pure essential oils, aloe, and zinc oxide.

Deodorant Paste

Underarm pastes have become really popular. They come in a jar, so you have to scoop the goop and rub it into your pits. Most of them are formulated with baking soda or arrowroot, which helps to minimize wetness, and a blend of essential oils, which help to combat bacteria and provide a beautiful smell. If you want to make your own, check out my DIY recipe on page 384.

Cleansing, Moisturizing, and Exfoliating

Aside from the things we've already talked about, caring for the beauty of your body falls into a similar vein as taking care of your face, neck, and chest. You should cleanse, moisturize, and exfoliate it on a regular basis using products that nourish your skin—products that don't contain the harsh chemicals I laid out in Chapter 1.

Bodywash and Hand and Body Soap

Washes and soaps are the hand and body products you'll encounter most often as you go through your day. In fact, you'll likely use them every day—or, in the case of hand soap, multiple times each day. Because their use is so common, and because they often contain so many harsh and toxic chemicals, I recommend that you switch to a cleaner alternative right away.

Two of the most common, yet unwanted, ingredients that you'll find in these products are:

1. **SLS (sodium lauryl sulfate):** strips your body of its natural oils. This is one of the ingredients I avoid for toxicity reasons (see page 28 for more information).

2. **Fragrance/Parfum:** This nonspecific ingredient often implies harsh chemicals . . . but companies are not required to disclose what they are.

Don't get me wrong. I adore beautiful soaps and amazing-smelling washes. Even if I don't use them, I like to smell them. And I love to display those cute soaps on my bathroom sink. Luckily, natural artisan soap-making has exploded, so you'll actually be spoiled for choice when looking for a truly natural soap. But be careful when shopping for bodywash and soaps; many companies now use packaging that implies a natural product to disguise what may be not so natural.

Aside from the usual culprits (pages 24–29), never buy "antibacterial" soaps because they likely contain the toxic chemical triclosan. And remember, you can easily make your own soaps. Check out my Liquid Hand and Body Soap recipe (pages 381–382), which is very easy to make.

Your Skin's Worst Enemy

Many of us filter chlorine out of our drinking water, but what about your shower or bath water? The negative effects of chlorine go way beyond the fact that it dries out our skin and hair. There is a link between chlorine and skin cancer.

Chlorine Absorption

You absorb more toxins from chlorine during a five-minute shower than you do from drinking a day's worth of chlorinated water. The toxin in question is carcinogenic chloroform. The whole-house filtration system that I invested in a few years ago was a game changer for my skin and hair—no more dry skin and scalp, and my hair color lasts twice as long.

Luckily, there are things you can do to minimize your exposure, the best of which is to get a whole-house water filtration system installed. A granular activated carbon filtration system is the best because it keeps the valuable minerals in your water and takes the bad stuff out. It's also way more eco-friendly than reverse osmosis. If you can't afford a whole-house system or if you live in a condo or apartment, your best bet is to install a filtering showerhead, which can really help. If you don't have a whole-home filtration system and you like to take baths, look for a dechlorinating bath ball, which will remove most of the chlorine.

What about Hand Sanitizers?

You may well ask about hand sanitizers. My daughter has always been obsessed with the crazy synthetic scents (like double chocolate cookie dough) that are loaded into cute-looking, mini hand sanitizers. Most of them, however, contain toxic triclosan. Fortunately, a few great companies have come out with all kinds of wonderful alternatives that contain antibacterial essential oils such as lavender or tea tree oil. If you use hand sanitizer, look for one that doesn't include the dicey ingredients I listed in Chapter 1.

Moisturizing with Lotions, Balms, Butters, and Oils

Body Lotion: Whatever you smear over the largest expanse of your skin every day is the first thing you need to investigate for toxic chemicals. Most of us reach for a lotion because it's easy to apply, absorbs quickly, and smells good. However, there's a huge difference between the myriad body lotions in drugstores and those in health-food stores—many of the drugstore lotions are chock full of synthetic chemicals that make your skin feel moisturized for a few seconds, along with tons of preservatives to extend shelf life for years. On the other hand, the healthier versions you may find in health-food stores can feel watery and ineffectual. What you really need to look for is a body lotion, balm, or oil that is crammed full of ingredients that can actually "feed" your skin. This is how I shop for a lotion:

- **Consider the fragrance:** I'm a sucker for a great fragrance; however, I do steer clear of synthetically fragranced lotions because I don't want all those phthalates. In these cases, you'll spot the term *fragrance* or *parfum* on the ingredient list. Instead, I look for lotions that use essential oil blends. And I never buy a lotion without testing it on my hand or arm and having a good sniff. Fragrance is so personal. Where one woman may love fresh citrus notes, another may want something more floral. You might even prefer an unscented lotion, especially if you apply your own perfume.

- **Consider the texture:** I have a huge issue with watery lotions. A lotion, as opposed to a body oil or balm, almost always contains water. However, how *much* water is the issue! I always squeeze a sample onto my arm, rub it in, and walk around the store. I can usually tell right away if a formulation is too watery, but I give it a few minutes to see how well it performs once it's been absorbed.

ARNICA

Supercharged Body Lotions: If you shop in a health-food store, you're likely to find body lotions that are supercharged with various supplements, medicinal remedies, or homeopathic remedies. My favorite ingredients here include:

- **MSM:** This is a "natural beauty mineral" with powerful anti-inflammatory properties. It can help joint and muscle pain, so it's great for arthritis, fibromyalgia, and muscle strain. It also helps build collagen.

- **Alpha lipoic acid:** This is a powerful antioxidant, so it helps with potential free-radical damage.

- **DMAE:** This compound can help firm your skin and curb inflammation.

- **Arnica:** Arnica is a homeopathic remedy that is great for swelling, bruising, aches, and pains.

- **CoQ10:** This is a great antioxidant, so it helps with potential free-radical damage.

- **AHAs:** Alpha hydroxy acids aim to exfoliate your skin.

- **Ayurvedic oils:** These are intended to balance your Ayurvedic *dosha*. According to the ancient Ayurvedic system of medicine originating in India, each of us has a predominant body type (*dosha*) that can become unbalanced, leading to ill health. The system works to address imbalances through diet and therapeutic practices such as yoga, meditation, medicinal herbs, and oils.

Body Butter and Body Balm: The advantage of butters and balms is that for the most part, they do not require too many preservatives because of their fruit butter or oil content, if kept in a cool, dark spot, even for months. Body butters and balms can be so delicious smelling that you want to eat them! They are typically

Keep in cool dark place

A must in Body Butters .

made with a variety of plant oils (olive, grape seed, avocado, and so on) and plant butters (shea, cocoa, mango, and so on). Again, always make sure that any added fragrance is from pure essential oils, which should be clearly marked on the ingredient list.

I love to make my own balms and butters because it saves me money, and it's very, very easy to do. Check out my recipes in Chapter 13.

Yummy Butters

Look for the following butters in your body lotion and butter formulations. I have used many of these butters in varying combinations for my DIY body butters, too.

- **Cocoa butter:** Pressed from cacao seeds, this is full of antioxidants, smells chocolaty, and melts into your skin. It's great for softening rough, dry skin.
- **Mango butter:** Pressed from the seed kernels of the mango tree, this is very high in essential fatty acids and contains loads of antioxidants. It helps to restore your skin's elasticity and even contains a little natural sun protection.
- **Shea butter:** This is my go-to for dry skin. Shea butter is extracted from the nut of the African shea tree. It's intensely moisturizing and full of vitamins A and E. There are two different kinds of shea butter. One is Nilotica shea, which is found in East Africa. It is soft and buttery and melts straight into your skin. The other, West African shea, is hard and waxy. I use this one for DIY skin care because it melts when heated and then firms up when cool, which means it's very easy to work with.
- **Kokum, Cupuacu, and Tucuma butters**: These are all deeply moisturizing and healing butters from the Amazon.

Exfoliating Your Body

Just like on your face, neck, and chest, exfoliating is one of the best things for glowing skin everywhere. You can use a number of different tools and products for exfoliation. All of the below products should be used with a liquid soap or shower gel as opposed to bar soap, which doesn't have the same "slip" or sudsy action as a liquid soap.

Here are your choices:

- **Loofahs:** A loofah is made from a dried, marrow-like, fibrous fruit. Its coarse fibers are good for skin exfoliation; however, the nooks and crannies are a great place for yesterday's dirt and bacteria to gather. If you are wedded to your loofah, make sure you dry it out completely between washes and replace it every month.

- **Poufs:** Exfoliating poufs are usually made from nylon mesh. They are extremely inexpensive, which is why you see them hanging out in the dollar store. I don't think they are wonderful at exfoliating because, although abrasive, they tend to have a slippery finish, so they don't do as good a job as some of the other products listed here. Be sure to recycle your pouf when you're done with it, because it is plastic.

- **Exfoliating gloves or mitt:** Most exfoliating gloves and mitts are made from a synthetic, nylon kind of material. They are created with hundreds of little abrasive fibers, which do a great job of exfoliating your skin. If you are against using a man-made fiber that is petroleum derived, you could try a silk mitt or a Turkish cloth mitt (*kese*)—both feel great.

- **Exfoliating body towel:** Most body towels are made from a thin, coarsely fibered nylon type of material. They usually measure about three feet by one foot, making exfoliating your entire body really easy. An exfoliating towel can reach your entire back, which is often neglected with other exfoliating products. Because it's so thin, it dries out really quickly when hung in your shower, which is a big advantage for keeping it bacteria free.

- **Exfoliating sisal strap:** A sisal strap often comes with plastic handles on either end for ease of use. Although I love the fact that sisal is a natural, biodegradable material, it does take longer to dry out, so it should be washed regularly and completely dried between uses.

- **Electric body-polishing brush:** Much like deep-cleansing facial brushes, electric brushes are available for your body, too. Many of them come with a bunch of attachments, including brush heads of various sizes and/or a pumice stone.

Body Scrubs and Polishes

There are so many scrubs and polishes on the market that it's hard to choose. By and large, I like to make my own so that I can save money and control exactly what goes in it. I don't advise using a body scrub or polish along with any of the body exfoliating devices listed above because the little granules can get stuck in the tiny fibers—and they are really hard to remove.

The advantage of using a scrub or polish over an exfoliating device is that you moisturize your skin at the same time, because they are usually formulated with cold-pressed plant oils. Your decision is whether to use a salt or sugar scrub. There are advantages to either, but here are some things to consider:

Salt Scrub: A salt scrub is more abrasive than a sugar scrub because the crystals are larger and have sharper edges. If you have a lot of dry skin that needs to be removed, salt may be the better choice for you. One big benefit of a salt scrub is that the salts that are commonly used in good-quality ones mineralize your skin with trace minerals such as calcium, magnesium, and potassium. Look for scrubs that are formulated with Dead Sea salt, Himalayan salt, Epsom salt, or Hawaiian salt.

Sugar Scrub: A sugar scrub is a better choice if you have sensitive skin because the crystals are more rounded, and they melt in the heat of the shower water. Sugar also has conditioning and exfoliating properties because of its glycolic content. A sugar scrub will leave your skin feeling less dry but will still do a good job of removing dead skin cells.

Having chosen your scrub type, it's important to be aware of the other ingredients in the formulation. Check that:

- The scrub uses natural plant oils (sweet almond, grape seed, olive, and so on), not mineral oils.

- The oils used to fragrance the scrub are pure essential oils, not artificial fragrances.

Beware: A salt or sugar scrub can make your bath or shower stall very slippery. Make sure you have a slip-proof mat in the bottom of your shower, and when you are done, spritz the bath or stall with a sprayer of white vinegar and wipe it out with an old (clean) rag or paper towel to prevent the next person (or yourself) from slipping.

Treating Yourself at the Spa

Who doesn't adore a spa visit? These relaxing establishments can help you take care of all the work we've been discussing—both for your face and for your body overall. When you visit a spa, however, you need to check that you are getting what you pay for and that they are using beautiful organic ingredients. I'm amazed that some "health" spas still offer treatments using products that contain toxic ingredients.

Before you book a spa appointment, ask the following questions:

1. What product lines do they use for their facials?
2. What product lines (essential oils, etc.) do they use for their massages?
3. How many product lines do they sell?
4. Are their aestheticians licensed and accredited?

The menus for services at these places range far and wide, from the relatively common aromatherapy facial, body wraps, and salt scrubs to the less frequent oxygenating facials, silk peels, and even vampire facials. With all of these services, the important thing is to do your research. Get recommendations from people who have received them. Look into the licensing and practices of the spa. And remember, there are a number of procedures, such as scrubs, that are easy (and much more affordable) to do yourself.

Part Two

. . . AND MOVING IN

Chapter 6

Beauty from Within

When I think of the inspiring and beautiful women in my life who have been mentors to me in one way or another, there are a few traits that they all share: they are fearless, curious, funny, self-deprecating, generous, and on fire! In short, all of them have fantastic personalities. If you don't have these kinds of role models, think about a well-known woman who has inspired you at some time in your life. It could be Maya Angelou, a personal favorite who overcame a torturous childhood to find something so beautiful in her soul that she shared it with the world through her arresting poetry. Marianne Williamson, Maria Shriver, Oprah Winfrey, Joanna Lumley, and Angelina Jolie are others who have had the courage to step up on a platform to express their truth in the hope that we might all learn to do the same. These are all women who inspire me to become a better person.

In ancient cultures, wisdom was passed down to a woman from a guru, a mentor, or a grandmother. This kind of wisdom empowered us to stay true to our purpose in life. Ironically, I think that one of my greatest strengths is the knowledge that most of the time I have no idea what all the answers are. This understanding keeps me humble enough to receive wisdom from people who have mastered certain areas of their lives in which I could use some help. I learned this early in life after a few years of being a very troubled teenager. I needed mentors, and when the student is ready, the teacher always arrives. Many women, including my beautiful mother, have been powerful inspirations to me at different moments in my life.

I was only 19 when I met a very wise woman who has been a mentor of sorts for my entire adult life. The reason I sought out her guidance was because she seemed deeply contented while having seemingly very little—she intrigued me because her spirit shined so brightly. One day, I called her up in tears—I was about 21 years old and a struggling actress—because I couldn't get an acting job to save my life. To make ends meet, I was forced to do a few humiliating (in my grandiose opinion) and soul-destroying jobs.

On this particular day, when my feet hurt from walking around a depressing store for hours, handing out toxic cleaning product samples, I phoned her during my 15-minute lunch break, thinking she would advise me to quit. In her serene tone, she reminded me that the job in question was a perfect opportunity for spiritual growth and that I was exactly where I was meant to be. I was stunned. I wanted sympathy and a way out. She went on to ask me if I thought I could live the rest of my day "beautifully." At first I was appalled, but as she continued in her soothing tone, my shoulders slowly dropped, and I began to feel excited by the challenge that she'd presented. Yes, of course, I could live the rest of the day *beautifully*—moreover, I knew exactly what she meant by this. I could get through the rest of the day with grace, dignity, and love despite my aching feet and the toxic cleaning supply samples. I knew I could, and I tackled the afternoon with a renewed sense of purpose.

That night, I fell into bed with the exquisite satisfaction of a day well lived. This experience was one of the many lessons that I learned about living "gorgeously"—that it's less about the circumstances of my life and much more about how I *respond* to them; finding this kind of purpose in my everyday life is what makes me feel truly gorgeous. You might be able to buy great face creams, but you can't buy a great personality or outlook on life. Good character has to be earned. The hard knocks of life shape us—they serve to soften our edges and often force us to dig deeper and find out who we truly are. Pain and suffering are part of life, but the great news is that they're also the medium for spiritual growth.

The more I began to explore this concept, the more I realized that taking care of your insides—your physical, mental, and spiritual health—is essential to not just looking beautiful, but feeling beautiful. To be truly gorgeous is a holistic endeavor. Sadly, many people don't see it this way; they separate physical body, mental and emotional life, and spirituality, looking at each as completely unrelated, yet they are all 100 percent integrated. Think about it. If you aren't feeling well, you don't look your best. If you're confident about what you're doing, you're more likely to shine brightly. If you feel spiritually lost, you won't embody your true self. This is why I feel it is so important to consider our whole being in the beauty equation and why I believe inner work to be so important. I can squeeze into the skinniest jeans on earth or have the best hair day I've ever had, but if I don't feel really good about who I am as a person, I'm never going to feel—or look—truly gorgeous.

This doesn't mean that I have to sit for hours in therapy or read a million self-help books. It doesn't mean that I have to find a spiritual guru or take myself off to an ashram—it simply means that I have to be willing to take some time out to become quiet and connect to who I really am. I have to know what foods make my body feel good. I have to know what actions will truly make me happy. I have to know what kind of movements will make me feel alive. In essence, I have to be deeply in tune with myself—and this isn't easy in our modern, always-connected society.

Busyness and Disconnection

We are getting busier, there's no doubt about it. But I actually remember a time when I didn't even have an e-mail account. Can you imagine? Sure, I was a super-busy yoga teacher running here and there, but when I got home, that stopped. I was fully present.

But nowadays, when I get home at the end of the day, I'm literally checking my texts as I walk in the front door, and then I have my laptop open on the kitchen counter while I'm cooking dinner. If I let it, this constant barrage of mostly unwanted correspondence will keep on going until I lay my head on my pillow. And then—first thing in the morning—ooh, better check my e-mail, Facebook, and texts before I get to anything else, right?

The scary thing is how all this craziness crept up on us. We didn't even realize what was happening, but it gathered more and more momentum until it took over our lives. Sure, to be increasingly connected to everything and everyone 24/7 is a pretty amazing thing; however, it can also lead to a state of chronic underlying stress and disconnection from who we really are.

I must admit that to some degree, I have always thrived on stress. I don't mean that jittery feeling of underlying anxiety; I mean in-the-moment, deadline-driven stress. I kind of dig that rush of adrenaline when I have to get somewhere fast, do something crazily challenging, or feel pressured by a timeline. I think a lot of people feel this way, but the awful truth is that for many of us, we're living in a world of the other kind of stress. An underlying state of chronic stress is becoming the norm. And this is aging us faster than is natural. We suffer in our health, our emotional well-being, and our beauty.

Recently, I was lucky enough to interview Thea Singer, author of *Stress Less,* which delves deeply into the scientific theories exploring the connection between stress and aging. According to Thea, the theory of telomere shortening may explain why and how we age.

Put simply, some of our cells divide and some do not; for example, skeletal cells do not, but skin cells do. When a cell divides, the "daughter cell" has a shorter telomere. What's a telomere? It's the casing at the end of a strand of DNA, much like the protective plastic seal on the end of a shoelace. Eventually, after years of cell division, the telomere might be as little as a nub. The surrounding cells tend to go into panic mode because they hate damaged DNA—they try everything they can to repair what they perceive to be a possible break in the chromosome. The problem with this is that when they try to "fuse" the chromosome, a mutation could arise, which is where cancer comes into the picture. So nature, as always, comes to the rescue by telling the cells to chill out or even go to sleep. Such "sleeping" cells are called *senescent* cells. But before you think everything is A-Okay with that, it's not! Although the senescent cells are "sleeping," chemical processes still continue inside of them, which cause them to spew out toxins. These very toxins break down elastin—and elastin breakdown literally causes saggy skin and jowls! So what does stress have to do with this? It's all cell division, right? Nope. One theory holds that stress can actually chew away at the telomeres. Also, the production of telomerase, the enzyme that can help lengthen a telomere, may be inhibited by stress.

And stress doesn't only affect your health and beauty in this way. It can actually throw off your digestive system so that your body isn't able to absorb the nutrients it needs to stay healthy.

So what's the answer to all of this? Living a life of mindful balance.

Mindful Balance

A few days ago, my Internet went down—and after a moment of panic—I actually found myself breathing a sigh of relief. I began to feel my body softening and my mind slowing down, and I was able to be more present for my husband and daughter than I've been in months. Instead of checking e-mails and texts while cooking dinner, I listened to music and became wholly involved with the job at hand—it felt great. It was just another reminder about the connection, both to ourselves and others, that our busy lives often take away.

Living a life of mindful balance means consciously choosing to let go of the busyness. It's so important to our health and beauty to step away from the hustle and bustle of life to focus on the present moment, to focus on the people and the world around us. Quiet time gives us the opportunity to know ourselves better.

It helps us understand what truly nourishes us—in the realms of food, movement, and spiritual connection.

Your intuition is an essential way of knowing what you need to feel healthy and fulfilled. If you are living in a world of stress, you lose access to this part of yourself, which means that you won't be able to make decisions about the best path to take. You won't be inspired to take in the nutrients you need. You'll simply be looking for quick fixes for problems you are experiencing *right now.* I need cake *now* because I'm tired. I need to sit in front of the TV *now* because I'm stressed. I need to check Facebook *now* because I feel sad. But none of this does anything for your overall health and well-being, which means that it also does nothing to help you feel and look beautiful.

Taking the time to really get to know yourself and what makes you feel good is essential to accessing your intuition. Living mindfully will give you the opportunity to do this. Focusing on the present takes you out of the "shoulds," "if onlys," and "I betters." Knowing what is supposed to be good for you is important, but so is listening to your own body and soul. I know this may sound New Agey to a lot of you, but your body truly will tell you what it needs; you just have to listen.

In the next few chapters, I'll lay out some of the practices that have helped me heal and get in touch with myself. I'll also lay out the "supposed tos"—because there are things that have been shown scientifically to be healthy and to combat aging. With all this information, you can find out what feels the best for you. Remember, though, don't stress out about it; that only leads to further illness and aging.

Chapter 7

Eat Gorgeously

We all know those annoying girls who live off Snickers bars and Lay's chips and who still look stunning, but what we need to remember is that most of them *are* girls—meaning that they are either in their teens or early 20s. We can get away with unhealthy habits when we are younger because our digestion and all our bodily functions are firing on full-cylinder strength. However, as we age, everything becomes weaker, including our digestive fire. Over a certain age, if we don't start eating really well, we will pay a big price both in our health and in our appearance.

One of the most proactive steps you can take toward juicing up your skin is to load up your diet with tons of fresh veggies, juices, and smoothies. An organic, primarily plant-based diet will pay off in a bright, glowing complexion and improved health. It's almost too simple to be true.

Do You Have the Guts to Be Gorgeous?

Before we jump in to a discussion of what to eat and what not to eat, we have to look at an important part of our health: enzymes, which are the life force of our energy. Our bodies naturally produce digestive and metabolic enzymes, and they are critical for optimal health and a strong immune system. However, life—with its stress, aging, poor diet, illness, medications, and so on—often gets in the way and has a very negative impact on these little energy "spark plugs." So before you go to work to combat aging internally from a nutritional perspective, you must first ask yourself: do I have the "guts" to be gorgeous?

Digestive Enzymes 101

We eat food, but our digestive system doesn't absorb food; it absorbs nutrients. Digestive enzymes, which are produced in the salivary glands, stomach, pancreas, and small intestine, break down our food into nutrients so that our bodies can absorb them to build healthy cells and tissue. A digestive enzyme deficiency prevents us from breaking down the foods we eat, thus preventing our bodies from absorbing the nutrients we need for healthy skin, healthy hair, and a strong immune system. How can we expect to have great skin if our bodies don't have the raw materials to create it? That said, what causes digestive enzymes to stop working correctly in the body? Such conditions include:

- Chronic stress, the most common reason for digestive enzyme problems. Our body has two modes: sympathetic fight-or-flight and parasympathetic rest-and-digest. When we're in fight-or-flight mode, digestion is given a very low priority, which means digestive function (including digestive enzyme output) is dialed down. Chronic stress leads to a constant fight-or-flight mode.

- Low-grade inflammation in the digestive tract, such as that caused by food allergies, Crohn's and celiac disease, intestinal permeability, parasitic infection, and so on.

- Age-related lower levels of hydrochloric acid (which is necessary to digest protein).

- Age-related decrease in digestive function (though I personally wonder whether this is a result of aging or aging badly).

- A poor diet of overcooked and overprocessed foods.

If you have an enzyme deficiency, you probably know it—even though you don't know that it's the problem. For people with this issue, common symptoms include:

- Acid reflux

- Gas and bloating after meals

- The sensation that you have food sitting in your stomach (a rock in your gut)

- Feeling full after eating a few bites of food

- Heartburn and indigestion

- Acne breakouts—especially along the jawline

- Rosacea and reactive skin conditions

Correcting an Enzyme Deficiency

The first thing you need for correcting a problem with digestive enzymes is a whole-foods diet that includes these enzymes. Dietary interventions work by reducing inflammation in the body and the digestive tract, improving nutrient deficiencies, removing enzyme inhibitors (processed foods, artificial ingredients, and too many grains, for example) and replenishing the friendly flora, your good gut bacteria.

However, it is important to understand that diet alone may not solve a damaged digestive system. Managing chronic stress is vitally important to restoring healthy digestive function. Most of us cram food into our faces at our desks or while we're on the go, and then we're off to do the next thing on our lists. No wonder we have digestive issues! Once you begin healthier dietary and lifestyle practices, digestive enzyme supplementation may be necessary to help your body properly break down your food; however, it's best to try to get the enzymes by eating as much of your food raw as possible. If food is cooked above 47 degrees Celsius—that's basically all cooked food—its enzymes are destroyed. For most of us, adhering to a 100 percent raw-food diet is challenging or unappealing, so I recommend just *adding* as many raw foods to your diet as you can. Eating a crunchy, fresh salad with every meal is a good way to go, as is drinking cold-pressed vegetable juices.

Also, remember that the *way* you eat is just as important as *what* you eat. You can eat all the health foods in the world, but if your body is unable to digest them properly, it will do little good. Eating mindfully is often the last thing on our to-do lists when we feel crazed. But it really is important, so here are my top tips for eating mindfully:

- **Never eat when you are angry**. If you are engaged in a heated discussion, put your fork down and don't resume eating until you have given yourself some time to breathe and cool down.

- **Chew each mouthful thoroughly**. I cannot stress this enough, because digestion begins in the mouth—where valuable enzymes begin to break down food as we chew. If you miss this step, you are missing a vital part of the digestion process.

- **Slow down**. As our lives get faster, so does every activity we engage in, including eating. Take time to enjoy your food.

- **Never eat in front of a screen!** Eating in front of a computer, phone, or TV screen seems like the logical thing to do when you need to grab every moment you have to watch a show, check Facebook, or just chill out. The problem is that we never *really* chill out when we are watching TV; our minds are going a mile a minute. But the worst aspect of staring at a screen (big or small) while eating is that you are eating unconsciously. This is how many of us overeat. I am totally guilty on this one. I often try to save time by eating my lunch while checking e-mail, but I keep trying to minimize this unhealthy habit and train myself to slow down and appreciate the smells, tastes, and textures of what's in front of me.

- **Drink a large glass of warm water before your meal.** This is ingenious, because it not only stops you from feeling as if you need to devour an entire buffet table to assuage your hunger, but it also activates the digestive enzymes in your stomach, signaling it to prepare for the delicacies coming its way.

- **Say a blessing.** This doesn't have to be a full-on religious blessing (although great if it is); neither does it have to be a New-Agey joining of hands (although that's great, too). It can simply be a moment to silently thank everyone and everything involved in bringing the food to your plate.

- **Take a moment to actually look at what's on your plate.** Notice the vibrant colors, shapes, and energy of the food. I know this might sound a bit esoteric to some of you, but I bet you'll notice a difference in energy between a plate of bright green, crunchy beans—and a plate of grayish green beans with a slab of dead flesh that has been cooked within an inch of its life.

So now, let's get to the food . . .

The Mediterranean Versus American

A recent study conducted by Dr. David Katz, the lead researcher at Yale University's Prevention Research Center, compared many of the most popular mainstream diets over the past two decades, and the unequivocal winner for best diet was the Mediterranean diet, which consists of simply eating real foods—minimally processed and mainly plant based. The study didn't look at the efficacy of the diet for losing weight; instead, it focused on long-term health results.

The great thing about this diet is that it makes sense, and it only asks that we eat *real,* whole foods, rather than obsess over individual nutrients—making it easier to stick to and understand.

While extreme diets promise us everything from quick weight loss to cancer remission, keep in mind that these are often a flash in the pan. Diet books promoting them sell really well, often making their way onto bestseller lists, because they offer a quick fix and a lot of hope. And most of these quick fixes and cleanses do work short term (wow, the pounds are falling off!), but ask someone a couple of years, even months, down the line, and it's extremely unlikely that they will have stuck with it. Moreover, all this yo-yo weight gain and loss can take its toll on your body—including your skin.

So, what exactly is the Mediterranean diet? Well, it's more of a *lifestyle* than a "diet." For the people of Ikaria, an island off the coast of Italy that is home to some of the oldest, healthiest, and happiest folks on earth, living a long, happy life isn't just about what they eat; it's about getting enough exercise and about community. But the way they eat is as follows: whole foods (predominantly fruits, vegetables, and grains), three meals a day of modest portion sizes, and way less meat. They get their healthy oils from olives and olive oil, but in *modest* amounts. Contrary to what we extra-virgin olive oil–loving Americans believe, they use small amounts to finish off dishes as opposed to sloshing it in frying pans to sauté everything. They get their sugar from the naturally occurring sugar in the fresh fruit that they eat.

In America, we've dug ourselves into a reductionist hole. We isolate and reduce nutrients down to what we think they can do individually. For example, we are told we should eats tons of omega-3 fatty acids, so we go on a mad hunt for foods with these essential fats. We get crazy over it. However, if we are eating a well-balanced, varied diet of whole fruits, veggies, grains, seeds, and legumes, we really don't need to pop supplements or eat specific foods that are ostensibly loaded with this particular nutrient. We simply get enough of it because of the way we eat.

Our other pitfall is that as soon as we hear a certain food has "amazing" health benefits, we eat way too much of it. For example, most of us have heard of the benefits of consuming raw virgin coconut oil, but to shove it into smoothies, baked goods, and everything we eat is a mistake because, much like olive oil, it's still a fat, and too much fat isn't good for us. Too much of *anything* isn't good for us. The key to a healthy diet is balance, a word that I don't love—because, like most people, I'm always on the lookout for a miracle food, and I'm drawn toward extremes. A "balanced" diet sounds boring and uneventful, but the truth is that it doesn't have to be. Once we slow down to appreciate the incredible colors, textures, and tastes of whole foods that come straight from nature, our palates come alive.

Feeling Full

One thing that many diets have in common is that they don't make you feel full. This goes completely against nature. Our stomachs are designed to feel full. They respond to a "stretch," which acts as a built-in radar that tells us when we are full. Small, calorie-counted meals leave you hungry because your stomach doesn't stretch. And on the other end of the spectrum, high-calorie foods that are devoid of fiber and water (chocolate, potato chips, baked goods, and so on) don't stretch the stomach, either. So, we're completely unsatisfied on either low-calorie or high-calorie diets.

Fortunately, there's a really easy way to fix this: eat tons of foods that are full of water and fiber (almost all fruits and veggies), and you'll feel really full and satisfied after eating. When you're eating out, ask them to hold the breadbasket and serve up a plate of cut-up raw veggies instead.

The "Detox" Cleanse

Many popular diets of late have included a "detox" juice cleanse in consumers' quests to get healthy and/or thin. I'd like to discuss this concept, because this kind of work can be helpful if you feel that your diet is in need of an extreme, boot-camp kind of push in the right direction. But keep in mind that juices do not contain fiber, which is one of the most important elements of a detox regimen. The best way to detox is simply to stop eating toxin-laden food for good, and load your diet with plenty of organic fruits, veggies, grains, and legumes. There is no point doing a juice cleanse and then eating and drinking unhealthy beverages and food as soon as you're done. If you learn to detoxify your diet and keep it that way, you probably won't need to cleanse so often.

As far as the weight-loss benefits of cleansing, if you drink only juices for a week, you'll obviously lose a certain amount of weight; however, you will put it all back on again in just a couple of weeks. If you are juice cleansing simply to lose a few extra pounds, try indulging instead in all the beautiful, whole foods that I recommend in this program, and you will reach and maintain your perfect weight.

One cleanse that made a lot of sense to me was a holistic one that I did a few years ago with Ayurvedic physician Dr. John Douillard, who is the author of six books on creating a healthy diet and lifestyle and the director of the LifeSpa Institute in Colorado. At the time I went there, I was experiencing some digestive issues and wanted to do a carefully guided cleanse. It was a great experience physically, mentally, and spiritually.

I asked Dr. Douillard what to look for in a good cleanse. He said that the most important thing is not the content of the cleanse itself—what you eat or drink during the cleanse—but rather any work done beforehand to address why you got toxic in the first place. The world has become increasingly toxic, and he explained that the body has a detoxification system that happens to use the same pathways as the digestive system. "If your digestion breaks down, so will your ability to detox," says Dr. Douillard. "Weak digestion forces the body to store toxins in the fat, instead of properly processing and removing them from the body. If you force the body into a sudden cleanse, the liver—which is the detoxifier—may react and say, *Why are you pulling those toxins out of my fat? I put them there for a reason! I am way too busy to process those toxins right now!* And then it might never quite complete the process of moving the toxins out. As a result, many cleanses merely move toxins from one fat cell to another, and they may end up in your brain, which is forty percent fat." Dr. Douillard went on to remind me that our ability to process hard-to-digest foods such as wheat, dairy, and fatty foods is reflective of whether or not we can detox well, and that if we experience our digestive strength weakening over the years, we are probably accumulating fat-soluble environmental toxins in our fat cells, including the cells in our brains.

Sadly, most over-the-counter cleanses are not well thought out and make promises they cannot keep, so be sure to look for a well-designed cleanse that can be supervised by a trained health professional.

How to Detoxify Your Shopping List!

When you're cruising around the store, list in hand, try to avoid:

- Foods that contain artificial dyes, flavors, or preservatives

- Any food that contains artificial sweeteners

- Any food that contains high-fructose corn syrup

- Highly processed foods such as faux meat and cheese

- All meat and dairy (for a short time if need be).

- All fish, especially swordfish, tuna, and grouper because of high mercury content

- Any foods containing added sugar

- Hydrogenated and fractionated oils (mainly palm and palm kernel oil found in a variety of sweets and baked goods)

- Foods that contain wheat or gluten (especially if you think you might be gluten intolerant)
- Foods that contain dairy products
- Nonorganic produce in specific items (see the "Mean 15" on page 182)

"What am I going to eat, then?" is the complaint I hear from many a friend I teach this to. My reply is that they are going to eat bucketloads of the most feel-good foods on earth. It takes a little while for some families to adjust their palates, especially if they are accustomed to eating a lot of sugar, salt, and fat (particularly fat from animal products). But we humans are extremely adaptable, and after a few short weeks, anyone who follows these guidelines will crave beautiful, fresh foods more than the toxin-laden food they may be used to. Trust me on this.

Why Meat and Fish?

Aside from ethical and sustainability concerns, meat and fish can contain a lot of environmental toxins, which is why I suggest avoiding both for your 30-day program, and beyond if you feel better from going without. If, however, you are dying for a piece of fish (which does contain healthy Omega 3 fatty acids), choose wild salmon. Fish and meat are very often contaminated with:

- Heavy metals, such as mercury and lead
- Antibiotics, which are routinely added to animal feed
- Growth hormones, which are routinely implanted into cattle
- Bacteria such as E. coli and salmonella
- Dioxin, which is a carcinogen from industrial pollution, and which lodges in animal fat.

The Gorgeous for Good Eating Strategy

My healthy eating philosophy is really quite simple. While it parallels the Mediterranean diet, I have added a few additional pieces for you to focus on. Here are the basic tenets. You should eat foods that are:

- Mainly plant based
- As fresh as possible
- Minimally processed
- Organic (or at least nontoxic)
- Anti-inflammatory
- Alkaline forming

Let's dive into these qualities a bit more.

Mainly Plant-Based Foods

Next up: eat a mainly plant-based diet. It sounds like a new fad, right? It's not; this is how ancient cultures subsisted for thousands of years. When we look at some of the healthiest and longest-living people on earth, we see that they eat meat occasionally (maybe two or three times a month), fish every week, and fruits and veggies for all other meals. However, keep in mind that modern-day fish and meat are very different from what they were even a hundred years ago. Our meat and fish products today, even if sustainably and responsibly farmed, may be loaded with environmental toxins because the toxins in our air, food, and water slowly make their way up the food chain and sequester in animal fat. The American meat- and dairy-eating culture is one of the prime reasons why our life expectancy is shorter than in any other industrialized nation.

If you cannot go without meat, make sure it is USDA-certified organic, grass-fed. Also try to cut your portion sizes in half and load up the space on your plate with beautiful, fresh veggies. And remember that the American Dietetic Association says that a portion of meat shouldn't be larger than a deck of cards. For the purposes of your 30-day program, I invite you to go meat free for the most part. A clean, animal-flesh-free diet will be easier on your whole system and might inspire you to lessen your meat consumption in the future. Health issues aside, eating meat is not sustainable for the planet.

But what about getting enough protein? Don't we need to eat a lot of it? Actually, most of us eat too much, mainly in the form of meat. Protein is composed of 20 amino acids, 8 of which are essential, meaning that we need to get them from our food. Many people believe that we can only get these from meat, but this is not true. The American Dietetic Association states that when a variety of plant foods are consumed over the course of a day, the diet will provide all of the necessary amino acids. This statement also indicates that vegetarians don't need to combine certain plant foods to create a complete protein at every meal. The key is to try to eat as big a variety of plant foods as possible. I recommend that you pack your daily diet with beans, peas, lentils, nuts, and tofu, which is easy to do when you utilize all the plant-based recipes that I include in Chapter 12.

The World Health Organization says that we need to get 5 percent of our daily calories from meat. While I don't recommend eating meat, we can do a quick calculation of how much protein we need based on this recommendation. Proteins have 4 calories per gram, so if I eat around 2300 calories a day, I need about 29 grams of protein daily. This is pretty easy to get (and even overdo) by eating whole plant foods. Look at the charts below.

Beans and Nuts
1 cup soybeans, 29 grams
1 cup lentils, 18 grams
1 cup refried beans, 15.5 grams
1 cup black beans, 15 grams
1 cup garbanzo beans, 14.5 grams
1 cup pinto beans, 12 grams
½ cup almonds, 8 grams

Fruits and Vegetables
1 avocado, 10 grams
1 cup peas, 9 grams
1 cup broccoli, 5 grams
1 cup spinach, 5 grams

1 cup asparagus, 5 grams
1 medium artichoke, 4 grams

Grains
1 cup cooked quinoa, 9 grams
1 medium bagel, 9 grams
1 cup cooked spaghetti, 8 grams
1 cup oatmeal, 6 grams
2 slices whole wheat bread, 5 grams
1 cup cooked brown rice, 5 grams

Meat Substitutes
1 cup tempeh, 41 grams
3 ounces seitan, 31 grams
1 cup tofu, 22 grams
2 tablespoons peanut butter, 8 grams

Getting Enough Lysine

Lysine is one of the essential amino acids that you need for good health. It is important for the production of carnitine, which is essential for turning fat into energy. Lysine also helps boost calcium absorption and manage and reduce severity of herpes simplex symptoms. When eliminating meat and dairy products from your diet, it's important that you make sure you get enough of it. You can easily achieve this by eating peas, tofu, tempeh, lentils, pistachio nuts, and pumpkin seeds.

Foods as Fresh as Possible

Along the same lines, I recommend eating foods that are as fresh as possible for the best nutrition. A fruit or vegetable begins to lose its nutritional value as soon as it's picked. This is why you want to eat food as close to its source as you possibly can. I make it a priority to get to my farmers' market every Sunday morning because many of the farmers pick their produce the night before to bring it to the city. If my green beans or red bell peppers have been trucked in from another state or, even worse, flown in from another country, I'm not going to get the full nutrient profile that nature intended for me. Beautiful fruits and veggies that are as fresh as possible are the mainstay of a really healthy diet.

Minimally Processed Foods

Food processing often removes the good and leaves the not so good. The easiest way to avoid highly processed foods is to cook from scratch. This doesn't mean that you have to tune in to the Food Network or buy exotic and expensive ingredients. On the contrary—a beautiful Greek salad with vine-ripened tomatoes, crispy Persian cucumbers, tangy red onions, and plump Kalamata olives is a stunning example of "cooking" from scratch.

It can be difficult to tell if many of our supermarket products contain highly processed, unhealthy ingredients because many of America's leading brands load their foods with ingredients to enhance flavor and texture and to extend shelf life, and they look good on the outside.

An obvious example is a loaf of whole-grain bread. This is the ingredient list taken from a loaf of sprouted whole wheat bread (which you can find in the refrigerated section of most grocery stores):

> Sprouted Organic Whole Wheat Berries, Filtered Water, Wheat Gluten, Sprouted Organic Whole Flax Seeds, Oat Fiber, Cultured Wheat, Organic Dates, Fresh Yeast, Organic Raisins, Soy Based Lecithin, Sea Salt

This is the ingredient list from a popular supermarket brand of whole wheat bread:

> Unbromated Stone Ground 100% Whole Wheat Flour, Water, Crushed Wheat, High Fructose Corn Syrup, Partially Hydrogenated Vegetable Shortening (Soybean and Cottonseed Oils), Raisin Juice Concentrate, Wheat Gluten, Yeast, Whole Wheat Flakes, Unsulphured Molasses, Salt, Honey, Vinegar, Enzyme Modified Soy Lecithin, Cultured Whey, Wheat Starch, Unbleached Wheat Flour and Soy Lecithin

Both of these breads are marketed as extremely healthy, whole-grain breads; however, the second list includes two highly processed ingredients: high-fructose corn syrup and partially hydrogenated vegetable shortening—neither is found in nature, and neither is good for your health. Heavily processed ingredients can find their way into many foods, including yogurts, frozen and prepackaged meals, cereal bars, pizzas, sauces, dressings, canned fruits, and even applesauce. To stay away from highly processed foods that your body doesn't recognize as real food, you need to get good at label reading.

When looking at a label, one thing to remember is that many soy products are highly processed. Hydrolyzed soy protein, isolated soy protein, soy protein concentrates, textured vegetable protein, soy lecithin, and soybean oil are unhealthy processed substances found in all kinds of "convenience" foods, including protein bars, energy bars, protein shakes, smoothie mixes, and so on. Many fake meat and cheese products also contain these highly processed ingredients, so be sure to read your labels.

Organic and Nontoxic Foods

You are way better off eating organic food, because if it's USDA-certified organic, it means more than just the absence of synthetic pesticides; it means that your food is not genetically modified, has not been irradiated, and has not been covered in sewage sludge. With so many environmental toxins in and around us every day, food is a very powerful area in which we can make some seriously healthy changes.

Also be aware of the toxins in food packaging: many companies still use can linings that contain the hormone disruptor bisphenol A (BPA), and toxic chemicals leach from plastic coverings and polystyrene.

Finally, beware of all the toxic chemicals that can be found in processed foods such as preservatives, additives, texturing agents, dyes, and so on. If you stick to whole, minimally processed foods, you won't have to drive yourself crazy looking for all these sneaky little ingredients.

The Mean and the Clean 15!

If you're worried about the cost of moving to all-organic food, check out the lists from the Environmental Working Group about which ones it's most important to buy. First is what I call the Mean 15—an expanded version of EWG's original "Dirty Dozen." These are the fruits and vegetables found to contain the highest amounts of pesticide residue when grown conventionally:

1. Apples
2. Strawberries
3. Grapes
4. Celery
5. Peaches
6. Spinach
7. Sweet bell peppers
8. Nectarines (imported)
9. Cucumbers
10. Cherry tomatoes
11. Snap peas (imported)
12. Potatoes
13. Hot peppers
14. Blueberries (domestic)
15. Lettuce

And here are those with the *least* pesticide residue—the Clean 15:

1. Avocados
2. Sweet corn
3. Pineapples
4. Cabbage
5. Sweet peas (frozen)
6. Onions
7. Asparagus
8. Mangoes
9. Papayas
10. Kiwi
11. Eggplant
12. Grapefruit
13. Cantaloupe
14. Cauliflower
15. Sweet potatoes

Anti-Inflammatory Foods

It's now been discovered that chronic, low-grade systemic inflammation is a common manifestation of premature aging. Diet isn't the only factor that contributes to inflammatory conditions, but it's certainly a very large part of them. So, what are inflammatory foods? The main culprits are sugar, cheap (not expeller-pressed) cooking oils, trans fats, dairy products (particularly cow's milk), feedlot-raised poultry and pork, red meat, refined grains, gluten, and food additives.

I include gluten in my "inflammatory foods" list because it often creates digestive issues such as bloating, gas, and irregularities in the bathroom department. Even if you don't have an autoimmune disease such as celiac disease, where you absolutely cannot eat any kind of gluten, you may experience some uncomfortable symptoms after eating bread, pasta, or anything with gluten in it. If you aren't feeling vibrant and full of energy, if your skin has any inflammatory issues such as rashes, rosacea, or extreme sensitivity, you might want to avoid gluten. My brother suffered from rosacea for years and saw a complete transformation in his skin when he eliminated gluten, dairy, and meat from his diet.

I encourage you to load up your plate with as many of these anti-inflammatory foods as you can:

1. Kelp (you can add this seaweed to soups and salads or take a kelp supplement)

2. Cruciferous veggies (such as cauliflower and broccoli)

3. Blueberries

4. Turmeric

5. Garlic

6. Sweet potatoes

7. Cooked Asian mushrooms (such as maitake and shiitake)

Also look out for any foods you might be allergic to, as food allergies can add a great deal to inflammation. The following foods account for more than 90 percent of all food allergies in the world:

- Peanuts
- Tree nuts
- Milk
- Eggs
- Wheat
- Soy
- Fish
- Shellfish

Miraculous Turmeric

India has one of the lowest rates of Alzheimer's disease in the world, and it was recently discovered that turmeric might be the reason for this. A specific compound found in turmeric, curcumin, is a potent antioxidant that reduces inflammation and may be extremely helpful in many degenerative diseases, including Alzheimer's. These findings are helpful because turmeric is an inexpensive spice (a root from the ginger family) that we can add to a variety of dishes. Here are my favorite ways to use turmeric:

- Sprinkled on egg or potato salad
- Added to soups, stews, and tagines
- Added to salad dressings
- Mixed with extra virgin olive oil and salt, drizzled onto steamed veggies
- Added to smoothies

I also love to make turmeric tea by simmering 1 teaspoon ground turmeric in 4 cups of boiling water for 10 minutes. Then I pour this over a cup containing 1 teaspoon of raw honey and a couple slices of raw ginger root.

Alkaline-Forming Foods

Our cells and blood must stay at a pH balance of around 7.4 to sustain life. So, our bodies miraculously regulate the foods we eat to make sure that this pH level is maintained. Some studies, however, suggest that if we eat more acid-forming foods, our bodies have to work harder to neutralize the acid by releasing minerals into our bloodstream. The theory goes that these minerals have to be pulled from our bones to carry out this heavy lifting, so we aren't getting the benefit we should from them.

Since most of the foods considered alkaline forming are also the healthy, anti-inflammatory foods, it makes sense to follow the alkaline/anti-inflammatory diet protocol. Keep in mind here that protein, by virtue of being made up of amino *acids*, is acid forming, which is why it makes a lot of sense, particularly in the case of meat and fish, to reduce the amount we eat.

Foods to Eat

Taking all the above into account, I want to lay out a list of some staples that I keep on hand at all times. If you stock your pantry with these things, you'll be well on the way to eating well.

- **Seeds:** Flax, hemp, sesame, pumpkin, and sunflower seeds. It's best to soak or grind your seeds before using them because it makes them more digestible.

- **Nuts:** Chestnuts, almonds, cashews, and macadamia nuts. I recommend buying raw nuts and then soaking or roasting before eating them whole, or soaking before cooking or blending them.

- **Nongluten grains:** Brown and wild rice, millet, teff, quinoa, buckwheat, and tapioca.

- **Veggie protein:** Lentils, split peas, legumes, and beans.

- **Dairy substitutes:** Nut milks, rice milk, hemp milk, coconut milk, coconut oil, and butter.

- **Veggies:** Particularly spinach, kale, cabbage, cauliflower, artichokes, carrots, cucumbers, radishes, onions, leeks, garlic, and sweet potatoes.

- **Fruits:** Particularly apples, pears, bananas, kiwi, melons, mangoes, blueberries, and papaya.

- **Spices:** Particularly turmeric and ginger.

- **Soy:** This should always be in traditional form, such as tempeh, tofu, soy milk, edamame, miso, and tamari. Always make sure that your soy products are certified organic. Also, be mindful that condiments such as soy, tamari, and shoyu sauce can sometimes contain sugar, wheat, gluten, and artificial additives and flavors. Always read the ingredient list.

Mercury and Our Fish

Our oceans are unfortunately polluted with many contaminants, especially mercury, which can affect our neurological and reproductive health. This is one of the main reasons why I recommend you go without fish for 30 days, so your body has a chance to detoxify itself. If you really want to include some fish, try to avoid tuna, swordfish, and lobster because of their high mercury content.

If you eat a lot of fish, particularly sushi (which is heavy on the tuna), I urge you to check out the National Resource Defense Council's mercury calculator (www.nrdc.org/health/effects/mercury /calculator/start.asp) to see if, based on what you are eating, your intake of mercury is below the safety alert level.

Because of very high levels of mercury, I suggest you:

- **Completely avoid:** Chilean sea bass, swordfish, orange roughy, and ahi, yellowfin, and albacore tuna.
- **Eat in moderation:** Wild Alaskan salmon (canned or fresh), sardines, scallops, shrimp, sole, and freshwater trout.

If you are a tuna lover, stick to canned chunk light or skipjack tuna, and eat it no more than once a week.

What about Fats?

Now I'd like to talk about something a lot of women worry about: fats. Most of us know that there are "healthy" fats and "unhealthy" fats. Dr. Dean Ornish, best-selling author and clinical professor at the University of California–San Francisco, states that saturated fat, which is found largely in animal products, is converted by the liver to cholesterol and raises the blood cholesterol level. But saturated fat is also found in some plant oils such as palm and coconut oil, which some people claim is healthier. For overall health, it is much better to try to dramatically reduce the amount of saturated fat in the diet, even from the "healthier" saturated fats. The only fats that we actually *need* are two essential fatty acids: omega-3 and omega-6. They are called "essential" because, unlike other fats, we have to get them from our diet—our bodies don't produce them at all. However, as in the case of all "good" things, we can take this a bit too far by downing bucketloads of omega supplements.

Remember what I said at the beginning of this chapter: in America, we tend to fixate on one or two nutrients and separate them from their food sources. That's not the goal of this section. I just want to bring to light the fact that according to the National Academy of Sciences, the adequate daily intake of omega-3 fatty acids is only 1.1 grams for women and 1.6 grams for men (this translates to about one-quarter teaspoon per day). The important thing to understand about fats is that it's not about packing in more omegas; it's all about getting the right ratio of omega-3 to omega-6 fatty acids. Since the standard American diet is very heavy on the omega-6s, most of us need to pack a lot more omega-3s into our diets.

There are different kinds of omega-3 fatty acids:

- **EPA and DHA:** Long-chain fatty acids that confer the greatest health benefits and are found exclusively in seafood and marine algae.

- **ALA:** Short-chain fatty acids that can be found
  in many plant foods such as flax, walnuts, hemp,
  soybeans, and pumpkin seeds. However, ALA has
  to be synthesized into EPA or DHA in order to be
  used by the body, and the conversion rate in plant
  foods is very limited. This is why many vegans and
  vegetarians are deficient in valuable omega-3 fatty
  acids.

While eating loads of oily seafood is a good way to get your
omega-3 fatty acids, it can come with a huge toxic price tag because much of our seafood is contaminated with heavy metals
and other pollutants.

The Best Source of Omega-3 Fatty Acids

One of the best ways to get your omega-3 fatty acids, especially
if you are vegan, is to supplement with algae-based supplements.
Algae (golden algae as opposed to blue-green algae) is the base of
the food chain for fish, and when they eat it, it concentrates in their
tissues, providing fish eaters with EPA and DHA. However, if you go
straight to the source (algae), you bypass the middleman (fish) and all
the inherent contaminants.

Glycemic Load

Another term that comes up a lot in discussions of nutrition
is *glycemic index* (GI). This refers to how quickly a food will spike
your blood sugar. When your blood sugar spikes, your pancreas
goes into overdrive, pumping insulin into your blood to get it to
where it might be needed. However, if you are sitting behind a
desk instead of hunting a wild boar, your muscles likely won't
need that extra energy from the sugar, so it will be stored as fat—
pretty simple, right?

While GI measurements are definitely useful, I prefer to look
at the glycemic *load* of a food instead. This statistic takes into

account the carbs *and* the glycemic index, thus giving you a more rounded understanding of how that food will impact your blood sugar. Generally speaking, the more fiber a food contains, the lower its glycemic load. For example, an orange has a lower glycemic load than a glass of orange juice because the whole fruit contains fiber.

- **Low-glycemic-load foods** (10 or less): Beans, fibrous veggies and fruits (such as carrots, peas, and apples), 100 percent bran cereals, lentils, cashews, whole-grain bread, and tomato juice.

- **Medium-glycemic-load foods** (11–19): Whole wheat pasta, rolled oats, brown rice cakes, no-added-sugar fruit juice, brown rice, and sweet potatoes.

- **High-glycemic foods** (20 or more): Sugar-added drinks, white rice and pasta, bagels, pizza, baked potatoes, raisins, and French fries.

To help keep the fat off and to heal your body, skin, and soul, it's smart to stick with foods that rank lower in glycemic load. If you can't cook, don't despair; the best foods are simple to prepare—scrumptious salads, soups, and slow-cooker stews are easy enough for a ten-year-old child to prepare (my daughter is learning fast!). If you'd like to see more foods and their glycemic load values, many institutions have created lists and databases. Just Google "glycemic index of foods," and you should find the information you are looking for.

Sugar: Beware!

Sugar is not good for us. It spikes our blood sugar and not only packs on the pounds but can also compromise our immune systems and prematurely age our skin. And, unfortunately, your body doesn't recognize the difference between brown sugar and dehydrated cane juice—sugar is sugar. So it's best to avoid it as much as you can, which can be difficult because it goes by so many names. Here are some of the many:

Agave nectar, barley malt, beet sugar, brown sugar, buttered syrup, cane juice, cane juice crystals, cane juice solids, caramel, carob syrup, corn syrup, corn syrup solids, crystalline fructose, date sugar, dehydrated cane juice, dehydrated fruit juice, dextran, dextrin, dextrose, diatase, diatastic malt, ethyl maltol, florinda crystals, fructose, fruit juice concentrate, fruit juice, fruit juice crystals, galactose, glucose, glucose solids, golden syrup, high fructose corn syrup, lactose, malt syrup, maltodextrin, maltose, maple syrup, molasses, refiner's syrup, rice malt syrup, sorbitol, sorghum syrup, sucrose, treacle, turbinado, yellow sugar.

If you need a bit of sweet in your tea, on your cereal, or in a particular recipe, choose a natural sweetener that won't spike your blood sugar, such as monk fruit powder, xylitol, or stevia.

Glycation

Glycation has become a bit of a buzzword in the antiaging space, because this unfortunate process has been found to be the cause of prematurely aging and yellowing skin—did you ever notice that older people who smoke and eat predominantly processed foods have a yellow tinge to their skin?

So, what is this glycation thing, and how does it affect you? I'll spare you an in-depth science lesson by giving you the basics: when we eat certain foods, particularly sugar, fats, and processed foods, their molecules stick to protein and fat molecules in our bodies without the assistance of a moderating enzyme. The result is a rogue molecule that is called an AGE (advanced glycation end product). These lovely AGEs cause protein fibers, such as collagen and elastin, to become stiff and malformed. This is especially the case with elastin, the elasticlike structure that gives shape and elasticity to your skin.

It's commonly understood that sugars, particularly fructose (fruit juice and honey), are the main culprits as far as glycation is concerned, but there are other foods that are just as bad. Studies have found that foods cooked at high temperatures (such as fried and seared foods) exacerbate the glycation process considerably, which is why a predominantly raw diet is a great thing, as is a diet that is free of processed foods. Remember, processed foods are subject to extremely high temperatures in their manufacture. It's also been discovered that high temperatures used in cooking are worse than the *length* of time something is cooked. So ditch your deep fryer and purchase a slow cooker instead.

Here are a few ways to combat glycation:

- Eat tons of fiber, which helps absorb glycation products.

- Dramatically minimize the amount of fried foods you eat.

- Minimize the amount of foods you eat from a barbecue.

- Switch to low-fat dairy products or give up dairy completely.

- Eat whole grains.

- Eat raw foods.

Aside from cutting out all the food culprits, one of the most healthy and proactive steps you can take is to rethink how you cook your food. Given that cooking at high temperatures (particularly frying) not only causes glycation but also releases damaging free radicals, it makes sense to cook at way lower temperatures and without oil where possible. My favorite way of cooking is to steam sauté using water instead of oil.

Stress ⟶ Cortisol Release ⟶ Sugar Levels Rise ⟶ Glycation ⟶ Damaged Collagen ⟶ Sagging and Prematurely Winkled Skin

Juices and Smoothies

A great way to get raw vegetables and fruits into your diet—and thus help prevent glycation—is through drinking fresh juices and smoothies. Yes, it's a bit of a pain, but only because you have to clean the darn juicer or blender out. If you have a good one, cleanup can be more than bearable.

I sometimes purchase organic smoothies or pressed juices when I'm on the fly, but they are so expensive that I regard them as a special treat. In Chapter 12, I've shared some of my favorite juice and smoothie blends with you. Here are just a few of the pros and cons of each:

Pros of Juice:

- You get an instant shot of energy
- You get an instant and concentrated shot of nutrients
- Juices are refreshing and hydrating
- You can juice up veggies that you wouldn't usually put together (such as beets and lime)

Cons of Juice:

- Juices that are predominantly made with fruit can raise blood sugar levels fast
- There is no fiber in juice
- Juice doesn't fill you up as much as a smoothie

Pros of Smoothies:

- A large smoothie makes you feel full and can replace a meal
- They're a great way to get your daily protein and fiber in one blast
- They're a fun way to introduce new foods, especially super-foods, into your diet

Cons of Smoothies:

- Smoothies that are loaded with fruits, dates, and honey can pack a high-sugar punch
- Commercial, premade smoothies can be filled with sugary juice and added concentrates and preservatives

Superfoods

Let's look at another trend that's been out there lately: superfoods. There's much been said about these densely nutritious foods of late—so much so that they're beginning to fill the shelves of more mainstream stores. But do we need them? Well, no, we don't. And by that I mean we definitely won't die if we don't get them, but I believe that they can do only good things.

The advantage of superfoods over supplements is that they are whole foods as opposed to isolated nutrients, so your body can better digest and absorb them than supplements.

The ones that I love and use regularly are:

Chia Seeds: These tiny, black seeds are crazy high in the good omegas. I soak them overnight before tossing a tablespoon of them into my smoothie. Soaking them makes them easier to digest.

Coconut Oil: I regard this as a superfood because it is full of lauric and capric acids, which have so many health benefits. Coconut oil also helps boost your metabolism. It must be raw and virgin—even better if it's organic and fair trade. I sometimes add one teaspoon to my morning oatmeal. But don't go overboard—remember, it's still a saturated fat.

Goji Berries: These look like mini rust-colored raisins, and they are slightly less sweet. I don't love eating them on their own (they're a bit dry and tasteless), but they add a wonderful, chewy texture and nutty taste to a smoothie. When I have them around, I toss in a good handful.

Greens and Protein Powders: Greens and protein powders are great if you are traveling and can't easily incorporate loads of fresh greens into your smoothie. Because you are ingesting a very concentrated source of nutrients, it's vital that you choose a powder that is certified organic, GMO free, gluten free, vegan, and 100 percent free of all additives, solvents, and preservatives. May favorite protein powders are made from hemp, pea, or brown rice protein. If, however, I am at home, it's healthier and more economical to get my greens and proteins from dark leafy green veggies, nuts, and seeds.

Maca: This is a Peruvian root that not only gives energy but also helps to balance your hormones and thyroid. It has a slightly astringent, nutty taste and comes as a beige powder. You can add it to virtually anything, but it does really well in smoothies. I add a good tablespoon to every smoothie.

Sesame Seeds: These tiny seeds are powerhouses because they are so full of nutrients, particularly calcium. A quarter cup of sesame seeds contains more calcium than 1 cup of whole milk. And toasting them releases even more calcium, and pulverizing them (as in making tahini paste) makes them easier to digest.

Supplements

I'm a firm believer that the best way to get my vitamins and minerals is through my food. If I eat a varied diet of fresh and preferably organic foods, I probably don't need to pop hundreds of supplements. Rather than focus on which supplement we think we need to take to address a specific problem, it's way better to focus on optimizing every aspect of our health, because all the different areas affect one another. A multivitamin is no substitute for a balanced diet; moreover, trying to control an isolated nutrient at an often much higher dosage than we need can completely upset the body's natural balance. For the most part, supplements should only be taken as a last resort and should be prescribed by a holistic nutritionist or registered dietician when possible. However, there are two supplements that you may want to take because of the fact that they aren't found in many foods: vitamins B12 and D.

Vitamin B12: If you are a vegetarian or vegan, you may need to supplement with B12 because it is generally found in animal flesh. The reason for this is interesting: B12 is made from bacteria. Animals eat bacteria along with their other foods and thus accumulate B12 in their flesh. If, like us, animals only ate triple-washed grass and sanitized, irradiated food, they wouldn't get the bacteria or the vitamin B12 into their systems. The only reason humans don't get it from plants is that we don't eat bacteria-laden plants—which is smart because, obviously, doing that could be dangerous.

Vitamin D: Vitamin D is essential for human health. Low levels are associated with heart disease and cancer. Vitamin D can and should be obtained through natural sources (the sun) whenever possible. Sun exposure, as opposed to sun overexposure, has been shown to be extremely good for our health. However, if you live in a cool climate or just know you're not getting enough sun, you might want to get your vitamin D level checked by a simple blood test. If it is low, supplement accordingly.

Gratitude

We've covered a lot about what is good and bad for us, but sometimes you need to take a step back. Remember what I said at the beginning of the chapter? That the *way* you eat is just as important as *what* you eat? Sometimes I need to switch my focus from obsessing about what I can and can't eat to being incredibly grateful for even having a choice in the matter. The reality is that a large percentage of the world is, at this very moment, hungry— many people are actually dying of starvation—while in America, we continue to obsess about squeezing ourselves into ever teenier skinny jeans. The truth is that many of us in the U.S. not only have access to clean, healthy food, but we also have choices that are absolutely staggering. Maybe this is the problem. My fridge, on any given day, boasts a selection of four different kinds of milk (rice, almond, coconut, and 2 percent cow's milk) because each family member ostensibly *needs* something different (like they'll die if they don't get it).

Yes, I totally fall into the group of people weighing my goji berries in the bulk bin section and filling my cart with organic kale; however, a day doesn't go by that I'm not acutely aware of what a privilege this is.

Chapter 8

Moving Your Body

The importance of moving your body for beauty cannot be overstated—and I'm not just talking about moving in the quest to lose weight. That's a beautiful side effect of movement, but it shouldn't be your only goal. Movement is all about feeling good. Not only does it help you tone your physique, it helps you reduce stress and fall in love with your body. Moving helps you realize just how much you're capable of. It gives you an appreciation for yourself, even with your "imperfections."

Our bodies were designed to move, not to sit at a computer all day. It's pretty simple—when we don't do what our bodies are meant to do, ill health sets in. A sedentary lifestyle wreaks havoc on our systems physically, mentally, and spiritually. You know how great you feel after a workout? Well, you're supposed to feel that way most of the time—full of energy, with all the feel-good chemicals buzzing around your brain. But, unfortunately, we've gotten rather used to feeling sluggish and even depressed most of the time. This is the main reason that we reach for buckets of caffeine laced with sugary syrups in the early morning and midafternoon. It's also why many of us comfort-eat—if we feel terrible in our own bodies, maybe downing a pint of ice cream or mowing through a bag of corn chips will soothe the ache of not feeling vibrant and alive. Seriously, the benefits of moving our bodies and getting the right amount of heart-pumping exercise go way beyond losing a few pounds.

My Inspiration

My parents are role models when it comes to exercise: my father is almost 90 years old and is in startlingly good health. His muscles are rock solid, and, despite being a bit wobbly on his feet, he manages to clock in an astonishing amount of daily exercise (with tennis, hiking, weights, and so on) that would make men half his age weak at the knees. He told me that he never feels like exercising, because at his ripe old age, he rises out of bed feeling less than sprightly; however, he also says that just ten minutes into his workouts, he feels 20 years younger. Moreover, he explained to me that his exercise regimen has allowed him to retain a sharp mind. "Once this goes," he said, pointing to his body, "the rest," he continued, pointing to his brain, "goes right along with it!"

My mother is in her mid-70s and despises conventional exercise because she's a nature girl. "Why walk on a treadmill in a gym," she queried, "when I can pull on my boots and take the dogs for a gorgeous walk in the woods?" She's got a point, but the real reason that she looks and moves in a way that's so young for her age is that she doesn't shy away from hard physical labor—a day isn't a good day if she hasn't dragged heavy branches or hauled piles of garden rocks or shoveled snow. Sweating in her yard makes her feel energized, useful, and connected to her surroundings. So, I have two great role models: one who pushes himself no matter what, and one who only does what she loves.

Loving It

You need to get pleasure from your exercise—whether it's pleasure from the feeling exercise gives you or pleasure from the activity itself—or you'll set yourself up to fail because you'll find too many excuses not to do it. Honestly, I don't love all the exercise I do, but I *love* how I feel the minute it's over—much like when I'm downing a rather unpleasant shot of wheatgrass juice, I sometimes have to grit my teeth to get to the good part. Here's my approach to keeping myself in tip-top condition:

- I do a variety of different exercise programs, including yoga, hiking, Pilates, kettlebells, and weights. I love some of them and have to take a deep breath before others, but I feel fantastic after any and all of them.

- The reason I force myself to do workouts that aren't entirely . . . let's say . . . "joyous" is because I know that if I want to see quantifiable results—which I most certainly do—my body has to push through its comfort zone into unfamiliar territory.

- I understand that 80 percent of my resistance to pushing myself comes from my mind, not from my body. My mind begins to freak out way before my body does, telling my body that it can't possibly do one more push-up. I've learned to tune out that voice and replace it with the simple mantra: "You can!"

- I always work out mindfully, which means that I am in tune with my body and my breath and understand that there is a big difference between pushing myself and hurting myself. As I get older, my joints and muscles aren't as strong and resilient as they used to be. Moreover, a lifetime of sometimes crazy exercise and way too many marathons comes back to haunt me with unhappy knees and creaky hips. I have learned how to take care of my body and to listen to the difference between mental and physical discomfort and pain. In yoga, the Sanskrit term *ahimsa* means not harming ourselves mentally or physically. I always try to practice this.

Conquering Resistance

We wouldn't be human if we didn't have a certain amount of resistance toward doing anything that's good for us, and in the case of physical exercise, this resistance can be strong. My resistance is always greater when I don't exercise regularly because when I feel that there's a huge gap between my couch-potato state and having buns of steel, I kind of give up. I just have no idea how I'm going to get there from here. If I haven't exercised for a while, the trick for me is to start small: a short, 15-minute workout is all it takes. Maybe I'll pull out my kettlebell weight and do a quick workout or try that exercise app that's been sitting idle on my home screen for months. The beauty is that by starting small, each day builds on the next, and as my body slowly becomes stronger and I feel more energetic and alive, my ability to conquer the enemy-thought army that tells me that I can't grows, too.

Taking Charge

One simple way to take charge of your health is to walk for at least 30 minutes a day. Even if this is all you do, if you are postmenopausal, you will be cutting your risk of developing breast cancer by at least 10 percent. Keep this in the forefront of your mind when you're tempted to curl up on the couch instead of putting your running shoes on.

A great way to make sure you get this walking in is to rescue a dog. I've had to step up my walking by at least 50 percent since a lively, black Chihuahua found his forever home with us. It's the pleading eyes.

How Much Is Really Enough?

Are two hard workout sessions a week enough, or is it okay to just do yoga every day? The answer depends on so many different things: your age, the type of exercise you do, and your physical condition are just some of the things that determine how much exercise you need to do on a daily basis. But the biggest question you have to ask yourself is: how much is enough for *what?* If you want to do the bare minimum to maintain basic good health, you'll have very different goals than someone who wants buns of steel and a six-pack—it all depends on what you really want.

I want to be in the best physical condition possible for a woman of my age. This means that I have to exercise my heart with cardio, my muscles with weights, and my bones with whatever weight-bearing exercises I choose. Also, I want to look toned and feel strong and empowered. I've found that a good choice for getting and staying in shape and healthy is to structure your workout routine like this:

1. **Exercise almost every day.** I exercise six days a week, come rain or shine—even if it's just a brisk walk with my dog—unless, of course, I am sick. I take the seventh day off, which is normally a Sunday, to let my body recharge.

2. **Challenge yourself.** I challenge myself each day to do a little more than I did the day before. This approach allows you to start off slowly and move up as you feel ready. Remember that it's important to listen to your body as you ramp up your workouts.

3. **Say good-bye to resistance.** I don't listen to my mind because it gives me all kinds of inviting excuses. My default is to always resist what's best for me. That little monkey sits on my shoulder, telling me that I'm too tired or I haven't got time. I've learned to tell him to buzz off—I move my body, and my mind follows. I always end up feeling amazing afterward.

One thing I like to do to keep myself on track is to schedule my exercise. If it's not in my schedule, it won't happen. I'd recommend that you try this, too. Look at the week ahead on your calendar and schedule in each session. You may need to book a couple of classes, or you may simply need to add a calendar entry. Be specific about the amount of time you intend to take for your exercise session. For example, if you are walking, you need to specify: is it a 40-minute walk? Make sure that you also allocate enough time to get ready for the gym, class, or walk and that you have carved out enough time to shower afterward and get wherever you need to go.

Sleeping Beauty

Getting enough sleep is imperative for beauty, especially when you are upping the ante in your daily exercise. Here are my top tips for getting a full night's beauty sleep:

- **Digital detox two hours before bed:** If you have trouble getting to sleep at night, turn off your phone, tablet, and TV two hours before you plan to go to bed. Studies have found that self-luminous screens (particularly on tablets and phones) cause a 23 percent drop in melatonin production. Melatonin is a hormone that signals your brain and body that it's time to sleep.
- **A hot bath or shower an hour before bed:** Although it's not very eco-friendly due to the amount of water used, a hot bath filled with 1 cup of Epsom salts is just the ticket if you're stressed and have trouble falling asleep. In the bath, the mix of hot water and magnesium will relax your muscles; in the shower, the relaxation comes solely from the heat.
- **Take some tea:** Start sipping a "sleepy-time" herbal tea after dinner. Most of the herbs in these teas are also great for digestion. Make your own homemade "sleeping beauty" tea easily: for the dried mix, combine 4 tablespoons dried lemon balm or valerian root, 4 tablespoons dried chamomile flowers, and 2 tablespoons dried lavender flowers. You can keep this mix in an airtight tin for up to 12 months—so all you'll have to do is steep 2 teaspoons of the mix in boiled water for 3 to 4 minutes.

- **Maintain optimum magnesium levels:** Load up on dark, leafy greens, nuts, and seeds. If I am traveling, I take a magnesium supplement. Most people benefit from taking 400–1,000 mg daily. Make sure you take the absorbable forms, which are magnesium citrate, glycinate taurate, or aspartate.

Exercise Addiction

On the flip side of resistance is exercise addiction. This is a serious problem for a growing number of women who believe that the only way they can function and feel even remotely okay is to push exercise past the healthy point. I have a friend who had a serious exercise addiction. We used to hike up a very steep canyon together. It was a tough, one-hour hike, and at the end she would say good-bye to me and set off to do the whole thing again. She stopped calling me to hike, and a few months later, I saw her *running* the whole thing—*twice*—with her knees strapped up in bandages. A mutual friend told me that a few weeks later, this woman had slipped on one of her marathon run-hikes and fractured her ankle, but she wouldn't stop exercising. She purchased a treadmill so that she could "keep in shape" until she could get back to her running.

According to a few friends of mine who are yoga and fitness instructors at studios and gyms, a lot of women double- or triple-dip, meaning that they'll go from a hardcore sculpting class to a spinning class to another hardcore aerobics class. The problem is that there is more pressure than ever for women to get the kinds of bodies they see on celebrities, models, and athletes, but for most women, this is unattainable. Social media can also fuel this obsession with photos of running shoes or six-pack abs accompanied by hashtags such as #3aday. It's become a badge of honor for some women to push themselves beyond healthy limitations.

To figure out whether or not you have an exercise addiction, simply ask yourself the following question: "How do I feel on a day when I cannot exercise?" If your answer is along the lines of "stressed," "anxious," "gross," or "guilty," you might have a problem. Similarly, if you take a day off and then push yourself to do double the following day, you might fall into the addiction category.

Exercise addiction is unlike most other addictions, such as those to alcohol, food, or drugs, because exercise seems virtuous. Friends will admire you when you go to the gym at 4 A.M. and then again straight after work. However, exercise addiction almost always leads to signs of imbalance such as lowered immunity, recurring injuries, and extreme anxiety. Too much exercise won't keep you gorgeous for good, either—the women I know who overexercise look older than they actually are because of the physical stress they put themselves through. Most exercise-dependent women I know look a bit haggard.

Just as in every other part of your life, it all comes back to balance. Whether we're talking about eating, exercising, or working, a healthy balance makes for a beautiful mind, body, and spirit.

Technique

Before we get into exercises themselves, I have to throw a note in about technique. Your technique is everything when it comes to exercise. Having taught yoga for 15 years, I am a stickler for good technique, because poor technique can not only diminish the efficacy of an exercise, but also cause serious injury. How do you know if your technique is okay? The key is to have a professional teacher or trainer watch you doing the exercise. This doesn't necessarily mean that you need to book a private trainer. You can join a class (strength training with weights, yoga, floor Pilates, and so on) and ask the teacher before class to keep a keen eye on your technique because you are not sure you are doing it correctly. I used to love it when a student came up to me at the start of class with this kind of request, because it gave me permission to freely correct them as needed—and I'd always give that student extra attention. Stand in the front, and don't be afraid to ask for what you need. Once armed with good technique, your workout will be way more efficient, and you'll be less likely to injure yourself.

Posture

Being in shape gives you the ability to combat one of the things that ages you more than anything else: bad posture. You could be virtually wrinkleless, but if you walk around hunched over with rounded shoulders, you'll look at least ten years older than you are. Interestingly, in Iyengar yoga, it's believed that posture—especially in the areas of the chest and shoulders—affects our emotions. They say that someone whose shoulders are back and whose chest is open will rarely be depressed. Perhaps this is why good posture adds to our youthful glow.

Here's a magical tip for good posture that I learned from an internationally acclaimed Rolfing teacher: Stand up and bring your mind's eye to a spot in the center of your back, just above your bra line. Gently draw that spot in and up toward your heart. This is a *subtle* action. You will feel the natural curve in your lumbar spine softening inward as it should; your shoulders will soften back, and your head will move into the correct position. Your counter action is to gently draw your lower belly in so you don't overextend your lower back.

The key is to remember to do this at least a few times each day. I recommend choosing a certain time or place that will trigger you to remember. For example, when I pass a certain garage while walking my dog, I remember to perform this simple action, and it changes the way I walk. Also, if you are very new to this, Post-It notes in choice locations around the house will help!

If you are looking for some professional help, you can always hire a trainer—either on an ongoing basis or for just a few sessions. But choose a teacher or trainer very carefully. I have worked with some amazing—and some terrible—trainers over the years. The latter either pushed me way beyond my capability or didn't teach me any technique.

Make sure you:

- Check out their credentials. Don't be afraid to ask about their qualifications.

- Ask what they specialize in and enjoy teaching most. If a trainer is passionate about a certain discipline, he or she is more likely to be good at teaching it.

- Always get a personal recommendation. This is an investment of your time and money, and you should speak to at least three people who have worked with the teacher or trainer you have in mind. Don't be afraid to ask the gym or studio if you can speak to a couple of the teacher's or trainer's past or present clients. A good gym should be able to work this out for you.

Four Strengths

There are four different areas of our health that we can focus on while working out. And structuring our exercise to take all of these into account is very important—especially as we age. Those four areas are:

1. **Heart strength:** The heart is a muscle that needs to be strengthened every day.

2. **Bone and muscle strength**: Weak bones and muscles lead to increased risk of injury.

3. **Flexibility:** We need to be flexible to function optimally throughout the day and to prevent injury. Flexibility diminishes very quickly as we age, but with consistent stretching, it comes back quickly.

4. **Balance:** One of the most neglected areas in terms of fitness is balance and yet in many ways, it's the most important because a bad slip or fall can take us out of the game for weeks, if not months. Balance is a motor skill that begins to diminish in our 30s.

All four of these components get weaker as the years roll by unless we intervene with regular contrary action. In the following pages, I lay out exercises that address all of these, and in your 30-day program, I note when to focus on each element. Please note that many of the exercises listed in this chapter address more than one area of training. In fact, there's a great deal of crossover—running can improve strength and heart health, while yoga can address every area. The exercises are listed in categories based on the area of health on which they seem to have the greatest effect.

Heart Strength (aka "Cardio")

A "cardio" workout is simply a heart-strengthening workout. The heart is a muscle, and like any other muscle in the body, it will lose its strength if not worked out regularly. We strengthen our heart muscle by making it work harder—this is achieved by engaging in any exercise that raises the rate at which it has to pump blood through the body. We should aim to raise our heart rate in some way each day. This doesn't mean we have to do a crazy aerobics class or run a half marathon. Almost any exercise, including a strong yoga practice, can effectively increase your heart rate. The benefits of a good cardio workout include:

- Improved cholesterol and fat levels in the blood
- Reduced inflammation in the arteries
- Open and flexible blood vessels
- Weight loss
- Elevated levels of serotonin (a natural, feel-good chemical in the brain)

The other benefit of getting in some cardio is that it helps to cleanse and detoxify your body by way of stimulating your lymphatic system through making you sweat. Your lymphatic system is a network of glands, nodes, and lymphatic pathways that rid your body of its toxins. Unlike your blood, the lymph has no pump to assist its flow, so you have to stimulate this on your own. This is why something like dry brushing is helpful: it assists in mechanically moving the lymph up toward the heart. In the same way, cardio may provide a pumplike action similar to that of the heart itself.

To work out the heart muscle—and your lymph system—it's useful to figure out what your "training zone" is. This depends on your age, weight, and current level of fitness. I recommend downloading one of many free apps that can help you to discover your resting heart rate, your maximum heart rate, and how to measure when you are in your training zone.

The following are some of my favorite cardio workouts.

Don't Push Too Hard!

Studies have shown that a moderate-intensity workout might be more beneficial than a high-intensity workout, especially for those with high blood pressure. In one study, it was found that by jogging—not running—two miles a day, 50 percent of participants with high blood pressure were able to come off their meds. If jogging for two miles seems totally out of the question for you, try jogging for a quarter of a mile and slowly work your way up.

Rebounder

In my opinion, the rebounder (aka mini trampoline) is pretty much the best thing to come along since sliced bread. A rebounder is a great way to get some cardio in, especially if you don't have much time. Rebounding is simply jogging on a trampoline. In the 1980s, a famous study by NASA found that rebounding is twice as efficient, in terms of cardio, as running on a treadmill. It is also much safer for your joints. The super-convenient thing about a rebounder is that you can do your daily exercise in bite-size increments. If I have a day at the computer, I might stop every hour or so to vigorously rebound for ten minutes. Not only am I getting my exercise, but it also helps relax my neck and shoulder muscles, and it makes me feel great.

I have a rebounder that folds and stores neatly under my bed. If you buy one—which I highly recommend—look for a model that is well made. The cheaper, 40-buck models don't last long.

Mindful Running

I love running because it makes me feel good instantly; however, because I have a couple of old injuries, not to mention a very tight hip, I rarely run anymore. Running is very hard on your joints. I have two friends who have been completely addicted to running for years—one blows her knee out monthly and has to sit with an ice pack strapped to it, and the other is about to face a second surgery on her Achilles tendon. To me, this is too high a price to pay for a feel-good run, so I recommend practicing "mindful running." This helps you not only enjoy your run more, but also keeps you from getting injured. Here's how I do it—feel free to take this method for yourself:

1. I do a few yoga stretches before setting off. While practicing these poses, I tune into my breath and "ask" my body if it's up for running that day. When I connect to my breath, it's easier to listen to my body. I become hyperaware of any aches, pains, or injuries. I try to honor what's going on, and if my body is screaming not to run, I choose another exercise.

2. If I feel that my body can cope with a run, I start really slowly by doing a run-walk-run for the first quarter of a mile. This is a good test to further check if my body is ready and warmed up enough.

3. Once I get going, I pay great attention to my feet, making sure that I use the whole of my foot and spread my toes wide to minimize impact.

4. I create a rhythm for my breath: I inhale for four steps and exhale for four steps. You'll find your own rhythm, but make sure you try to inhale and exhale

through your nose, because it's a more effective way of utilizing your oxygen intake.

5. As I get into my rhythm, I constantly check in with my body, making sure that my facial muscles, shoulders, and upper back are relaxed.

Walking and Hiking

I often feel I'm copping out by just walking. Is walking really an exercise? I think it can be, but you need to work up some speed. There's a big difference between a stroll and a walk that counts as a workout. The American College of Sports Medicine recommends that regular healthy adults walk at moderate intensity for a minimum of 30 minutes, five days a week. How do we know what moderate intensity is? You need to feel your heart beating faster than it normally does and break a sweat. However, you know you're going too hard if you can't carry on a conversation.

Depending on your fitness level, you may not be able to raise your heart rate by just walking. You might want to invest in a small heart-rate monitor to be sure you get into your training zone. For me to break a sweat, I need to go on a hike that has a pretty steep incline for a good mile or so. This may sound obvious, but when you're hiking, watch for loose rocks, uneven ground, and fallen branches. I know two women who have twisted their ankles so badly from not seeing a loose rock on a hike—and these injuries put them out of the game for at least six weeks.

Cycling and Spinning

I love my bicycle, but I have to admit that tootling to and from the farmers' market barely raises my heart rate a notch. In order to get enough decent exercise from a bicycle, I need to spin or at least train on one of those ghastly stationary bikes at the gym. I say "ghastly" because I find stationary bicycling insufferable unless it's in a spin class with a killer soundtrack and an overly enthusiastic teacher. I rarely love these workouts, but they put my heart rate through the roof, which is a good thing. A great indoor-cycling teacher told me that the one pitfall of spinning is that students can easily plateau after a few months of training. This is why he changes up the routine every week. If you are an avid spinner, just make sure you are shocking your body off its plateau by giving it what it least expects.

Cardio Machines

Cardio machines such as ellipticals can be great, but only if used in the right way. It's also important that you don't plateau on one of these machines. A couple of my girlfriends go to the gym every morning, stuff in their earbuds, and pound away for almost an hour, yet both women struggle with weight issues consistently, which may be due to them not following these important guidelines:

- Always enter your personal stats, because machines are usually calibrated for someone weighing around 150 pounds. Although it's sometimes laborious to enter all your stats, you'll get a much better workout if you do.

- Bump up the resistance, not the speed. Many women go like the clappers on these machines, thinking that speed equals calorie burn, but it doesn't. It's way more effective to increase the resistance to a point at which you are seriously challenged.

- Good posture is very important. If you slouch over your machine, you'll end up hurting your back and not working the leg and gluteal muscles that you think you are targeting.

- Use the whole of your foot, not just your toes. We have a tendency to push into the balls of our feet and our toes on these machines.

- The most important tip is to challenge yourself by changing up your routine. It's easy to plateau on a cardio machine, which means that you will stop seeing results. Maybe give that equipment a rest for a couple of weeks and choose a different machine (such as the rowing machine) or ramp up the resistance—or at least change the program that you've become used to.

Dancing

Here's an exercise that a lot of people don't consider: dancing. I have seen goddesslike bodies emerge on friends who later in life decided to embark on a journey of dance. Most proper dance classes are a massive workout, which requires mental as well as physical agility. Ballroom-style dance studios have mushroomed all over the country as a result of *Dancing with the Stars* or *Strictly Ballroom* (in the U.K.). Women over a certain age are pulling on high-heeled pumps to shimmy across the floor. My BFF in the U.K. has transformed her body this way, and she's addicted to dancing. However, if ballroom isn't your bag, there's Zumba, jazz, tap, and ballet, among various others. Taught well, all of these disciplines will give you a great cardio workout—not to mention improve your strength, flexibility, and balance.

Bone and Muscle Building

It's now common knowledge that we lose at least 5 percent of our muscle mass per decade after the age of 35. So, by the age of 55, we may have lost a whopping 10 percent of our lean muscle mass. Not only is this not so attractive, it also has the added effect of making it harder to lose weight. Without lean muscle mass, fewer calories are burned while you work out—and while you rest. With your muscle, it's a use-it-or-lose-it situation, so I suggest you "use it" six days a week. This doesn't mean that you have to go pump iron all the time. It just means that you have to challenge your muscle strength, and there are many ways that you can do this.

Strength (resistance) training means that you are training yourself to become stronger every day by having your muscles work against resistance. This resistance could be a huge barbell or the floor when you are doing a push-up—or it could be a steep incline on a hike you're doing.

Strengthening your muscles is vital as you age, not just for beauty, but also for optimum functionality. Remember, you want to strengthen all the major muscle groups in your body—some people just work on their thighs or their arms, but to be optimally healthy, you've got to work the whole enchilada. It's amazing what you can accomplish in your living room with a couple of weights and a chair.

Here are some of the most effective methods for building strength:

Weights

There are two different kinds of weights you can use:

- **Free weights:** I love to use free weights for sculpting my arms. I invested in 3- and 5-pound weights, which sit in my hall closet along with yoga mats, blocks, straps, and a foam roller. If I can't find time to do anything else in a day, I might whip out my weights and do five to ten minutes of triceps, biceps, or shoulder sculpting. I've picked up my favorite exercises from the odd personal training session and DVDs. With free weights, form is very important. If you are in any doubt as to exactly how you should perform free-weight exercises, it might behoove you to invest in a one-on-one, 30-minute session with a trainer to help you craft your "home" session. I also love my kettlebell weights (see next page).

- **Machines:** I've never been a big gym machine girl because I find them a bit boring; however, loads of women love them because once you've got the hang of them, you can stick in your earbuds and just get on with it. It's imperative that you do at least one personal training session when creating a workout using weight machines at the gym—as with free weights, form is very important.

Kettlebells

I'm obsessed with my kettlebells—sounds a bit raunchy, right? Actually, there's nothing remotely sexy about a Russian kettlebell other than the fact that it will lift and tone your behind like nothing else. A kettlebell is a large, cast-iron ball weight with a single handle. You work out with just one bell, and you get to choose your weight. For beginners, I recommend a 5-pound weight; for intermediates, a 10-pound weight; and for advanced or very strong kettlebellers, try a 15-pounder.

Kettlebells are really easy to use: you mostly perform a series of squats while gripping the bell with both hands, swinging it between your legs and then up above your head. Technique is very important, because you need to take great care of your lower back and shoulders. Make sure you get a good DVD to follow for a detailed workout.

Pilates

With Pilates, you will likely have the option of doing a private or semi-private class with an instructor or a group "floor" class. If you choose the latter, you will be trained on a traditional reformer, which will help to gently and safely strengthen and stretch your muscles. This option is an excellent idea if you have injuries or physical limitations, because the instructor will be able to customize accordingly.

Pilates on Steroids

Sebastien Lagree developed his own form of Pilates by way of his patented Proformer and Megaformer machines. This workout (www.lagreefitness.com) is like no other workout I've ever done. The machines themselves are quite different, and you typically work out in a class of other students to a rocking playlist. The Lagree method uses resistance and counter-resistance to maximize exertion and minimize injury. I've never exercised so hard in my life. These machines have taken my physical fitness to a whole new level. Sadly, studios that use this method are somewhat sparse, but if you can find one near you, go.

Beautiful Behind

There are two weight-training exercises that just have to be done as often as humanly possible if you want to create or maintain a firm derriere. The beauty of both squats and lunges is that they can be done anywhere and at any time of the day. They can be part of a yoga, gym, or cardio practice and can be done with or without weights. You can get up right now and practice a couple of rounds of reps. I'll join you!

Squats: With or without weights, squats are one of the best exercises that you can do for toning your derriere and thighs. What is key is that you perform a deep enough squat. To do a proper squat, stand with your feet a little more than hip distance apart, with your toes turned slightly outward. Bend your knees as if you are trying to sit on a tiny chair behind you. Drop your bottom to below your knee height, and use your glutes to bring you back up. Focus all your weight into your heels. Do 20 reps, rest, and then do 20 more. Holding a couple of weights will make it even more challenging.

Lunges: For maximum glute and thigh toning, I like to combo squats with lunges. A well-executed back lunge can do wonders for that tough area where your glute meets your thighs. To lunge, stand with your feet a few inches apart, making sure you feel well balanced (I like to wear stable training shoes). Step your right foot all the way back while bending the back knee. Pause for a moment and check that your left knee is stacked directly above your left ankle (you may need to scoot your right foot back a tiny bit). As you exhale, bring your right foot back to its starting position. Repeat 12 times and then move on to your left leg.

Your Core

The word *core* in the fitness space has become ubiquitous because fitness professionals have realized how strong abdominal muscles affect almost every physical action we take. I have a massive, restaurant-capacity KitchenAid stand mixer, which I keep on a high shelf in my pantry. I have to really think twice before hauling this monster down to bake muffins, and if it weren't for my pretty well-worked-out core, I probably would've been seriously injured by the darn thing crashing down on top of me. I employ literally every single abdominal muscle to keep me from teetering over, metal monstrosity in hand.

Without a strong core, we can also really hurt our backs, particularly our lower backs, because the muscles overstretch to compensate for the lack of strength in the front of the body. So, whatever it takes, get those muscles as strong as you can. Two of my favorite core workouts are the plank and exercises using the fitness ball.

Fitness Ball: Fitness balls are great because they're very supportive for abdominal crunches. To work your abs with a fitness ball, simply sit on the ball with your knees bent and your hands gently supporting the back of your neck. On your inhale, lean back until you feel your abs fully engage. As you exhale, use your lower abs to raise your chest up toward your thighs. It's very important that you keep your elbows wide at all times, because it will prevent you from pulling at your head or neck. Try ten repetitions, rest, and then try ten more. You can slowly work your way up to 50. When you are done, stretch out your abs by lying back across the ball, with the ball supporting the lumbar region of your spine. If possible, gently stretch your arms overhead.

Plank: Plank pose (aka a push-up) is a great core and full-body strengthener that won't hurt your neck or lower back if performed correctly. Simply get onto the floor on all fours. Make sure your hands are directly in line with your shoulders and your fingers are spread out and facing forward. Curl your toes under, straighten your knees, and edge your feet back until your legs are fully extended. Focus on these three things: keep your shoulders away from your ears, draw your low belly up to your spine, and use your leg and glute muscles to keep you in the pose—don't push your butt up. Then simply hold, with your body straight, like a plank. I recommend trying to stay in plank for a minute at a time, preferably a few times a day. Like squats and lunges, you can do this anywhere.

Quick Five Minutes

You can create a quick, five-minute workout any time of the day by simply moving back and forth between plank and the yoga position called downward facing dog (see page 278 for explanation of how to do this). This transition is both strengthening and energizing.

Flexibility and Balance

I cannot stress enough the importance of working on your flexibility and balance on a daily basis because a lack of these will inevitably lead to an injury somewhere along the line.

Yoga

Although there are other practices that can help you with flexibility and balance, yoga is truly the best choice. In addition, yoga also helps you with cardio and strength training. It is also a deeply spiritual practice—and you don't have to be associated with any particular religion to get this benefit from it.

The word *yoga* is derived from a Sanskrit word that means to bind, attach, and yoke. It also means union or communion. A wise yogi, Mahadev Desai, said that yoga is "the yoking of all the powers of the body, mind, and soul to God." Yoga is just one of the six orthodox systems of Indian philosophy that was systemized by Patanjali in his classical text *The Yoga Sutras*.

The beauty of yoga is that many of us are drawn to it as a purely physical practice because, let's face it, some of the most beautiful bodies we see are "yoga bodies." However, by practicing with a good teacher, you can be drawn into the deep spiritual nature of the practice as well, and this takes it to a whole different level. I love that yoga is a mind-body-spirit workout for everyone: on one end of the scale, I have taught male athletes who want a hard workout (and I always sneaked in a bit of meditation), and on the other end, I have taught women who just wanted to mentally escape from the hellish stress in their lives. Either way, if you practice regularly, you will be led to a better place physically, mentally, and spiritually.

If you are interested in yoga as your primary form of exercise, make sure to choose the right kind for you. There are so many different yoga traditions: Ashtanga, Bikram, Flow, hot yoga, and Iyengar, to name a few. Realize that not every school of yoga is going to be right for you. Here are some of the main schools of yoga, many of which I have practiced and/or taught; they include some of the most common kinds you'll see if you're looking for a class.

Anusara: *Anusara* means to "step into the current of the Divine Will." And in this type of yoga, there is an equal focus on spiritual and physical alignment. I love the open invocation that is often used at the beginning of an Anusara class. A translation from Sanskrit to English is:

I offer myself to the Light, the Auspicious Lord,

Who is the True Teacher within and without,

Who assumes the forms of Reality, Consciousness, and Bliss,

Who is never absent and is full of peace,

Independent in His existence, He is the vital essence of illumination.

Ashtanga: This form of yoga is extremely athletic and, when taught in its pure form, is very challenging. You need to be athletic, fit, and free of injuries to pursue this kind of yoga. Ashtanga was founded by Sri K. Pattabhi Jois, who taught it to adolescent male athletes in India. When practicing, you are encouraged to synchronize your breath with a progressive series of postures that you move through without stopping. Given that most of us are not young athletes, I recommend exercising extreme caution if you are drawn toward this strenuous practice. I have experienced and seen many Ashtanga-induced injuries over the years. However, if you're up to it, strengthening and challenging your body to go way beyond what might feel comfortable can be exhilarating.

Bikram: Bikram was the first hot yoga practice to hit America. The founder, Bikram Choudhury, turned the heat in his studios up to 100 degrees to replicate the climate in India, yoga's birthplace. He created a sequence of 26 postures that are practiced under very sweaty circumstances. While this is probably obvious, I only recommend this to people who can handle heat really well. Many of us can get really agitated by the intense heat even though we think we can handle it, so be careful. Also, be aware that you have to be super careful that you don't overdo it, because the heat makes you feel that you can stretch further than your body is really able to.

Flow: *Flow* is a name given to a hybrid yoga practice where you move, or flow, from pose to pose without resting. In many ways, it's a watered-down (and a less strenuous) version of Ashtanga yoga. I recommend Flow yoga for those of you who have the basics of a yoga practice down and enjoy a more fast-paced class.

Hatha: You'll see the term *Hatha yoga* on many studio and spa schedules. The word *Hatha* in Sanskrit means "sun and moon," referring to the balancing of male (sun) and female (moon) energies. Hatha yoga is a term often used to describe a generic yoga class that uses a series of postures (asanas) to build strength and flexibility. The breathing and spiritual aspects of the class depend on who is teaching it.

Hot Yoga: This is where the yoga studio is heated up to the point at which you break out in a sweat before you've even begun to move. Inspired by Bikram, there are now a number of hot yoga schools that have developed their own signature philosophies. It's not for everyone. The same warnings go for hot yoga as for Bikram: don't do it if you can't handle intense heat, and don't overwork yourself—remember, the heat can trick you, making you feel that you can stretch your muscles way further than usual, and this can sometimes result in injury.

Iyengar: Iyengar yoga was founded by the late B. K. S. Iyengar, who penned the legendary *Light on Yoga*—the bible of modern yoga. Iyengar believed that yoga is a technique ideally suited to prevent physical injury and mental illness and to generally protect the body. This is why this style might be a wise choice if you have injuries or physical limitations—the teacher will tailor the practice to your needs. Iyengar is a slow, detailed practice that focuses on technique and form. If you want a quick, sweaty workout, this isn't the practice for you. Each pose is held for an extended period while detailed instructions force you to focus on every bone, muscle, and ligament.

Integrative Yoga Therapy

While not technically a tradition of yoga, Integrative Yoga Therapy is gaining in popularity, especially among health professionals who now realize the tremendous benefits of yoga for healing. Most of the people who study this kind of yoga wind up teaching it.

Integrative Yoga Therapy was founded in 1993 by Joseph Le Page, a yoga teacher in the Kripalu tradition, which focuses on energy healing. He has created a number of comprehensive teacher training programs for use in medical settings and individually customized sessions.

Jivamukti: Although Jivamukti yoga incorporates a lot of chanting, meditation, music, and ancient and modern spiritual prayer and affirmations, it is not for the faint of heart physically! Cofounders David Life and Sharon Gannon combine an Ashtanga style of practice that also integrates all the beautiful spiritual aspects of a well-thought-out yoga practice.

Kripalu: Kripalu yoga was developed at Kripalu Center, which is North America's largest facility for holistic education. This form of yoga combines focus, meditation, yoga poses, and breath work to help you develop a "quiet mind" and induce deep relaxation. Kripalu emphasizes following the flow of *prana* (life force) in the body and practicing compassionate self-acceptance.

Kundalini: Kundalini yoga has an almost cultlike following in Los Angeles, with many celebrities flocking to a large studio a mile from where I live. It's based on the teachings of the late Yogi Bhajan, who bought his yogic teachings with him to the U.S. in 1969. Kundalini yoga classes include chanting, meditation, breathing, and a sequence of postures that all lead to the awakening of our flow of "energy" and a fusing of our consciousness with the Divine. Kundalini is a gentler form of yoga, physically speaking, so it might be great for a beginner, and it's perfect as a prenatal yoga practice.

Power Yoga: Power yoga was developed by Bender Birch as her Western spin on Ashtanga yoga. It is very similar to Flow or hot yoga in that you move swiftly from pose to pose while integrating your breath with each movement. When I have a lot of energy, I crave this kind of class.

Viniyoga: Viniyoga was created by T. K. V. Desikachar, who believed that yoga really needs to be customized to the individual because each of us is completely different in our needs, limitations, and goals. As part of my teaching training, I studied Viniyoga and found it to be an invaluable practice for taking care of myself, especially when I am super achy or have injuries. It is also a wonderful practice for seniors and anyone with physical limitation or a serious injury. You can visit www.viniyoga.com to find out if there is a teacher or class in your city or country.

Testing Balance

One in three Americans over the age of 65 falls every year, and that fall can lead to a debilitating injury or death. If you want to find out how good your balance is at this point in your life, try the following simple exercise.:

1. Have a stopwatch handy.
2. Stand with your feet shoulder width apart in either flat shoes or bare feet.
3. Cross your arms over your chest.
4. Lift one knee to a 45-degree angle.
5. Begin the stopwatch and close your eyes.
6. If you uncross your arms or tilt to the side more than 45 degrees, stop the watch and start again.

Now, compare how you did with the averages below:

- 20–49 years of age: 24 to 28 seconds
- 50–59 years: 21 seconds
- 60–69: 10 seconds
- 70–79: 4 seconds
- 80 and older: most cannot even perform the test for a few seconds

You want to strive for a time that is way above the average for your age.

Yoga is one of the best practices for improving your balance. A handful of yoga asanas (poses) are especially geared toward improving your balance. Any pose that requires you to stand on one leg (such as tree or eagle pose) is an excellent way to start, and when you've mastered the pose with your eyes open, try it with your eyes closed.

Fountain of Youth

Aside from yoga, a workout I love for enhancing flexibility is the Five Tibetan Rites, also known as the "Fountain of Youth"—because this practice effectively strengthens and stretches all the main muscles in your body. It also helps with balance. I know at least five elderly women (over 80) who keep themselves limber and strong by performing these rites daily. I recommend you learn this simple practice, which you can do in just ten minutes.

I recommend doing the rites in the morning rather than the evening, because they do stoke your energy. Begin by practicing 5 to 7 repetitions of each rite, and build up to 21.

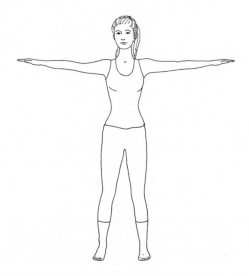

Rite 1: Stand with your arms outstretched and horizontal to the floor, palms facing down. Make sure your arms are in line with your shoulders. Your feet should be about hip distance apart. Draw the crown of your head up toward the ceiling. Focus on a spot in front of you so that you can count your rotations. Spin around clockwise until you become a little dizzy. Gradually increase the number of spins from 2 to 21. When I first started, I could only do about 7 rotations; I'm now up to 14.

Breathing: Inhale and exhale deeply as you spin.

Tip: If you feel super dizzy, interlace your fingers at your heart and stare at your thumbs. Also, have a chair very nearby to grab onto to steady yourself if you feel as if you are going to fall.

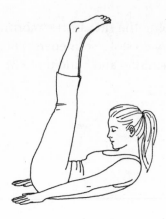

Rite 2: Lie flat on the floor. Fully extend your arms along your sides and place the palms of your hands against the floor. If you have lower back issues, place your fingers underneath your sacrum. As you inhale, raise your head off the floor, tucking your chin into your chest. Simultaneously lift your legs, knees straight, into a vertical position. If possible, extend your legs over your body toward your head. Then slowly exhale, lowering your legs and head to the floor, keeping your knees straight and your big toes together.

Breathing: Breathe in deeply as you lift your head and legs, and exhale as you lower them.

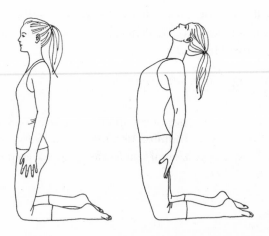

Rite 3: Kneel on the floor with your toes curled under. Place your hands on the backs of your thigh muscles. Tuck your chin in toward your chest. Slide your hands down the backs of your thighs as you draw your shoulders back and your head up toward the sky. Keep in mind that you are arching your upper back more than your lower back. Move your head back as if you were drawing a line with your nose on the ceiling. Slowly return to an upright position and repeat.

> **Breathing:** Inhale as you arch your spine and exhale as you return to an erect position.

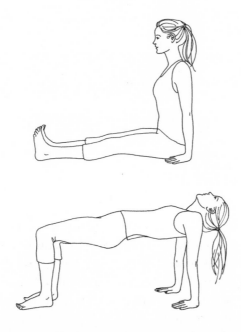

Rite 4: Sit down on the floor with your legs straight out in front of you and your feet about 12 inches apart. Place your palms on the floor alongside your sitz bones. As you gently drop your head back, raise your torso so that your knees bend while your arms remain straight. You are basically in a tabletop position. Slowly

return to your original sitting position. Rest for a few seconds before repeating this rite.

> **Breathing:** Breathe in as you rise up into the pose, hold your breath as you tense your muscles, and breathe out fully as you come down.

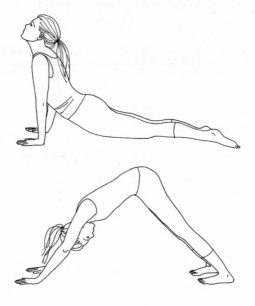

Rite 5: Lie down on your belly with your palms face down and in line with your bra strap. Press up into an upward-facing dog by curling your toes under, lifting your heart, and drawing your shoulders back. Your arms should be straight. Look straight ahead of you, or, if you are a little more flexible, gently draw your head back, taking your eyes toward the sky. Then draw your hips up and back, extending your spine, into downward-facing dog pose. Repeat by moving back and forth between downward- and upward-facing dog.

> **Breathing:** Breathe in as you rise up into upward-facing dog; breathe out as you push back into downward-facing dog.

Body Rolling

The final activity that I recommend for improving flexibility is body rolling using a body roller. If you are very sensitive, you might want to go with a foam roller, but if you prefer something harder, you can go with a piece of PVC pipe or order one of the many great body rollers online.

Why I love rolling out: it stretches the muscles and tendons and helps release the fascia (structure of connective tissue surrounding muscles, joints, and tendons). Rolling before a hard workout increases blood flow to your soft tissue, and rolling after a workout helps release your muscles. While body rolling isn't a workout in and of itself, it is invaluable for keeping your muscles soft and pliable.

One Last Note

Unless you have a medical condition that requires you to own a bathroom scale, I highly recommend that you donate it to the local thrift store. Being obsessed with how much you weigh is unhealthy and counterproductive. If your mood is determined by whether or not you've lost a few pounds, all the more reason to get rid of the darn thing. Aside from the fact that scales give not at all accurate portrayals of how you look or how much fat versus muscle you are carrying around, they can lead to an unhealthy obsession that bleeds into the rest of your life. I trust myself, not a scale, because my weight is just a small part of the whole picture. If I've been overeating or not working out, I don't need a scale to track my progress—I can *feel* it. My body doesn't feel strong and full of vigor, and my jeans are tighter—sometimes much tighter! I'll weigh myself maybe two or three times a year—when I find myself either in the doctor's office or at a fancy hotel or spa. But I refuse to let a scale have any power over me.

Chapter 9

Getting to Know You

As you are fully aware by now, being gorgeous is both an internal and an external job. We've started learning about the internal things that really do help us feel and look better—nutrition and movement. These two things take you to a new level of health, but now we're going to explore even one level deeper—your mind, emotions, and spirit. This is the realm of true, deep-down beauty. Authenticity—truly knowing who you are, what you want, and how you want to be in this world—makes you glow from the inside. It helps you come across as a confident woman—sure in yourself, sure in your beliefs, and sure in your ability to express yourself honestly in the world.

This self-belief is not something that just happens. Like all other things that greatly benefit us, it takes work. And I won't lie—you can't just do this for a few weeks and then stop, if you want your inner beauty to keep glowing. Knowing yourself is an ongoing process, but it's so rewarding that the work of it often doesn't feel like work. Think of it as getting to know a good friend; it's just, in this case, that the friend is you.

The practices I lay out in this chapter will help you slow your mind and become familiar with your thoughts. They will give you the ability to dig down into yourself to see which beliefs and thoughts guide your life. They will also help you see which of these beliefs and thoughts come from a place of truth in you and which ones come from societal or familial beliefs and expectations. This work should help you see the areas in your life that would benefit from some change—and I also give you suggestions on how to work toward this change.

Meditation Practice

One of the most profound practices that I've come upon in my work of getting to know myself is meditation. There has been so much research done on this powerful technique that I can't even dream of covering it all here. It ranges from studies on focus and concentration to compassion and kindness. A regular meditation practice has been shown to calm the mind and help people think clearly in stressful situations. In fact, even the military has found proven success using meditation programs—both in battle and after a soldier's return home. Learning and practicing basic meditation techniques before going into battle has led to soldiers being more balanced and less reactive when they do get into combat situations. And training in meditation afterward has been shown to have impressive results in alleviating post-traumatic stress disorder.

While my life is hardly as stressful as a combat zone, I have experienced similar benefits during my own chaotic periods. I've been meditating (almost daily) for nearly 25 years, and over that time, I've noticed that I have a much greater capacity to cut through the craziness of the world around me to both focus on what's important and stay true to who I am.

So, if you only get one thing from this book, I hope it's that you learn to create a short daily meditation practice. Meditation is really the only way that I can counteract the stress in my own life. Once you've created a short practice, you can take it with you anywhere.

No-Stress Meditation

To do basic meditation, all you really need is a quiet space and some determination. The goal is to sit silently for a set amount of time, during which you observe your thoughts—which, believe me, is not an easy thing to do, but you will learn how.

For a lot of people, the mind can go off on a negative tangent when they begin to meditate: "Okay. Time to meditate. I'm going to be calm and switch off the thoughts in my mind. But how can I do that? I'm so busy. Wait. Did I respond to Kristin? Crap, I really need to send that e-mail. I'll do that after . . . wait . . . no . . . I'm meditating. Why can't I focus? What's wrong with me? Okay. I have to calm my mind. Calm. Calm. Breathe. Calm. Calm like a beautiful, serene lake. Which reminds me, I need to buy a bathing suit. Ugh. I hate buying bathing suits, and I so need to stop this meditating nonsense so I can do a hundred million squats to face trying on a bathing suit . . ." And on and on your mind will go. This is 100 percent normal! Don't worry. The thing to do when your mind wanders is simply to be aware of it. When you separate the "you" from your racing mind, you are meditating.

Noticing the script of your mind opens your eyes to just how many thoughts go through your head each day. It helps you see the noise in your mind. And bringing your mind back to focus helps you gain control over this "monkey mind." If you are able to do that, you have a solid foundation from which to operate. You know how to recognize when your mind is spiraling out of control. But, more important, you know how to bring your mind back to a place of peace, which will help you make better decisions and act in ways that are truer to how you want to be in the world.

The thing about meditation is that it's a practice. It's referred to in this way because, much like piano or dance, you have to practice it to get good at it. You can't just sit down on day one and expect to get comfortable and still your mind. You may find it virtually impossible at first. It's still a work in progress for me, but the great news is that it's definitely gotten easier over the years. And that's how it works for everyone who's brought this practice into their lives: the more they do it, the easier it becomes.

One of the secrets of learning to meditate successfully is to start small. There is no way that you can expect yourself to sit easily and mindfully for 20 minutes if you've never done it before. It would be like asking a small child to sit still for 20 minutes without moving a muscle—it just won't work. Most people who try to meditate get put off initially because they find it too torturous to sit and not peek at the clock. Just like the mind running wild, this is normal. The mistake is to set yourself up to fail by believing that you are only meditating if you sit for a minimum of 20 minutes and if your mind is completely still that whole time. I recommend that you start with five minutes. Five minutes is doable for practically everyone, and you can extend the time from there. Once you are able to sit without stress for five minutes, try ten. Then 15. Then 20. You will be able to build up your endurance quickly, so don't worry if it's hard at first.

I will say that, even though I have been meditating regularly for more than two decades, it's sometimes still easy for me to sprint through my day and realize, as I fall into bed at night, that I hadn't gotten around to meditating that day. Such days can mount up, and I'll find that a week goes by with no meditation. Because I understand how different I feel when I do meditate regularly, a week without it leaves me feeling very stressed—and my husband is definitely the first to notice!

The Balance

Over the years, I have found that my deepest and most satisfying meditation sessions occur when I find the perfect balance between focusing and letting go. My mind absolutely slows down when I give it something to focus on, such as a mantra or a breathing practice (both of which we'll cover in this chapter). However, there is a very fine line between forcing my mind to focus and gently letting go. Finding this balance is a skill that takes time. Be patient with yourself and know that the key to learning balance is simply to notice if and when you are forcing your mind to focus. Think of *guiding*, rather than forcing. Watch how much easier the whole thing becomes when you let go.

The Mechanics of Meditation

To start a meditation practice, the first thing you need to do is find a space where you will be undisturbed by kids, pets, and partners. Try a few different spots in your home, as each has a different feel to it. I like to make sure that I am facing east when I sit to meditate. Most of the spiritual traditions in the world state that it is best to face the east, too. In the Kundalini tradition, subtle magnetic currents are said to flow from east to west, so by facing east, you can take advantage of the very subtle currents flowing into you.

The next thing you'll need to do is figure out how to sit comfortably. Some people sit on the floor, and some sit on a cushion. However, if you suffer from hip, leg, or back pain, you might be better off sitting in a chair. Never force yourself to sit in a cross-legged lotus pose if it doesn't feel right—even though this is the pose you see in almost all depictions of meditation. While lotus is the optimal meditation position because this pose encourages your spine to extend naturally, it doesn't work for everyone.

Here are a few hints for different sitting positions:

Cushion or Floor Sitting: I like a proper, round meditation cushion because it is way firmer than a scatter cushion (like the ones on your couch). On the floor or on a cushion, you sit cross-legged. You need to make sure that your hips are higher than your knees, though, as this protects your knee joints from excess pressure. If your knees rise up above the level of your hips, you may not be flexible enough for this position and thus should sit on a higher cushion (or a chair). You can also try to further protect your knees by placing a small cushion under each outer thigh. When you relax your hips, there should be no pain or stiffness, and your knees should feel well supported rather than hang in the air. To finish off this position, extend your spine upward and let your hands rest on your thighs.

Chair Sitting: If you sit in a chair, make sure that you are either supported by a cushion in the lumbar region of your back or that the back of the chair is upright enough to support you in sitting with an extended spine. You need to have your feet firmly planted on the floor in front of you. Rest your hands on your thighs with your palms facing either down or up toward the sky, with your fingers in a mudra (see below). Feel your sitz bones pressing into the seat of the chair, and extend your spine upward. Imagine you have a cord attached to the crown of your head that is pulling you up toward the sky. Soften your shoulders away from your ears.

Hand Mudra

You may want to use a mudra (hand gesture) when you meditate. I love the basic hand gesture of resting my hands on my knees, palms facing up, and bringing my thumbs and middle fingers together. It feels as if I'm sealing in my energy.

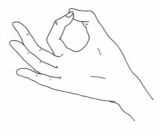

Mantra Meditation

While meditation doesn't require a specific point of focus, there are a few tools that can help you get control of an out-of-control mind. Breathing practices are one of these, but another very simple one is the use of a mantra, which is basically just a phrase or word that you repeat silently to yourself as you sit quietly. A mantra can give the mind a little something extra to hook onto. You don't need to be affiliated with any philosophy or religion to have a mantra. If you are Christian, you might want to repeat a simple phrase such as, "Be still and know that I am God." If you are not affiliated with any particular religion or yoga school, you may want to try using the mantra *so'ham* (pronounced "so hum"). In Sanskrit, this means

"I am that," and it's a powerful mantra for connecting your consciousness or your soul to its source.

You use a mantra by simply closing your eyes and focusing on your breathing first. As your breath deepens, start saying your phrase mentally, repeating either the whole thing or part of it on both the inhale and the exhale. For example, with *so'ham*, you silently say *So* as you inhale and *Hum* as you exhale.

When repeating a mantra, it's imperative that you don't try to force anything. Repeating a mantra should feel effortless and easy. If you find yourself wrangling your thoughts like naughty preschoolers so you can focus on your mantra (the teacher), let it go and simply watch your breath.

The Golden Moment

The magical moment of my meditation practice always seems to come toward the end of a session, when I let go of my point of focus (my breath or my mantra) and allow my mind to do whatever it wants to do. I simply watch it without bringing it back to center. During this time, I not only learn a lot about myself but also find some blissful moments of space between my thoughts. It's as if an attention-grabbing child (your thoughts) has been bugging you for hours, and you suddenly turn to him/her and say, "Okay, you have my full attention. Go for it. Do whatever you want to do!" In that moment, the child may rattle off a load of nonsense to you, and then become quiet—absolutely silent. This is the golden moment, the gap, if you like, between your thoughts. It will only be a fleeting moment, so don't try to hold on to it; simply acknowledge that for a moment you may have experienced a deep peace. The voices/thoughts will have piped up again, but now you can watch them with a little more objectivity and compassion.

Me Time

I try to meditate each day, but that doesn't always happen. So I've actually created something I refer to as "me time," which is a 15-minute routine that acts as an insurance policy in case I don't get to my meditation later in the day.

This "me time" has become the most valuable part of my day. It's when I can momentarily quiet the negative mental chatter, which, unless I get objective about it, I can mistake for reality. If I don't take time in the morning to take care of this crazy monkey mind, I can rush headlong into my day being unconsciously motivated by fear, anger, and/or self-pity. I would so much rather be motivated by acceptance, hope, and love—but I need to wipe the slate clean on a daily basis by practicing a short meditation. I'll walk you through just how to create this morning routine for yourself in the 30-day program, but I want to introduce you to it here.

I recommend doing your "me time" routine as soon as you wake up. If I leave it until later in the day, I rarely get around to it. Part of establishing a routine is to do it at the same time every day. So, if you usually pull yourself out of bed at 6:30 A.M., set your alarm for 6:15. If you usually reach for your cell phone to check texts and Facebook before you have time to even gather your thoughts, resist! All of it will be waiting for you when you're done taking care of yourself.

My 15-minute routine includes:

- Mindfully drinking warm lemon or ginger water

- Practicing three to five basic yoga poses

- Practicing a five-minute meditation

You can probably do all this in 10 minutes, but I give myself 15 just to be safe.

If you don't think you have time for this "me time" routine, simply ask yourself this question: would you rather spend ten minutes per day erasing junk mail from your phone and computer, or doing something that will transform your life? Our time is so precious, and it is often stolen by silly things like junk mail or some other activity that is useless, annoying, and stressful. So, if you ever tell yourself that you don't have time to take care of yourself, consider your priorities. And remember, you can always erase the junk mail while you're on the toilet or chatting to a work colleague.

Digital Detox

A digital detox is a wonderful practice that will help you find some peace in your day. Our crazy, connected world is often one of the reasons people find themselves so overwhelmed and their minds so out of control. So think of this as a meditation addendum. Try to do a mini digital detox once a day—shut everything down for a short slice of time (15 minutes is good) and go for a walk (no phone required) or sit and listen to music—something without a phone or computer involved. Your nanny, boss, or BFF can live without you for 15 minutes while you go and clear your head by being 100 percent present for something that brings you relaxation and joy.

If possible, do an annual or semiannual digital detox where you spend an entire weekend without phones or computers. This can be self-imposed (if you have the willpower) or imposed by a retreat or vacation. My husband and I often take a weekend out where we both decide to switch off our phones. Work can wait, friends can wait, the world can wait—while we take the time out to soothe our spirits and recover our souls.

No Big Deal!

Let me just wrap up our discussion of meditation with a simple reminder: you don't need to make a big deal about it—as in, "Okay. Now I've got to close my eyes and *stop my thoughts.*" You will *never* be able to stop them, so don't even try! As you begin your meditation practice, just look to these three magical keys to successful meditation:

1. **Stay short:** Set yourself up for success by creating a shorter meditation time than you think you can manage. If you think that five minutes is impossible for you, then start with three minutes.

2. **Breathe:** You can always begin your meditation with a couple of breathing exercises (see below) because these exercises always serve to slow down your racing mind.

3. **Watch:** Don't try to *stop* thinking! You will drive yourself crazy if you try to control or stop your thoughts, and meditation isn't about trying to control your thoughts. Let them do what they want to do (they will anyway). Your only job is to watch.

Breathing Exercises

Breathing practice and meditation go hand in hand, as both can help calm and center your mind. Paying attention to your breath means letting go of extraneous thoughts. It means putting the focus solely on you, right *now.* It brings you into the present moment by asking you to think about your physical self—the air in your lungs, the movement of wind through your nose.

As a yoga teacher, I've learned and taught many different breathing techniques. In yoga, breathing practice is called *pranayama*, which means "extension of the breath" or "extension of the life force." I love the latter definition because yogis believe our breath is intimately connected to our life force (aka our energy field within). Pranayama is a specific practice in which we subtly move this life force using our breath. Practicing pranayama has become a vital step of my meditation practice. It teaches me how to be mindful and to easily slip into a meditative state. There are myriad breathing exercises you can do, and I've outlined three of the simplest ones here: Basic Yoga Breathing, Ujjayi Breathing, and Alternate Nostril Breathing. When practicing these breathing techniques—or really any pranayama—it's important that you:

- Never force your breath. It should always be easy.

- Relax and soften your body, particularly the muscles around your face, jaw, neck, and shoulders.

Basic Yoga Breathing

The best way to learn this technique is to start by lying comfortably on the floor. This way, you can completely relax and allow your breath to flow easily. Simply lie on a carpet or yoga mat and place a firm pillow or bolster under your knees. Let your arms lie gently at your sides, with your palms facing upward. Once you are set, simply follow these steps:

1. Close your eyes and soften your face. Allow your whole body to release into the flow. Begin to breathe naturally through your nose.

2. Place your left hand on your abdomen, just below your belly button, and wrap your right hand around the lower part of your right ribcage.

3. Begin to focus your attention on your breath as it moves in and out of your body through the back of your nose. Your lips are lightly closed. Continue to breathe softly and naturally—in and out through the nose.

4. On your inhalations, feel the natural lift of your belly, followed by the expansion of your ribcage.

5. On your exhale, feel a slight compression of your ribs, followed by your belly softening and lowering.

6. Next, bring your left hand to your upper chest, just below your collarbones. When you inhale, feel the breath moving all the way up into this area. As you exhale, watch the breath flowing out of your chest, your ribs, and finally, your belly.

7. Release both your hands to the floor with your palms facing upward. Continue to breathe gently, watching your breath naturally move in and out of the three regions (belly, ribs, chest).

8. Finally, allow your breathing to come back to normal.

Ujjayi Breathing

Also known as "ocean breath" because of the sound it creates, *ujjayi* (oo-jai-ee) breathing technique is one of the most powerful tools that I've ever learned. It's enabled me to get through times of intense fear and stress in a way I never imagined possible. Here's how to do it:

1. Take a comfortable seat, either in a chair or cross-legged. Close your eyes and soften your jaw and facial muscles.

2. Begin to deepen your breath.

3. Inhale slowly through your nose, taking the breath over the back of your throat. This should create a gentle hissing sound in the base of the throat, much like the building of an ocean wave.

4. Exhale slowly through your nose, slightly closing off the back of your throat in order to better control the slow exhale. Again, you will be creating a slight hissing sound in the base of the throat. On the exhalation, the breath sounds like the crashing of a wave.

5. As you inhale, feel the breath travel over the back of the throat and into the lungs; allow the chest cavity to fully expand, while keeping your shoulders and face completely relaxed.

6. As you exhale, allow the belly to gently draw in, rather than allowing the chest cavity to collapse.

7. Continue your slow ujjayi breath, being mindful of the sound—always keeping it slow and even.

Try breathing in for three slow beats and out for three slow beats. Counting the beats of your inhale and exhale can calm you as you do this practice.

The beauty of the sound of this breath is that you can easily focus on it during meditation. It can also be your guide: when the sound is thin or ragged, it means that your mind has wandered off. When the sound is soft, even, and full, it means that you are connected to it. Practice developing your ujjayi breath—over time, you will learn to lengthen the inhale and the exhale and refine the beautiful sound.

Alternate Nostril Breathing

Alternate nostril breathing is said to powerfully balance the left and right sides of your brain. It's a wonderful breathing technique for beginners because it requires very little concentration and is instantaneously relaxing. Here's how to do it:

1. Sit in a comfortable position and relax your shoulders, jaw, and facial muscles.

2. Place your right thumb on your right nostril, pressing gently.

3. Inhale through your left nostril.

4. Place your ring finger on your left nostril, closing it off.

5. Exhale through your right nostril.

6. With your ring finger still closing off your left nostril, inhale through your right nostril.

7. Close off your right nostril with your thumb and exhale through your left nostril.

8. This is one round; repeat for another five rounds.

While breathing, slow the breath down by counting four slow beats for your inhale and four slow beats for your exhale.

After practicing this for a short while, you'll be able to practice anytime and anyplace with your eyes closed. If you are ever really stressed out or about to blow a fuse, excuse yourself and do a few rounds of this breathing. In about two minutes, you will become completely centered and able to handle the situation.

Body Scan

Another practice that I like to do to get in touch with how I'm feeling and to bring me into the present moment is the "body scan." This is perfect to do at the end of the day when you're exhausted. It not only helps release the stress of the day but also gives you a much-needed pick-me-up for the remainder of the evening.

To do the body scan, take a moment to get quiet. You may want to lie on the floor with a cushion under your head and another under your knees. Allow yourself to release by taking a few slow, deep breaths. Bring your awareness to the crown of your head. Imagine that your awareness is a powerful white light that is going to scan your entire body for blocks and imbalances. Draw this light of awareness slowly down across your head, neck, chest, torso, and all the way down to your feet, noticing how each area of your body feels. Then draw the "light" back up again. Go as slowly as you can, noticing any pockets of discomfort and consciously releasing them.

I have been doing this exercise for years, and I often catch something that I might have missed had I been rushing around. I might notice that my stomach feels a little bloated or that my hips are really tight. I might acknowledge that my shoulders are almost touching my ears or that the arches of my feet are sore. We rarely give this kind of attention to our bodies, and I've learned the importance of becoming still in order to find out what the heck might be going on with me.

Journaling

Everything we've covered up to this point has been part of an effort to calm your mind and bring you into the present moment—to make you familiar with your body, your thoughts, and your emotions. But how do you go deeper? How do you learn who you truly are? How do you figure out what you want out of this gorgeous life?

Many of us are so stressed out trying to take care of everything and everybody in our lives that we lose perspective on ourselves. Rather than connecting on a daily basis to our deeper purpose, which always makes us feel more valuable, we get pulled every which way and wonder who on earth we are, never mind our true purpose.

Journaling is one powerful way to shine a light on your life—both what it currently is and what it could be. Whenever I've felt spun out, drained, exhausted—which always leads to a kind of "what's the point" mentality—I've found this practice to be life changing.

By journaling, you get to discover who you really are. You can only really be authentic if you know your "truth." One dictionary definition of authenticity is "accurate representation of the facts." Are you representing the facts of who you really are? I'm not necessarily talking about your age, your job, or your ethnicity. I'm rather talking about who you really are deep down. Once you discover your truth, you can own it—and this is one of the things that makes you beautiful. You are unique, you have a special something to give to the world, and when you give your gift, it should feel effortless and bring you an enormous amount of joy. This will make you shine.

Journaling is especially important if you're feeling locked in a pattern or situation that's causing you to suffer. It could be a destructive relationship, a dead-end job, or a painful marriage. It could be loneliness or a depressing lack of purpose and drive. I've been in all of the above at one time or another, and the crashing realization that "This just isn't *me!*" was the first step toward moving away from people, places, or things that weren't supporting my truth. In hindsight, it seems obvious (I should've known), but when I was younger, I didn't have the wisdom or courage to express my truth. Actually, I'm not sure I had a clue what it was, but I knew when I was breathing the wrong air. Journaling can help you see just what's out of whack in your life.

There is no one way to journal; you can really do whatever you find useful. You can write down whatever is in your head. You can use journaling prompts to help you focus. You can simply choose a topic and start writing. Doing this kind of work will help you see just what is whirling around in your mind regarding your life in general or about a specific topic. You'll also start to notice themes and trends and ideas. Through these, you can better understand your values and dreams. In your 30-day program, I include a couple of journaling prompts that I've found to be incredibly helpful in my own life.

Stream-of-Consciousness Writing

A quote often attributed to Einstein clearly points out the need for knowing and changing our mind state when trying to change our lives: "We cannot solve a problem from the same level of consciousness that created it." This tells me that my "thinking" (chattering) mind hasn't a clue. To find the answers to whatever is plaguing you, you need to get below your usual operating system of consciousness and into your unconscious stream of mostly "meaningless" thoughts. It is here that you will find gold. A great tool to access this deeper level of consciousness is to write like a lunatic! Seriously, don't think . . . just write. I learned about stream-of-consciousness writing practice from my writing mentor, the brilliant Alan Watt, author of *The 90-Day Novel*. The idea is that when you don't allow your pen to stop, you get beyond your inner editor and access the deeper reaches of your consciousness.

To do some stream-of-consciousness writing:

- Open your notebook to a fresh, new page.
- Write the theme or problem at the top of the page, but always frame positively. For example: "If money and resources were not an issue, my dream life would look like . . . " or "When I look back at my life ten years from now, what I hope to have achieved is . . ." or "I am so blessed in my life because . . . "

- Use a pen that you love to write with (it's very important that it flows effortlessly across the page).

- Set a timer for a chosen period and start writing. Do not stop writing until the timer goes off. Even if you can't think of another word to write—even if you are writing, "this is BS" over and over again—it doesn't matter. The pen does not stop until the timer goes off.

Changing Your Thoughts—and Your Life

You may have heard of *affirmations* and *intentions* as tools you can use to make changes in your life. These two techniques are staples in the world of personal development, and the basic concept behind them is that they can help you train your mind to look at yourself and the world in a new way. They help change how you think about things, and this change then inspires you to act differently in the world—thus bringing about different outcomes in your life. Affirmations and intentions are about taking responsibility for your beliefs and making a conscious decision to change them. No one else is going to do that for you.

Affirmations are simple, positive statements that portray you and the world in a way that you would like it to be—rather than how you're experiencing it right now. Say, for example, you are afraid to give a speech. An affirmation to help change this negative thought pattern might be, "I am safe and my speech goes flawlessly." Affirmations are always stated in the present tense, as if they are already occurring in the intended way.

Intentions are slightly different from affirmations, and I think they are one of the best tools out there to change a stubborn belief. They pack a bit more of a punch and give you clear action to take to make desired changes in your life.

One definition of the word *intention* is "to mentally determine a course of action or a result." There's a big difference between this and an affirmation. For example, if you know you never drink enough water, you can say the following affirmation: "I am always perfectly hydrated"; however, this is clearly untrue if you can never remember to drink as much water as you need to. You can create an intention about this situation by saying something like: "Today I will drink two liters of filtered water." You are not only expressing a desired change but also giving yourself a goal to reach. For me, this makes it much more likely that I will do something. In creating a firm intention, I give the thought purpose, and I give myself a demonstrable action to take.

The best way to create an intention is to first tap into the negative beliefs that are holding you back or stressing you out. I call these negative beliefs "resisting thoughts." They are seriously like a resistance army that is out to stamp out my light. We all have them to some extent. It doesn't matter how we got them; what matters is what we do with them. Do we allow them to thwart our creativity? Or do we find a way of cutting through them so that we can be who we are actually supposed to be—beautiful, powerful women who shine from within?

Let's take a look at some examples of resisting thoughts and the intentions that work against them:

The resisting thought: I can't be bothered to meditate. I haven't got enough time, and it's way too hard, anyway.

The intention: Today I will carve out five minutes to sit down on my meditation cushion, close my eyes, and take a few deep breaths.

• • •

The resisting thought: I can't really be bothered to work out today. I'm too tired, and I've got way too much to do.

The intention: Today I will carve out 30 minutes at 2 P.M. to go for a hike.

The resisting thought: I can't get it together to write out that business plan today, because it's not really going to work out anyway. Nothing I do ever succeeds.

The intention: I will spend at least an hour this morning working on my plan, because every tiny step I take builds on the last.

• • •

The resisting thought: I'll never have enough money to afford that vacation.

The intention: I will create a vacation fund today and put 20 dollars in it on the last day of every month.

• • •

The resisting thought: I'll always be stressed out, because I have too much to do.

The intention: Today I will make a list of everything I need to do and only do the things that I need to do today.

• • •

The resisting thought: I'm too ugly and old to be able to . . . (fill in the blank: find the man of my dreams, get the career I want, etc.).

The intention: Today I will only focus on my strengths and what I love about myself.

The most powerful intentions for me are the ones that involve my going beyond my little self and finding out ways in which I can give to others and the world. You can never go wrong with an intention where your goal is to lift up others around you— whether it is simply to help them feel better about who they are or to figure out what you can do to help their physical/mental suffering. When I make an intention like this, it's as if the powers of the Universe align with me, so that opportunities to carry out my intention present themselves to me all through the day.

I always check my intentions to see if the endgame is going to serve my friends, my community, or the world in some way. For example, if your intention is to start a handmade soap company, checking in on the "why" may help you discover that your larger purpose is to provide beautiful, nontoxic products that will make people feel wonderful. You may even decide to give back in some way by donating some of your products or profits. Armed with this kind of purpose, your intention will have tremendous power.

My personal experience with setting intentions is that it's the only way I get things done. They might not work out exactly as I imagined—they might well turn out better than I could have ever dreamed possible—but at least I am moving in the right direction. When I had the idea to write my first book, *Gorgeously Green,* almost a decade ago, it started off as a thought: "Wouldn't it be great if there were a book that made green living accessible and fun? Hmmmm . . . why don't *I* write that book?" It was a good idea, right? But if I hadn't moved into making it into a firm intention, it would have stayed just a thought. So, over the next few days, I created the intention: "I am going to write the proposal for a book entitled *Gorgeously Green* by the end of July." I gave myself three months because I thought that was a realistic time frame. Notice that I didn't say, "I am going to write a book that will become a bestseller." Even though that might have been my dream, I would have been trying to force a result rather than staying in the process. I have no control over the result—only the action that I take today toward my goal. Setting an intention is all about working toward that goal.

While affirmations and intentions are probably the most popular techniques for changing your thoughts to change your life, there are many others. Writer and affirmation expert Noah St. John came up with the powerful idea of "Afformations," which is a clever concept: instead of repeating an affirmation, you turn it into a question. For example, instead of saying, "I am prosperous" when the evidence in your life clearly points to the fact that you aren't, you ask, *"How* am I so prosperous?"* This will get your subconscious working on a whole different level. It will start searching for all the many ways that you are prosperous ("I have a beautiful family," "I'm able to cook healthy, delicious food every day," "I have all the clothes I could possibly want," "I'm talented at what I do," and so on). This affirmation-turned-question nudges you to look for things that are true rather than believe something that perhaps doesn't seem to be. Give it a go and see if it works for you. Start off with: "How am I gorgeous?"

A great example of a powerful question—and a more powerful answer—is one asked by Marianne Williamson: "Who am I to be brilliant, gorgeous, talented, fabulous?" She then answers the question with another question: "Who am I *not* to be?" This is why questions are so powerful; they force us to inquire and move beyond our beliefs in the many labels we've given ourselves. This is why I think Noah St. John's approach is so powerful when you are working on changing deeply ingrained beliefs. Instead of asking why you hate yourself so much, ask why you love yourself so much. You will be forced to come up with at least a few answers ("I am kind, talented, funny," and so on) that are way more truthful than the false beliefs that you may have built into the "story" of who you are.

Another inspiring thought leader in the personal development space is the brilliant Byron Katie. She encourages you to take responsibility and do "The Work," which is, again, asking questions. She asks you to think of something in your life that causes you suffering and to ask the following four questions about it:

1. Is it true? (Yes or no? If no, move to question 3.)

2. Can you absolutely know that it's true? (Yes or no?)

3. How do you react? What happens when you believe the thought?

4. Who would you be without the thought?

This is powerful stuff! Katie is all about digging out those thoughts that we hang on to for dear life. "The Work" encourages you to release them, move out of being a victim, and empower yourself with the truth of who you really are. I highly recommend any of her books if you find yourself stuck in a seriously negative situation.

Getting to Know You

The world of meditation, breathing, and personal development is vast and overwhelming. Many people look at this stuff as New Age BS, but if you really look at what it's doing, you'll see that a lot of good can come from it. It's all about tapping into yourself so you can better understand what you want and who you are. Many of these teachings will help you find out what makes you feel happy and fulfilled, and give you tips and techniques to help you get there. Yes, there may be some . . . um . . . weird stuff out there, but trust yourself to filter out the crazies, and follow your gut to find the good stuff. And when you do—and you meet and embrace the real you—you will shine so brightly that there will be nothing stopping you from becoming your true gorgeous self and staying that way for good.

Part Three

THE GORGEOUS
FOR GOOD
30-DAY PROGRAM

Chapter 10

30-Day Program Primer

Beauty Primer

For some of you, changing your beauty regimen might be a full case of out with the old, in with the new. I'm afraid that's always how *I* do it. If I'm switching to a new protocol or product line, I can't even bear to look at my old stuff.

On the other hand, some of you might want or need to hang on for dear life to products that you've either recently purchased or just can't live without. This is totally fine, because if something's working for your skin, you should keep it in the mix. If you're now horrified because a recent, expensive purchase has been deemed useless or unsafe by yours truly, don't despair! Just use it up; a few more applications aren't going to strike you down with some terrible disease.

Having gotten all that out of the way, if you're in the market to purchase a few new products for the 30-day program, check out Part One of the book for information on what to look for—and what to look out for—when shopping. If you want a supply of specific product recommendations, visit my website at www.sophieuliano.com.

Below, I give very basic suggestions about what you'll need and what you might want for the 30-day program.

Five Techniques to Create Healthy and Gorgeous Skin

Technique 1: Precleanse and Decongest Pores. This is the most overlooked, misunderstood, and vitally important element of any results-focused skin treatment program. A creamy cleanser—yes, even if you have oily skin—that is rich in essential fatty acids will slice through cosmetic waxes and help the skin to actually "breathe." It will help dissolve the excess skin sebum that clogs pores and leads to breakouts. Be sure to avoid any kind of foaming cleanser that might contain SLS, because that will strip your skin and alter its natural pH balance, creating inflammation and irritation. I recommend that you use either a terry or muslin cloth with hot water to remove this cleanser. Look for a cleansing cream, cleansing lotion, cleansing oil or butter, or hot cloth cleanser.*

Technique 2: Deep Cleanse and Exfoliate. This step should be done with a cleansing bar, an emulsion, or a gel that will dig down deep to refine the skin's texture, help with skin discoloration, clear breakouts, and balance blotchy skin. Afterward, your skin should feel squeaky clean but not tight and dry. If your skin is mature, dry, and not particularly sensitive, you might want to look for a cleanser that contains one of these acids: AHA, BHA, or LHA. If your skin is sensitive or if you suffer from inflammation such as acne or rosacea, find a cleanser that contains next-generation flower acids along with antioxidants and minerals to help brighten and soften your skin. I recommend that you use an electric brush, your hot cloth, or your fingers to massage in and then rinse off this cleanser. Look for a purifying cleanser, gel cleanser, exfoliating cleanser, AHA cleanser, or clarifying cleanser.

Technique 3: Intensive Skin Nutrition. The application of pure, undiluted ingredients and skin nutrients is highly effective and allows you to "power up" the results of your program and match

---

*Often sold as a "hot cloth" cleanser, this creamy cleanser is supposed to be removed with a hot muslin or terry cloth.

individual ingredients to specific skin conditions. Your skin nutrition will likely come in the form of a serum, which should contain peptides, antioxidants, and vitamins, especially a stable form of vitamin C such as magnesium ascorbyl phosphate. For ultimate antiaging benefits, apply vitamin C crystals daily. Look for L-ascorbic acid (must be water-soluble powder). (See pages 108–110 to learn more about vitamin C.)

Technique 4: Hydrate, Nourish, and Replenish. An effective daily moisturizer should provide not only moisture but also vital nutrients to the skin. It should also be chock full of antioxidants, minerals, botanical extracts, and essential fatty acids (omega-3s). Hyaluronic acid is a superior moisturizing ingredient that is great for all skin types.

Technique 5: UV/Environmental Protection. Sun exposure, pollution, and daily environmental assaults accelerate skin aging, period. It is important to note that chemical sunscreens cannot provide the broad-spectrum protection necessary to prevent deeper environmental damage, and most of them are highly toxic. Effective, chemical-free ingredients such as titanium and zinc oxide act as "reflectors" to *physically* block UV rays, instead. Look for BB creams and chemical-free sunblocks that contain these wonderful ingredients.

Four Products for a Glowing Complexion

Now that you know the technique you'll need to implement, here are the must-have products for your program. Regardless of your age or skin type, these four products are the foundation of your new skin care protocol.

Product 1: A retinoid. If your skin is mature or dry and not sensitive, you might want to look for a retinoid formulation that contains retinol; however, if your skin is sensitive, you're better off looking for a retinol derivative or a plant-based bioretinol. (Go to page 106 for more information on retinols.)

Product 2: A serum. Your serum should contain vitamins, peptides, and antioxidants. Serums are very active skin care formulations with high concentrations of specific active ingredients.

Product 3: A peel. I recommend using a full-strength peel product throughout your program. If your skin is normal to dry or mature, look for a peel that contains alpha hydroxy acids such as malic, lactic, glycolic, citric, and tartaric acids (many of these are natural fruit acids). If you have an oily T-zone and/or blackheads, make sure your peel also contains beta hydroxy acids (such as salicylic acid). If your skin is sensitive, you can use gentler enzyme peels to provide a more natural, chemical-free way of refining skin texture, lightening pigmentation, and minimizing lines and wrinkles. Go to page 280 to learn more about peels.

Product 4: An electric facial cleansing brush. These brushes help to deep cleanse in a way that it's hard to do with a cloth. I recommend using your brush for the second step of the cleansing routine outlined in the program. The regularity with which you use it is up to you and your skin type. I tend to use mine about twice a week.

Five Useful Helpers

The following products aren't 100 percent necessary for the program; however, they're cheap and easy to buy, so I recommend you pick them up.

1. Small cosmetic sponges. I like to remove my first layer of makeup with these little sponges.

2. Inexpensive terry or muslin facecloths. I recommend having a bunch of these for both cleansing and drying your face. Use a fresh one for every cleanse and toss your used one in the laundry. You can use them as rags when they look too dingy.

3. A soft, terry-cloth bandana. I always shove my hair back in one of these before cleansing.

4. A brush for dry brushing of the skin and/or a body-exfoliating device.

5. A bottle of neroli, lavender, eucalyptus, or tea tree pure essential oil.

Towel Tip

I like to add a couple of drops of neroli, lavender, eucalyptus, or tea tree essential oil to my dry terry or muslin facecloths when I put them away after laundering. This not only makes my laundry closet smell wonderful but also infuses the cloths with aromatherapy so that when I soak them with hot water for cleansing, the scent is released.

Diet Primer

Here's the deal—I'm not going to get you to go out and buy all kinds of special "health" foods. There are tons of healthy breakfast, lunch, and dinner recipes in Chapter 12 that I've included in the program. I've listed specific recipes for each day of the program, but you don't have to use them. For some people, laying out meal plans removes a huge stress from their lives—planning meals can be overwhelming in and of itself. For other people, experimenting with food is fun. Either way, don't feel pressured to stick with exactly what I've laid out. Swap out smoothies or juices for others if you like. Maybe choose a different salad—or make up one of your own. If you hate mushrooms, choose a different veggie entirely. While some of you feel more comfortable with creating the same smoothie every morning (which is fine), others want variety—either way, go with what works for you and your lifestyle. If you don't love cooking, find a great juice/smoothie bar, and hit your local health food store for pre-prepared vegan salads or entrees. The thing to keep in mind is that each of the recipes I include goes along with my general eating guidelines of what to avoid:

- **Meat:** Most of us are better off without animal flesh—or at least cutting back on it dramatically. If you really want to include meat, stick to certified-organic, pasture-raised meat.

- **Fish:** Although oily fish, such as salmon and sardines, are a very valuable source of omega-3 fatty acids, they can also be contaminated with heavy metals and dioxins. I prefer to avoid them when I'm trying to really clean up my diet, but feel free to add in the odd piece of wild Alaskan salmon (fresh or canned), or a can of sardines. A cleaner way to obtain your omega fatty acids is by consuming ground flaxseeds or golden algae.

- **Sugar:** I suggest that you avoid all refined sugar and artificial sweeteners. Read the labels of any boxed, canned, or packaged foods you put in your cart to make sure you catch any sneaky ingredients. See pages 198–190 for a list of some names that sugar can go by. Remember, even "healthy" sweeteners, such as raw honey, maple syrup, and brown rice syrup, should be eaten in moderation.

- **Dairy:** Most of us are better off cutting out dairy. If you suffer from allergies or any digestive issues, cutting out dairy might really help you. The only exception I make is for fermented dairy products such as organic, plain yogurt, and kefir, because fermented foods are chock full of gut-friendly probiotics.

- **Refined grains and gluten:** Refined grains are devoid of healthy fiber and are very efficient at spiking your blood sugar. Avoiding refined grains means staying away from most baked goods. As for gluten, most people simply feel better when they exclude gluten from their diet, because even if you are not a diagnosed celiac, you may be sensitive to gluten, which could present itself as digestive issues, fatigue, or a weakened immune system. If nothing else, it would be interesting for you to see if certain symptoms disappear when you exclude gluten from your diet. Aside from wheat, also try to avoid spelt, barley, bulgur wheat, couscous, durum, farro, rye, and seitan.

- **Alcohol:** Even the rather benign sounding "a couple glasses of white wine" is a no-no for the 30 days. It's not that you have to forgo your alcohol forever, but remember that all alcoholic beverages turn to sugar in your body and make your liver, which is your main organ of detoxification, work way too hard. Alcohol also dehydrates you, taking away some of that glow in your skin.

- **Coffee:** Coffee is also very dehydrating, and since we want to juice up your skin, it's better to avoid it for the 30 days. Coffee is also extremely acidic, and because an alkaline system lends itself best to staying healthy and youthful, you're better off drinking tea. If, however, you are going to be miserable without your morning cup of joe, have just one, and drink it black or add a nondairy creamer such as almond or coconut milk. If you are a black tea drinker, limit yourself to three cups a day. If you drink green or white tea, up to five cups a day is fine, but make sure that you don't substitute your tea for your water.

- **Soda (diet soda, too):** Regular soda is loaded with sugar, and diet soda is loaded with chemicals. Both have been linked to a plethora of health issues, including obesity. It's best that you avoid them completely.

- **Fruit juice:** A little is allowed (organic), but keep in mind that it's loaded with fructose, which seriously spikes your blood sugar.

- **Corn and soy:** Although I recommend fermented soy in your program such as miso and Tempeh, it's preferable to minimize your intake of both corn and soy because they are the two crops that are most likely to be genetically modified. They are predominantly produced to feed animals. Corn is also acid-forming in the body.

To see and feel a difference within a month, you really do need to eat in specific ways. Remember, it's just 30 days. If you want to go back to all your old eating and drinking habits after this short period, you can. Keep in mind that you don't need to be fanatical. If you're at a wedding, go ahead and have a tiny piece of cake. If you can't stand it, have the occasional blueberry muffin, or sneak some cheese or turkey into your salad, but try to give the program's way of eating a shot. You won't regret it.

The most important thing to understand is that this is not a weight-loss diet where you have to count calories or control your portion size. Within reason, because you are eating whole plant-based foods, you can eat as much as you want. This may seem shocking to those of you who are accustomed to counting every half cup of anything you put on your plate, but trust me, if you are eating these beautiful whole foods, it's tough to overeat! This is a *Live-it*, as opposed to a Die-it, meaning that this way of eating will make you feel vibrant and alive instead of sluggish and sick.

Finally, if you do decide to cave in and eat a sugar-laden treat or burger and fries, it's no biggie—just pay attention to how you feel an hour later. This clean way of eating is not about being forced into a not-allowed box, it's more about helping you to make choices that help you feel strong, vibrant, and alive each and every day.

SHOPPING PLAN

Sometimes simply planning what to buy at the market is the most overwhelming part of starting a new way of eating. But there are some great websites that can help make this easier. I love www.plantoeat.com, a website that lets you download recipes that you're planning to make. Once you do this, it automatically generates a shopping list for you.

I've put all the recipes from this program online, so go to www.sophieuliano.com, click on the Kale Leaf and enter the following code: EATGORGEOUSLY. This way you can easily download the recipes into the plantoeat.com program—or any other that you use. I want this to be as easy as possible!

My Favorite Healthy Alternatives

If you find yourself craving any of the "bad" foods we're leaving out of the 30-day program, try substitutions for some of these:

- **Coffee:** Teeccino (delicious herbal "coffee"); black, white, green, red, oolong, and hibiscus tea.

- **Wheat bread/pasta:** Brown rice, quinoa, black bean or mung bean pasta, or kelp noodles; sprouted grain or gluten-free breads.

- **Dairy:** Nut milks or hemp, flax, rice, or coconut milk (make sure they are all unsweetened). Cashew cream or cheese.

- **Meat:** Tempeh, mushrooms, tofu (especially sprouted tofu), and beans.

- **Alcohol:** Kombucha (a delicious, sparkling drink that is as dry and refreshing as a glass of white wine).

- **Soda/diet soda:** Sparkling water with a little organic fruit juice concentrate. However, try to drink this in moderation, because all sparkling beverages contain carbonate, which is pretty acidic.

- **Sweetener:** Monk fruit, xylitol, stevia, and dates.

- **Cooking oils:** Instead of cooking with oil, try using veggie broth, low-sodium tamari, vegan Worcestershire sauce, and seasoned rice vingar.

- **Protein Bars:** Although not my first choice for snacks, they can be useful in a pinch. Make sure they are made with hemp/pea/whey protein, and that they don't contain any added sugars. Look for bars made with whole foods such as nuts, and superfoods.

- **Chips:** Look for Kale Chips, Sprouted Grain Chips, Rice Chips, and Seaweed Snacks.

CASHEW CREAM TWO WAYS

I'm obsessed with cashew cream, and I use it liberally for both sweet and savory dishes as a cream, as a dip, or to add texture and creaminess to soups and desserts. Here are my two favorite recipes.

Serves 4 to 6

CASHEW CREAM, SAVORY

1½ cups raw cashews, soaked overnight

2 teaspoons lemon juice

1 clove garlic

1 teaspoon onion powder

1 teaspoon nutritional yeast

½ teaspoon sea salt

CASHEW CREAM, SWEET

1½ cups raw cashews, soaked overnight

1 teaspoon vanilla extract

1 to 2 tablespoons maple syrup

For both versions, place all the ingredients plus ½ cup water in your high-speed blender and process until smooth. You get to control the thickness of your cream by the amount of water you add. The amount called for here will make a very thick cream; simply add more water slowly until the cream reaches the desired consistency.

Your cashew creams will keep in an airtight container in your fridge for up to three days.

What to Eat and Drink

Now that I've covered all of the things to cut out, here's a list of great healthy beauty foods to eat. These are loaded with vitamins and minerals that will help make you glow from the inside. Try to buy as many of them organic as possible.

The recipes in the program incorporate all of these, but if you're hungry beyond what's laid out each day and need to snack, reach for something listed here.

- **Leafy greens** such as steamed, raw, or sautéed spinach; chard, kale, collards, and dandelion.

- **Salad greens** including mixed baby lettuce, mesclun, romaine, watercress, bean sprouts, watercress, and pea shoots.

- **Fresh herbs**

- **Purple foods** such as blueberries, purple kale, red onion, purple broccoli, purple cauliflower, eggplant, and red cabbage.

- **Cruciferous veggies** such as cauliflower and broccoli.

- **Veggies** such as onions, leeks, bok choy, celery, daikon radish, mushrooms, peppers, asparagus, carrots, beets, green beans, squash, sweet potatoes, and kohlrabi.

- **Nuts and seeds** (Always soak prior to eating.)

- **Beans** such as kidney, red, lima, navy, garbanzo, and soy. (Organic canned beans are fine.)

- **Seaweed** usually comes dried, and you eat or cook it after soaking. (I suggest you avoid hijiki because it can contain high amounts of arsenic.)

- **Organic fruits** such as apples, pears, pineapple, plums, cantaloupe, bananas, blackberries, and blueberries.

- **Super foods** such as chia seeds (soaked), raw cacao powder, hemp, flaxseed (ground), and goji berries.

- **Grains** such as quinoa, millet buckwheat, teff, oats, and sprouted grains.

- **Spices**, especially cumin, cinnamon, and turmeric.

- **Healthy oils** such as certified virgin, cold-pressed olive oil, flaxseed oil, and raw coconut oil. (I recommend cutting as many oils out of your diet during the 30 days as you can because you will be getting plenty of healthy oils from nuts, seeds, and avocados.)

- **Filtered water** is important because you don't want to be drinking gallons of chlorine. If you don't have a whole house filter, make sure you purchase a filter jug.

Tips for Success

- Use a slow cooker. I use mine at least twice a week because I can toss a stew, veggie chili, or soup into it in the morning and come back to a hearty, healthy meal in the evening.
- Double a dinner recipe so you can freeze half of it for the following week.
- Chop and store/freeze all your veggies/fruits on the weekend, so that you're ready to go for smoothies, salads, and slow-cooked dishes during the week.
- Keep a bag of raw (and then home-roasted) almonds in your purse and the glove compartment of your car in case you get a sudden hunger attack.
- Make sure that you choose restaurants that offer a delicious vegan option.
- Involve your family in your new eating plan and invite them to join. If they are resistant, ask them to respect what you're trying to do and work with you. The key is never to force anyone to follow your way of eating, because they always rebel. Attraction rather than promotion is the way to go!
- Always have a plan for the day: make sure you can hit a healthy deli for lunch, and if you are going out after work, have a few snacks on hand to keep you from reaching for something unhealthy. Thinking ahead will set you up for success.

- Instead of thinking of three elements on your plate (meat/fish, veggie, and carb), think of five or six elements for variety. For example, I may include greens, beans, tofu, starchy veggies, rice, and a sauce on one plate. The more tastes, the better.

- Focus on bumping up the flavor while on this plan. Vegan foods such as tempeh and tofu need a bunch of seasoning to dial them up to the next level—and to make them carnivore friendly.

- In my program, I don't ask you to weigh out or measure your portions because this is not only annoying, but takes the pleasure out of eating. I will repeat, if you are loading your plate with healthy plant-based foods, it's hard to overeat—just enjoy! If you get tired of salads, cut up veggies and create loads of dips such as hummus and guacamole. You can eat the dips with veggies, on their own, or as part of a gluten-free or sprouted grain tortilla/wrap or warm whole wheat pita.

- Keep loads of healthy vegan options in the front of your fridge at eye level. Many of us habitually open the fridge to reach for a piece of cheese or ham. I make sure I have coconut yogurts, hummus, fruit "butters," baked tofu, and so on, all ready to go.

- Allow extra prep time in the mornings because you will be way more likely to eat healthy if you prepare a salad for lunch, and even make a start on dinner before you leave the house. I also have way more energy in the morning than in the evening when I get back from work. If everything is halfway prepared, I'm more likely to take it to the finish line instead of calling in for pizza.

- If you are in a rush, consider creating a "power bowl" for dinner by simply combining all the plant-based foods you love in one bowl (for example, roasted yam, quinoa, guacamole, and black beans). Get creative and combine as many different foods and spices as you please. Then top with your favorite dressing.

- If you are very busy, consider signing up for an organic/healthy grocery store delivery service—this way you can simply make your list and have it delivered to your front door. There are also a few great apps that offer store-to-door service from your new favorite stores.

Fitness Primer

As I mentioned in Chapter 8, I suggest that you exercise six days a week and have one rest day, so this is what I've set up in the 30-day program. Obviously, if you are exhausted or sick, you may choose to rest and/or do a little gentle yoga instead of what I recommend. Before you kick back, thinking *There's nooooooo way that I'm going to do hard-core exercise six days a week*, let me explain that by "exercise," I don't mean that you have to pump iron or train for a marathon. There are loads of different choices available to you, but remember these few tips (see pages 200–201 if you'd like more information on what these mean):

1. Exercise hard enough that you can feel your heart beating faster than usual.

2. You need to sweat.

3. Work beyond your comfort zone.

4. Remember that your workouts can be split if you are pressed for time.

What You Need

You don't really need to buy anything; however, if you want to add a couple of helpful boosters to your fitness program, here are my suggestions:

- **Rebounder:** I'm obsessed with my mini trampoline. It's one of the safest and most effective ways for me to get my daily cardio.

- **Kettlebell:** You can now buy these at most sports stores and many big-box stores. Snag yourself one, because a single ten-minute routine could push your heart rate through the roof. Start with a 5-pound bell if you are a beginner, 10 for intermediates, and 15 if you are strong, buff, and up for the big one!

- **Yoga mat:** You want one with just the right amount of "stick" to keep your hands and feet from slipping.

Mind-Body-Spirit Primer

In the mind-body-spirit part of the 30-day program, I'm going to offer up some suggestions to help you relieve your stress and get to know yourself better—because these are the things that lead to true beauty. It may seem overwhelming, but doing this doesn't have to take over your life—just a little time dedicated in pursuit of this will make a world of difference.

For this part of the program, which will consist of a morning routine and some writing exercises, I recommend you pick up:

- A timer (or use one on your phone)

- A yoga mat

- A meditation cushion (or simply identify a comfy chair in a quiet area of your home)

- A journal with plenty of space to write

I will slowly work you into your morning routine and then, beginning on day seven, I will share an intention with you that I have found to be extraordinarily effective. Creating an intention is a powerful way to set up your day. Whenever things go downhill or you get fearful or anxious, you can center yourself by bringing to mind the intention that you started the day with.

Aside from this, once each week, I will ask that you set aside some time to journal by way of some powerful stream-of-consciousness writing exercises. This will help you find what lies beneath the noise of your daily thoughts. There is gold to be mined, and all you need do is ask yourself the right question and get writing.

Treat Yourself

So, what do you do after the 30 days are up? Well, first of all— treat yourself! You did some amazing work. But make sure you don't do something that will completely compromise everything you've worked for. Consider a deep-tissue massage—one of my favorites. I always used to feel guilty about having massages because I felt they were way too indulgent. Then I started to realize the unbelievable benefit of a good deep-tissue massage. If resources are an issue, you might be able to find a masseuse who will barter with you for something that you have and she doesn't (homegrown veggies, babysitting, handcrafted jewelry, accounting or business advice, photography, and so on). Most of my friends trade our services—never be afraid to ask! If you can afford it, or find a way of bartering, I recommend treating yourself to a massage every month.

You can also do something like take yourself on a relaxing vacation—or schedule a "staycation," where you explore your own town. Sometimes it's hard to separate from the work that lives at your house, but it's essential to a good staycation. You have to give yourself permission to not work, to order food, to let those little tasks go. If you feel like you can do this, staying home on vacation can be seriously relaxing because you don't have to deal with the hassle of travel, and you have all the comforts of home.

Aside from treating yourself, the most important thing to do after your 30-day program is to evaluate what it's done for you so you can create a lifelong program of your own. What parts did you really love? What parts did you hate? Did you find any new foods you like? Did you find foods that you simply can't live without? It's all a matter of figuring out what makes you feel and look your best. Taking care of yourself shouldn't be a horrible hassle. I quite enjoy my morning ritual—in fact, I can't imagine my life without it now. And while I love a good croissant, I realize that I love it even more if it's a once-in-a-while treat rather than a frequent food. So make sure to look at your life postprogram and think critically about what you want in your future—and remember, it's all about balance.

Chapter 11

Get Gorgeous in 30 Days

DAY 1

Beauty

For the next 30 days, you will do a morning and evening beauty routine that involves cleansing, nourishing, and protecting the skin on your face, neck, and décolleté. Once you get it down, it should add a mere five minutes to your morning and evening routines. You will also moisturize your whole body daily.

We'll also incorporate a few peels throughout this program. And on many of the days, I'll have you add another task that will help you clean up your beauty routine. Today, we start by choosing and buying—or collecting, if you happen to already use them—all the products we'll need for this program.

You'll want to buy or make:

1.   An emulsifying cleanser for dissolving and removing makeup, dirt, and grime.

2. A brightening cleanser to deep clean and brighten.

3. A retinol product.

4. A nourishing, antioxidant- and/or peptide-packed serum (see recipe on pages 374–375 to make one at home).

5. A vitamin C serum or powdered vitamin C to add to your serum (see recipe on page 374 to make one at home).

6. A moisturizer that contains hyaluronic acid along with other proactive ingredients.

7. A mineral sunscreen with an SPF of 30 to 40.

8. A facial peel.

9. Lavender or tea tree essential oil.

10. Facial cloths (muslin or terry) or cleaning sponges.

11. A fat makeup brush or a fan brush (you can find these in the makeup department; they are typically used to apply bronzer or powder).

12. Organic, virgin coconut oil.

13. A good daily hand and body moisturizer.

14. A long-handled, natural-bristle brush.

You can find guidelines for choosing products in Part One of this book.

Diet

Prebreakfast Detox: Kick off day one with my Liver Cleanse Juice (page 324) before breakfast—but after you brush your teeth

Breakfast: Sliced seasonal fruit + unsweetened plain coconut yogurt or Raw Coconut Yogurt + granola (page 333)

Lunch: Spicy Vegetable Cocktail Juice (page 325) + sprouted grain or gluten-free toast topped with sliced tomato, avocado, fresh basil, and a little extra virgin olive oil

Afternoon Snack: Countess Coconut Smoothie (page 326)

Dinner: Steamed Green Veggies (page 367) + Baked Tempeh with Balsamic Glaze (page 341) + brown rice

Fitness

If you already have a routine in place that incorporates cardio, flexibility practices, and weight training, feel free to follow that. However, if you're new to exercise or simply want to get a more standard routine under your belt, follow the guidelines that I lay out here. Each day, we will do about 40 minutes of exercise—two days each week will be all cardio; two days will be cardio and weight training; and two days will be cardio and flexibility practices. And then there is that one blessed day of rest each week.

Today, we will start off slowly with some cardio and a little personal exploration.

Cardio: Walk at a brisk pace for 30 minutes, making sure to push your edge. Don't be afraid to get out of breath and sweat a bit. It's good for you!

Exploration: Go to Chapter 8 and read through the different types of exercises I discuss—and feel free to brainstorm more on your own. Make a list of activities that sound good to you, and use this program to try them out. Try at least one new cardio exercise, one new weight-training routine, and one new flexibility practice each week. This means that you should choose four new forms of each. List them now.

If you need to buy anything such as a kettlebell, a rebounder, or some hand weights, make doing that a part of your day today.

Morning ME Time

For the next 30 days, you will do a morning "me time" ritual that will help set the tone for each day. Throughout the routine, the goal is to be mindful and fully aware of what's happening in the present moment—not running through a to-do list in your head. The routine takes about 20 minutes in all, so just set your alarm clock a tiny bit earlier. The routine is:

1. Brush your teeth.

2. Prepare and mindfully sip warm lemon or ginger water.

3. Practice your five-minute mini yoga routine.

4. Meditate while focusing on your breath, body, and/or a specific topic for five to ten minutes.

5. Conclude with an intention.

I'll teach you about each aspect of the routine over the next few days, and then we'll put it all together. But, today, you are simply going to do a couple of things to prep yourself.

First, find a quiet space that you can go to every morning for your "me time" ritual. This doesn't mean you have to build an altar (although great if you do!); it's just a space where you can sit with your water, move through your yoga routine, and meditate without disturbance.

Next, you should choose how you will sit to do your breathing and meditation—on a yoga mat, a meditation cushion, or a chair. This morning, try out your seating options. See where you can sit comfortably for a few minutes without being disturbed.

DAY 2

Beauty

Now that you have your products, I'd like to explain an integral part of the nighttime routine that you will start tomorrow. I have found that a two-step nightly cleanse makes a huge difference in the quality of my skin. So here is the basic protocol for the technique:

Step 1: This first step cuts through oil, grime, and makeup to really clean deeply. Apply your emulsifying cleanser to your face, neck, and chest while your skin is dry. Massage it into your skin with circular motions, making sure you reach all the little nooks and crannies. To rinse it off, fill your sink with warm water and add about five drops of lavender or tea tree essential oil. Submerge your cloth or sponge, squeeze it out, and use it to remove the cleanser, rinsing as many times as needed. If you are in the shower, take your soaked cloth or sponge into the shower with you.

Step 2: The second step is simply washing with your brightening cleanser, which will not only strip off dead skin cells but also remove any traces of oil from Step 1. Splash your face with warm water, apply your cleanser to your face, neck, and chest, spend a couple of minutes massaging it into your skin, and rinse off thoroughly. No need to use your cloth or sponge here; simply splash with warm water.

Diet

Breakfast: Gorgeously Green Queen Smoothie (page 327) + sprouted grain or gluten-free English muffin/toast with almond butter and sliced banana

Lunch: Creamy Butternut Squash Soup (page 337) + brown rice + green side salad

Afternoon Snack: Ridiculously Healthy Muffin (page 334) or rice cake with almond butter + apple/cherry butter

Dinner: Vegan Pesto Millet Bowl (pages 351–352)

Fitness

Cardio: Try a cardio routine that you've never done before. Do it for 20 minutes.

Flexibility: Do 20 minutes of your choice of flexibility practice.

Morning ME Time

1. Brush your teeth.

I know it sounds silly, but this step is essential to do before you consume anything. After a night's sleep, your mouth is full of bacteria, and anything you put in your mouth—even the lemon or ginger in your water—will attract it. It also feels great to have a clean, fresh mouth before your yoga or meditation.

DAY 3

Beauty

Today, we start our morning and evening routines.

Morning Facial Routine:

Cleanse: Wash with your brightening cleanser. If you shower in the morning, simply use this in the shower and apply the rest when you get out.

Nourish:

- **Feed** with an antioxidant- or peptide-packed serum.

- **Boost** with vitamin C if it's not already in your serum (powdered crystals added to your serum are preferable).

- **Hydrate** with a moisturizer that contains hyaluronic acid along with other proactive ingredients.

Protect: Use a mineral sunscreen with an SPF of 30 to 40.

Evening Facial Routine:

Cleanse: Use my Two-Step Cleanse with emulsifying, make-up-melting cleanser followed by a brightening cleanser. If you shower at night, you can do this process in the shower and apply the rest of your products when you get out. If you have a facial cleansing brush, use it this evening to remove Step 2 of your cleanse.

Nourish:

- **Boost** collagen production and skin cell turnover with your retinol products applied straight onto cleansed skin.

- **Feed** your skin with an antioxidant- or peptide-packed serum.

- **Hydrate** with your moisturizer.

Daily Body Moisturizing: Apply your hand and body moisturizer liberally over your whole body before you leave the house.

Diet

Breakfast: Energy Booster Smoothie (page 326) + steel-cut oatmeal topped with Date Puree (page 331) and coconut oil

Lunch: Kelp Noodle Salad (page 364)

Afternoon Snack: Serenity Juice (page 325) or any smoothie

Dinner: Macro Bowl (pages 345–346)

Fitness

Cardio: Do 20 minutes of your choice of cardio.

Weight Training: Try a weight-training routine that you've never done before. Do it for 20 minutes. Hint: An at-home kettlebell workout is quick, easy, and fun!

Morning ME Time

1.   Brush your teeth.

2.   Prepare and mindfully sip warm lemon or ginger water.

After you've brushed your teeth, add a couple of slices of lemon or raw ginger root to a mug of boiling water. Let it steep for a minute before adding some cool water to make it drinkable. If you dislike lemon or ginger, just drink the hot water. If you take a daily probiotic or any supplements that are best taken on an empty stomach, take them with this drink. Remember to be mindful of what you are doing, which means slow down. Enjoy the process of warming the water, slicing the lemon or ginger, and sipping. Notice the subtle taste, sounds, and colors.

DAY 4

Beauty

Dry Brushing: Bring this refreshing practice into your pre-shower routine today. See pages 147–148 for more information.

Morning Facial Routine: Cleanse with brightening cleanser, nourish with serum, vitamin C, and moisturizer, and protect with mineral sunscreen.

Daily Body Moisturizing: Apply your hand and body moisturizer liberally over your whole body before you leave the house.

Evening Facial Routine: Cleanse using the Two-Step Cleanse and nourish with retinol, serum, and moisturizer.

Diet

Breakfast: Ridiculously Healthy Muffin (page 334) or rice cake with apple butter + Gorgeously Clean Greens Juice (page 324)

Lunch: Alkalizing Salad (page 356)

Afternoon Snack: Pipe Cleaner Smoothie (page 327)

Dinner: Creamy Vegan "Mac n' Cheese" (pages 344–345) and green salad

Fitness

Cardio: Do 40 minutes of your choice of cardio.

Morning ME Time

1. Brush your teeth.

2. Prepare and mindfully sip warm lemon or ginger water.

3. Practice your five-minute mini yoga routine.

After you brush your teeth and drink your water, it's time to gently get your body in motion. This is not a workout; rather, it's a simple practice to wake up your body that over time will create tremendous flexibility. These three poses will open and stretch out your spine and your hamstrings before you sit down to meditate. As you practice them, be mindful of your breath.

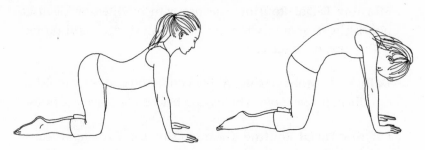

Cat (or Cow): On your hands and knees, gently inhale and press your belly toward the ground, arching your spine as you look up. Then exhale as you draw your bellybutton into your spine and release your head toward the ground. Go back and forth between these poses, breathing slowly and deeply, doing about ten sets.

Tip: When you inhale and arch your spine to look up, draw your shoulders away from your ears.

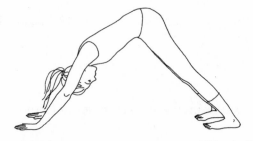

Downward-Facing Dog: From all fours, slowly bring yourself up to down dog. This is a beautiful inversion, meaning that your heart is above your head. Start with your knees bent and gently release your heels, one at a time, into the earth. If you're not able to do this right away, stay on your toes with your knees bent, and slowly stretch through your calves, with flat feet being a goal. Practice five slow full breaths in down dog.

Tip: Spread your fingers wide as you press your palms firmly into the floor.

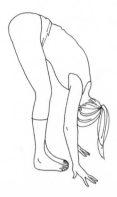

Standing Forward Bend: From down dog, walk your hands back toward your toes to come into this rejuvenating forward bend. If your hamstrings are tight, bend your knees. Gently nod your head back and forth to release your neck. Stay in this pose for three to five breaths. When you are ready to come up, gently bend your knees and roll up one vertebra at a time until you are standing. Take a moment in your standing pose to re-adjust your posture, making sure your tailbone points toward the earth and the crown of your head draws up toward the sky.

Tip: When you are in this pose, look at your feet. Spread your toes wide apart and lift the arches of your feet.

Practice this short sequence each morning. Or, if you feel a little more energetic, consider switching to the Fountain of Youth Practice (pages 222–226).

DAY 5

Beauty

Morning Facial Routine: Cleanse with brightening cleanser; nourish with serum, vitamin C, and moisturizer; and protect with mineral sunscreen.

Evening Facial Routine: Cleanse using the Two-Step Cleanse; peel; and nourish with retinol, serum, and moisturizer.

Peel 1: This is your first peel day; you'll do it at night after your Two-Step Cleanse. However, if you have rosacea, acne, or very sensitive skin, skip the peel.

Here's the drill:

1. Perform your Two-Step Cleanse as usual. Pay special attention to Step 2, making sure that every trace of grime, and especially oil and grease, is removed.

2. Apply your peel with a fat makeup brush or a fan brush, making sure to cover your entire face, neck, and décolleté with a thin layer of your peel.

3. Set a timer for five minutes and simply wait. You may feel some slight stinging (or, in some cases, a lot). Don't freak out; the stinging or burning sensation means it's doing its thing and will lessen the next time you peel.

4. Rinse thoroughly with warm water.

5. Apply your retinol, serum, and moisturizer.

Daily Body Moisturizing: Apply your hand and body moisturizer liberally over your whole body before you leave the house.

Diet

Breakfast: Coconut Chia Pudding (page 330) or steel cut oatmeal topped with Date Puree (page 331) + The Flow Juice (page 323)

Lunch: Curried Waldorf Salad (page 360)

Afternoon Snack: Super Crunch Granola (pages 334–335)

with or without an unsweetened, nondairy milk

Dinner: Quinoa and Black Bean Burger (page 349) + Kale and Seaweed Salad (page 363)

Fitness

Cardio: Do 20 minutes of your choice of cardio.

Flexibility: Try a flexibility practice that you've never done before. Do it for 20 minutes.

Morning ME Time

1. Brush your teeth.

2. Prepare and mindfully sip warm lemon or ginger water.

3. Practice your five-minute mini yoga routine.

4. Meditate while focusing on your breath for five minutes.

After you've finished your yoga routine, move gently into the sitting space that you identified on the first day of the program. Now spend a few moments getting into the optimum posture for meditation. If you are on a cushion or mat, you will sit cross-legged. In a chair, firmly plant both feet on the floor. Then, no matter where you are sitting, press your sitz bones firmly down into the chair or cushion or floor and feel your spine extending upward toward the sky. Follow the natural curves of your spine as you extend. Soften your shoulders away from your ears, and release your facial muscles. If you are in a chair, you may need a large cushion behind you to assist you in not slumping. Rest your palms gently on your thighs.

Once you're in the right position, set your timer for three minutes, close your eyes, and simply watch your breath. You don't need to control it, deepen it, or force it. Just notice it. Is it smooth or ragged? Does it make a sound? Is it deep or shallow? Is there a tiny pause between your inhale and your exhale? Your mind will wander off; this is normal—all you need to do is observe it wandering off and then gently bring your attention back to observing your breath. Focusing on your breath and expanding your awareness is the key to meditation. That's all you need do this morning. How easy is that?

DAY 6

Beauty

Dry Brushing: Bring this refreshing practice into your preshower routine today. See pages 147–148 for more information.

Morning Facial Routine: Cleanse with brightening cleanser; nourish with serum, vitamin C, and moisturizer; and protect with mineral sunscreen.

Daily Body Moisturizing: Apply your hand and body moisturizer liberally over your whole body before you leave the house.

Evening Facial Routine: Cleanse using the Two-Step Cleanse and nourish with retinol, serum, and moisturizer. If you have a facial cleansing brush, use it this evening to remove Step 2 of your cleanse.

Diet

Breakfast: Super Crunch Granola (pages 334–335) with unsweetened, nondairy milk + Gorgeously Green Queen Smoothie (page 327)

Lunch: Dandelion, Apple, and Chickpea Salad (page 361)

Afternoon Snack: Countess Coconut Smoothie (page 326) or gluten-free crackers + hummus

Dinner: Cauliflower and Leek Soup (page 336) + quinoa or brown rice and a green salad with sliced avocado

Fitness

Cardio: Do 20 minutes of your choice of cardio.

Weight Training: Do 20 minutes of your choice of weight training.

Morning ME Time

Today we will add just a bit more to your meditation routine.

1. Brush your teeth.

2. Prepare and mindfully sip warm lemon or ginger water.

3. Practice your five-minute mini yoga routine.

4. Meditate while focusing on your breath and body for five minutes.

After you've finished your yoga routine, move gently into the sitting space that you identified on the first day of the program. Now spend a few moments getting into the optimum posture for meditation. Set your timer for five minutes. Close your eyes and begin to watch your breath. After a few moments, begin to notice what's going on with your body. Are you clenching your jaw? Are your shoulders really tight? Are you tightening or softening your belly? What about your hips? You might be holding way more tension in one hip than the other. The important thing is that you start to tune in to your body by being mindful. Try not to judge—for example, "My hips are so tight because I don't do enough yoga"—just notice with a kind and compassionate attention.

Now see if you can tune in to how you feel—the underlying feelings behind these physical sensations. Are you anxious? Annoyed? Maybe you're excited or sad. If you are not used to checking in with your feelings, allow your body to be your guide. For example, I always know that I am fearful if my belly is clenched or tender. Just as with the focus on the breath, your mind will wander. Simply bring your attention back to your body.

When your timer goes off, conclude your meditation by allowing your thoughts to do whatever they want. Let go of focusing on the breath. Do not try to control or stop your thoughts. Give them free rein to go nuts if they want to. Just watch them. This is the most magical part of your entire meditation process because, ironically, when we allow our thoughts to run wild, they often don't! It's in these precious moments when you completely let go of control that you may experience moments of utter stillness.

DAY 7

Beauty

Morning Facial Routine: Cleanse with brightening cleanser; nourish with serum, vitamin C, and moisturizer; and protect with mineral sunscreen.

Daily Body Moisturizing: Apply your hand and body moisturizer liberally over your whole body before you leave the house.

Evening Facial Routine: Cleanse using the Two-Step Cleanse and nourish with retinol, serum, and moisturizer.

Product Purge: Today, in addition to your standard morning and evening routines, you'll also go through a product purge. Grab all the beauty products you have in your bathroom, your makeup bag, closet—wherever—and lay them out on your table. Then grab a large trash can, because if you're like most people, you'll be getting rid of a great deal of stuff. For each product:

1. Check the expiration date. If you can't find a date, you'll have to estimate how long you've had it. For cosmetics, throw it out if it's more than six months old. For skin care products, if vitamin C is an ingredient and you've had it for more than six months, toss it. For other products, you can look for the batch code (see page 73 for an explanation) or search online for the "period after opening" time.

2. For the products that haven't yet expired, check out the ingredients to see if they have any of the chemicals I've listed in Chapter 1. Remember, these aren't all outlawed, but you do have to determine which are most important for you.

3. If you want, you should also check out the credibility of the manufacturer in other areas, such as animal cruelty and environmental impact. Most of this research can be done online.

Diet

Breakfast: Gluten-Free Flax Pancakes with Blackberry Cashew Cream (page 332); you can purchase frozen, gluten-free pancakes in a pinch.

Lunch: Roasted Beet, Orange, and Hazelnut Salad (pages 365–366) + sprouted grain toast/pita topped with Artichoke-Olive Hummus (page 358)

Afternoon Snack: Apple + handful of almonds or pecans

Dinner: Spicy Veggie Chili (page 350) + brown rice + a green salad

Fitness

Day of rest.

Morning ME Time

1. Brush your teeth.

2. Prepare and mindfully sip warm lemon or ginger water.

3. Practice your five-minute mini yoga routine.

4. Meditate while focusing on your breath and body for five minutes.

5. Conclude with an intention.

The final step of your morning routine is to create an intention for the day. When I do this, I feel as if I am sealing in the benefits of my meditation and giving my mind a clear direction for the day. Plus, it gives me something to come back to if at any point I feel overwhelmed by the events of the day. If you'd like to create your own intentions, feel free; however, I have given you some of the ones I've found to be most powerful in my own life. They are listed at the end of each day.

Today's Intention: Today, I will be guided by love, not fear.

DAY 8

Beauty

Dry Brushing: Bring this refreshing practice into your preshower routine today. See pages 147–148 for more information.

Morning Facial Routine: Cleanse with brightening cleanser; nourish with serum, vitamin C, and moisturizer; and protect with mineral sunscreen.

Daily Body Moisturizing: Apply your hand and body moisturizer liberally over your whole body before you leave the house.

Evening Facial Routine: Cleanse using the Two-Step Cleanse and nourish with retinol, serum, and moisturizer.

Diet

Breakfast: Sprouted grain or gluten-free English muffin topped with almond butter and sliced banana + Rooty Fruity Smoothie (page 328)

Lunch: Hearty Provençal Soup (pages 337–338)

Afternoon Snack: Unsweetened plain coconut yogurt or Raw Coconut Yogurt (page 333) topped with berries

Dinner: Brown Rice, Asparagus, and Green Bean Risotto (pages 342–343)

Fitness

Cardio: Try a cardio routine that you've never done before. Do the new practice for at least 20 minutes, but make sure to do 40 minutes of cardio in all.

Morning ME Time

1. Brush your teeth.

2. Prepare and mindfully sip warm lemon or ginger water.

3. Practice your five-minute mini yoga routine.

4. Meditate while focusing on your breath and body for five minutes.

5. Conclude with the intention: *Today I will focus on my strong, healthy, and beautiful body and look for ways I can use it to be of*

service to others. (Example: Pick up bags or do housework for someone who is weaker than you are.)

DAY 9

Beauty

Morning Facial Routine: Cleanse with brightening cleanser; nourish with serum, vitamin C, and moisturizer; and protect with mineral sunscreen.

Daily Body Moisturizing: Apply your hand and body moisturizer liberally over your whole body before you leave the house.

Evening Facial Routine: Cleanse using the Two-Step Cleanse and nourish with retinol, serum, and moisturizer. If you have a facial cleansing brush, use it this evening to remove Step 2 of your cleanse.

Hair Mask: This hair mask is effective and cheap, and it makes your hair look amazing. Simply mash together 1 ripe avocado and 2 tablespoons melted coconut oil in a small bowl and apply to your hair after a light shampoo. Cover with a plastic cap and then make a towel turban over that. Let the mixture sit on your hair for at least 20 minutes. Use a gentle shampoo to remove mask. Finally, do a rinse made with 1 cup warm water and 1 cup apple cider vinegar.

Diet

Breakfast: Chocolate Brownie Oatmeal (pages 329–330) or steel-cut oatmeal topped with sliced banana

Lunch: Creamy Butternut Squash Soup (page 337) + Beet and Carrot Slaw (pages 358–359)

Afternoon Snack: Apple + a handful of Gorgeously Green Trail Mix (pages 361–362)

Dinner: Veggie and Portobello Mushroom Curry (page 353) + brown rice or quinoa

Fitness

Cardio: Do 20 minutes of your choice of cardio.

Flexibility: Do 20 minutes of your choice of flexibility practice.

Morning ME Time

1. Brush your teeth.

2. Prepare and mindfully sip warm lemon or ginger water.

3. Practice your five-minute mini yoga routine.

4. Meditate while focusing on your breath and body for five to ten minutes.

5. Conclude with the intention: *Today I will affirm the beauty, talent, and/or strength of at least three women in my life.*

DAY 10

Beauty

Dry Brushing: Bring this refreshing practice into your preshower routine today. See pages 147–148 for more information.

Morning Facial Routine: Cleanse with brightening cleanser; nourish with serum, vitamin C, and moisturizer; and protect with mineral sunscreen.

Daily Body Moisturizing: Apply your hand and body moisturizer liberally over your whole body before you leave the house.

Evening Facial Routine: Cleanse using the Two-Step Cleanse and nourish with retinol, serum, and moisturizer.

Diet

Breakfast: Energy Booster Smoothie (page 326) + Super Crunch Granola (pages 334–335) with unsweetened, nondairy milk

Lunch: Mock Tuna Salad Open-Faced Sandwich (pages 346–347)

Afternoon Snack: Spicy Vegetable Cocktail Juice (page 325) + sprouted grain crackers

Dinner: Vegan Lasagna (pages 350–351)

Fitness

Cardio: Do 20 minutes of your choice of cardio.

Weight Training: Try a weight-training routine you've never done before. Do it for 20 minutes.

Morning ME Time

1. Brush your teeth.

2. Prepare and mindfully sip warm lemon or ginger water.

3. Practice your five-minute mini yoga routine.

4. Meditate while focusing on your breath and body for five to ten minutes.

5. Conclude with the intention: *Today I will align myself with Divine Creative Intelligence to create my dream life.*

DAY 11

Beauty

Morning Facial Routine: Cleanse with brightening cleanser; nourish with serum, vitamin C, and moisturizer; and protect with mineral sunscreen.

Daily Body Moisturizing: Apply your hand and body moisturizer liberally over your whole body before you leave the house.

Evening Facial Routine: Cleanse using the Two-Step Cleanse and nourish with retinol, serum, and moisturizer.

Diet

Breakfast: Bircher Muesli (page 329) + Serenity Juice (page 325)

Lunch: Greek Salad (pages 362–363) + warm sprouted grain pita/wrap

Afternoon Snack: Sliced veggies + Artichoke-Olive Hummus (page 358)

Dinner: Hearty Provençal Soup + brown rice

Fitness

Cardio: Do 40 minutes of your choice of cardio.

Morning ME Time

1. Brush your teeth.

2. Prepare and mindfully sip warm lemon or ginger water.

3. Practice your five-minute mini yoga routine.

4. Meditate while focusing on your breath and body for five to ten minutes. Today, also tune in to your thoughts on the idea of control. How do you feel about the fact that you are not in control of everything in your life? Are you in touch with your intuition, a deeper knowing that will never lead you astray? Try to tune in to that still, small voice within.

5. Conclude with the intention: *Today I will surrender my little self and open up to the vast power and infinite possibilities of the Universe.*

DAY 12

Beauty

Morning Facial Routine: Cleanse with brightening cleanser; nourish with serum, vitamin C, and moisturizer; and protect with mineral sunscreen.

Daily Body Moisturizing: Apply your hand and body moisturizer liberally over your whole body before you leave the house.

Evening Facial Routine: Cleanse using the Two-Step Cleanse; peel; and nourish with retinol, serum, and moisturizer. If you have a facial cleansing brush, use it this evening to remove Step 2 of your cleanse.

Peel 2: Check out page 280 for detailed information on peels. However, this time, your skin should be a little more acclimated to it than the first time, so try to leave it on for eight to ten minutes. If it stings too much, just keep it on for five.

Diet

Breakfast: Coconut Chia Pudding (page 330) or steel-cut oatmeal with sliced banana + The Flow Juice (page 323)

Lunch: Quinoa-Millet Apricot Salad (pages 364–365)

Afternoon Snack: Rooty Fruity Smoothie (page 328)

Dinner: Veggie Hot Pot (pages 353–354)

Fitness

Cardio: Do 20 minutes of your choice of cardio.

Flexibility: Try a flexibility practice that you've never tried before. Do it for 20 minutes.

Morning ME Time

1. Brush your teeth.

2. Prepare and mindfully sip warm lemon or ginger water.

3. Practice your five-minute mini yoga routine.

4. Meditate while focusing on your breath and body for five to ten minutes.

5. Conclude with the intention: *Today I will take a pause before reacting to any person or situation that bothers me. I will breathe slowly and ask the Divine for guidance.*

DAY 13

Beauty

Dry Brushing: Bring this refreshing practice into your pre-shower routine today. See page 147 for more information.

Morning Facial Routine: Cleanse with brightening cleanser; nourish with serum, vitamin C, and moisturizer; and protect with mineral sunscreen.

Daily Body Moisturizing: Apply your hand and body moisturizer liberally over your whole body before you leave the house.

Evening Facial Routine: Cleanse using the Two-Step Cleanse and nourish with retinol, serum, and moisturizer.

Diet

Breakfast: Gorgeously Green Queen Smoothie (page 327) + Ridiculously Healthy Muffin (page 334) or sprouted grain muffin with apple butter

Lunch: Dandelion, Apple, and Chickpea Salad (page 361)

Afternoon Snack: seasonal sliced fruit + handful of Gorgeous Green Trail Mix (pages 361–362)

Dinner: Moroccan Stuffed Eggplant (pages 347–348) + a green salad

Fitness

Cardio: Do 20 minutes of your choice of cardio.

Weight Training: Do 20 minutes of your choice of weight training.

Morning ME Time

1. Brush your teeth.

2. Prepare and mindfully sip warm lemon or ginger water.

3. Practice your five-minute mini yoga routine.

4. Meditate while focusing on your breath and body for five to ten minutes. Today, specifically tune in to any part of you that might be experiencing physical pain. Breathe into the pain. If you pretend that it's not there, you will likely create more suffering. As you breathe into it, can you soften the affected area? What is the pain trying to tell you? By tuning in to your body and inquiring about the source of pain, you can often get useful information. Our bodies are designed to alert us when something is wrong or when we need to attend to any emotional or physical issue that has perhaps been ignored for too long.

5. Conclude with the intention: *Today I will quiet enough so that I can listen to the wise feedback of my miraculous body.*

DAY 14

Beauty

Morning Facial Routine: Cleanse with brightening cleanser; nourish with serum, vitamin C, and moisturizer; and protect with mineral sunscreen.

Daily Body Moisturizing: Apply your hand and body moisturizer liberally over your whole body before you leave the house.

Evening Facial Routine: Cleanse using the Two-Step Cleanse and nourish with retinol, serum, and moisturizer.

Heel and Elbow Peel: You can use the same peel you've been using for your face on your heels and elbows, too. You can experiment with how long to leave it on, but your heels will likely tolerate a good 20 minutes. Rinse off in the shower with a good exfoliating device such as a pumice stone or foot file. After your shower, massage coconut oil or shea butter into the areas you have treated. You may want to wear a pair of soft cotton socks for the next few hours so that the butter or oil has a chance to work its magic.

Diet

Breakfast: Coconut Chia Pudding (page 330) or steel-cut oatmeal topped with Date Puree (page 331)

Lunch: Alkalizing Salad (page 356)

Afternoon Snack: Ridiculously Healthy Muffin (page 334) or rice cake with apple butter

Dinner: Moroccan Beet Soup (page 339) + Steamed Green Veggies (page 367)

Fitness

Day of rest.

Morning ME Time

1. Brush your teeth.

2. Prepare and mindfully sip warm lemon or ginger water.

3. Practice your five-minute mini yoga routine.

4. Meditate while focusing on your breath and body for five to ten minutes.

5. Conclude with the intention: *Today I will open my heart to the Universe and trust that something way better than I could imagine is always happening.*

Today you will also add a 20-minute walking meditation into your day. To do a walking meditation, you simply take a short walk while simultaneously tuning in to every sensation in and around you. Start off by feeling the soles of your feet pressing into the ground. Do you walk with more weight on your heels or the balls of your feet? Is your pelvis tilted forward or back? What about your shoulders—are they hunched up to your ears? After scanning your body, become hyperaware of your surroundings. What are the temperature and light like? What are the sounds around you? How many different shades of green do you see? The point of a walking meditation is to teach yourself to enjoy the "now" by encouraging your mind to focus on what is present.

DAY 15

Beauty

Morning Facial Routine: Cleanse with brightening cleanser; nourish with serum, vitamin C, and moisturizer; and protect with mineral sunscreen.

Daily Body Moisturizing: Apply your hand and body moisturizer liberally over your whole body before you leave the house.

Evening Facial Routine: Cleanse using the Two-Step Cleanse and nourish with retinol, serum, and moisturizer. If you have a facial cleansing brush, use it this evening to remove Step 2 of your cleanse.

$\mathcal{D}$iet

Breakfast: Gorgeously Clean Greens Juice (page 324) + Bircher Muesli (page 329)

Lunch: Warm Lentil and Roasted Tomato Salad (pages 367–368)

Afternoon Snack: Apple or pear with handful of almonds or pecans

Dinner: Pecan-Stuffed Shiitake Mushrooms (page 348) + Cauliflower Mash (page 359)

$\mathcal{F}$itness

Cardio: Try a cardio routine that you've never done before. Do the new practice for at least 20 minutes, but make sure to do 40 minutes of cardio in all.

$\mathcal{M}$orning $\mathcal{ME}$ $\mathcal{T}$ime

1. Brush your teeth.

2. Prepare and mindfully sip warm lemon or ginger water.

3. Practice your five-minute mini yoga routine.

4. Meditate while focusing on your breath and body for five to ten minutes. Today, also focus on the common feeling that you don't have enough time to complete everything you need to do. Is this something you often feel? Do you cut your personal time short to focus solely on your to-do list? If your life is guided by the belief that you have no time, it will come true, and you will be in a perpetual rush. Meditate on the truth that there is always enough time for the important things; sometimes you just have to assess your priorities.

5. Conclude with the intention: *Today I will do one thing that frightens me.*

DAY 16

Beauty

Dry Brushing: Bring this refreshing practice into your pre-shower routine today. See page 147 for more information.

Morning Facial Routine: Cleanse with brightening cleanser; nourish with serum, vitamin C, and moisturizer; and protect with mineral sunscreen.

Daily Body Moisturizing: Apply your hand and body moisturizer liberally over your whole body before you leave the house.

Evening Facial Routine: Cleanse using the Two-Step Cleanse and nourish with retinol, serum, and moisturizer.

Diet

Breakfast: Chocolate Brownie Oatmeal (pages 329–330) or Coconut Quinoa Porridge (page 331)

Lunch: Hearty Provençal Soup (pages 337–338)

Afternoon Snack: Slice of toasted sprouted grain bread or rice cake topped with mashed avocado and a squeeze of fresh lemon juice.

Dinner: Creamy Mung Bean or Black Bean Pasta (pages 343–344)

Fitness

Cardio: Do 20 minutes of your choice of cardio.

Flexibility: Do 20 minutes of your choice of flexibility practice.

Morning ME Time

1. Brush your teeth.

2. Prepare and mindfully sip warm lemon or ginger water.

3. Practice your five-minute mini yoga routine.

4. Meditate while focusing on your breath and body for five to ten minutes.

5. Conclude with the intention: *Today I will take care of my inner and outer beauty by exercising, eating well, and taking care of my beautiful skin.*

DAY 17

Beauty

Morning Facial Routine: Cleanse with brightening cleanser; nourish with serum, vitamin C, and moisturizer; and protect with mineral sunscreen.

Daily Body Moisturizing: Apply your hand and body moisturizer liberally over your whole body before you leave the house.

Evening Facial Routine: Cleanse using the Two-Step Cleanse and nourish with retinol, serum, and moisturizer. If you have a facial cleansing brush, use it this evening to remove Step 2 of your cleanse.

Make Your Own Hand Soap: Since soap is something you use all the time, it's best to have the healthiest version possible.

Check out the recipe on pages 381–382 to make healthy and powerful soap.

Diet

Breakfast: Sprouted grain or gluten-free toast topped with almond/cashew butter and sliced banana

Lunch: Spicy Veggie Chili (page 350) + green salad

Afternoon Snack: Pipe Cleaner Smoothie (page 327)

Dinner: Baked Tempeh with Balsamic Glaze (page 341) + Steamed Green Veggies (page 367)

Fitness

Cardio: Do 20 minutes of your choice of cardio.

Weight Training: Try a weight-training routine you've never done before. Do it for 20 minutes.

Morning ME Time

1. Brush your teeth.

2. Prepare and mindfully sip warm lemon or ginger water.

3. Practice your five-minute mini yoga routine.

4. Meditate while focusing on your breath and body for five to ten minutes. Also, focus today on your view of your meandering mind and any judgments you may have about it or yourself. Today, when your mind wanders away from the topic of itself, simply smile to yourself and bring your focus back to watching your breath or meditating on the topic of meandering thoughts.

5. Conclude with the intention: *Today I will look for the Divine in every person who comes across my path.*

DAY 18

Beauty

Dry Brushing: Bring this refreshing practice into your pre-shower routine today. See page 147 for more information.

Morning Facial Routine: Cleanse with brightening cleanser; nourish with serum, vitamin C, and moisturizer; and protect with mineral sunscreen.

Daily Body Moisturizing: Apply your hand and body moisturizer liberally over your whole body before you leave the house.

Evening Facial Routine: Cleanse using the Two-Step Cleanse and nourish with retinol, serum, and moisturizer.

Diet

Breakfast: Serenity Juice (page 325) + sprouted grain or gluten-free toast topped with almond butter

Lunch: Macro Bowl (pages 345–346)

Afternoon Snack: Rice cake topped with almond butter + apple/cherry butter

Dinner: Cauliflower and Leek Soup (page 336) + Kale and Seaweed Salad (page 363)

Fitness

Cardio: Do 20 minutes of your choice of cardio.

Morning ME Time

1. Brush your teeth.

2. Prepare and mindfully sip warm lemon or ginger water.

3. Practice your five-minute mini yoga routine.

4. Meditate while focusing on your breath and body for five minutes, then let your thoughts go wild for five minutes without trying to bring your focus back to your breath. Allow yourself to be amused by your thoughts. Simply watch them and see what they do. Who knows what you'll learn about your mind?

5. Conclude with the intention: *Today I will make a list of three things that I have been putting off, and I will do all three.*

DAY 19

Beauty

Morning Facial Routine: Cleanse with brightening cleanser; nourish with serum, vitamin C, and moisturizer; and protect with mineral sunscreen.

Daily Body Moisturizing: Apply your hand and body moisturizer liberally over your whole body before you leave the house.

Evening Facial Routine: Cleanse using the Two-Step Cleanse; peel; and nourish with retinol, serum, and moisturizer.

Peel 3: Tonight is your third peel. Take a good look at your skin in a magnifying mirror. What is going on with it? If it is peeling, flaky, or red, you may want to give the peel a miss tonight and just continue with your usual P.M. routine. If your skin looks fine, go for it! Tonight you'll leave your peel on for 10 to 15 minutes.

Diet

Breakfast: Super Crunch Granola (pages 334–335) with unsweetened, nondairy milk + Rooty Fruity Smoothie (page 328)

Lunch: Warm Quinoa and Butternut Squash Salad (page 368)

Afternoon Snack: Sliced veggies + Artichoke-Olive Hummus (page 358)

Dinner: Veggie Tacos (page 355)

Fitness

Cardio: Do 20 minutes of your choice of cardio.

Flexibility: Try a flexibility practice that you've never done before. Do it for 20 minutes.

Morning ME Time

1. Brush your teeth.

2. Prepare and mindfully sip warm lemon or ginger water.

3. Practice your five-minute mini yoga routine.

4. Meditate while focusing on your breath and body for five minutes.

5. Conclude with the intention: *Today I will trust my gut instincts as they are ALWAYS right.*

In addition to your morning routine, I invite you to create an eating meditation today. This won't take much time out of your day; simply do it at lunch. Here's what you do: Eat your lunch alone, and be present with each bite. Turn off all your devices—phones, computers, and so on. Slow down and pay attention. Take the time to really look at your meal. What are its colors? How many steps were involved in bringing this food to your plate? Pick up the plate and smell your food; does it make your mouth water? What is the texture of the food? Allow your taste buds to really experience the first bite of food by feeling the food in your mouth, and then as you begin to chew, notice how the taste changes. How do you chew? Does the food require a lot of chomping and grinding, or does it dissolve in your mouth? Take a few moments before your next bite.

DAY 20

Beauty

Dry Brushing: Bring this refreshing practice into your pre-shower routine today. See page 147 for more information.

Morning Facial Routine: Cleanse with brightening cleanser; nourish with serum, vitamin C, and moisturizer; and protect with mineral sunscreen.

Daily Body Moisturizing: Apply your hand and body moisturizer liberally over your whole body before you leave the house.

Evening Facial Routine: Cleanse using the Two-Step Cleanse and nourish with retinol, serum, and moisturizer.

Diet

Breakfast: Coconut Quinoa Porridge (page 331) + The Flow Juice (page 323)

Lunch: Dandelion, Apple, and Chickpea Salad (page 361)

Afternoon Snack: Energy Booster Smoothie (page 326)

Dinner: Vegan Pesto Millet Bowl (pages 351–352)

Fitness

Cardio: Do 20 minutes of your choice of cardio.

Weight Training: Do 20 minutes of your choice of weight training.

Morning ME Time

1. Brush your teeth.

2. Prepare and mindfully sip warm lemon or ginger water.

3. Practice your five-minute mini yoga routine.

4. Meditate while focusing on your breath and body for five to ten minutes.

5. Conclude with the intention: *Today I will find my true strength by allowing myself to be vulnerable.*

DAY 21

Beauty

Morning Facial Routine: Cleanse with brightening cleanser; nourish with serum, vitamin C, and moisturizer; and protect with mineral sunscreen.

Daily Body Moisturizing: Apply your hand and body moisturizer liberally over your whole body before you leave the house.

Evening Facial Routine: Cleanse using the Two-Step Cleanse and nourish with retinol, serum, and moisturizer. If you have a facial cleansing brush, use it this evening to remove Step 2 of your cleanse.

Diet

Breakfast: Bircher Muesli (page 329) with Countess Coconut Smoothie (page 326)

Lunch: Sprouted grain or gluten-free toast topped with olive tapenade, avocado, tomato, and fresh basil

Afternoon Snack: Gorgeously Clean Greens Juice (page 324) + handful of Gorgeously Green Trail Mix (pages 361–362)

Dinner: Asian Mushroom Stir Fry (page 340) + brown rice or quinoa

Fitness

Day of rest.

Morning ME Time

1.   Brush your teeth.

2.   Prepare and mindfully sip warm lemon or ginger water.

3.   Practice your five-minute mini yoga routine.

4.   Meditate while focusing on your breath and body for five to ten minutes.

5.   Conclude with the intention: *Today I will take some quiet time to listen to the still, small voice within.*

In addition to your morning routine, today you will also do the following writing exercise:

Your Dream Life: We tend to impose so many limitations on ourselves—why we can't, shouldn't, or will never be able to realize our dreams. Today is the day that you are going to bust through the limitations by doing a stream-of-consciousness writing exercise.

Grab your notebook and write out the title: "My Dream Life." And then answer the question: If money and resources were no longer an issue, what would my dream life look like?

Set your timer for three minutes, and don't let your pen stop until the timer goes off.

This is one of the most powerful writing exercises I've ever done. It gives you permission to run wild with your hopes, wishes, and dreams.

DAY 22

Beauty

Dry Brushing: Bring this refreshing practice into your pre-shower routine today. See page 147 for more information.

Morning Facial Routine: Cleanse with brightening cleanser; nourish with serum, vitamin C, and moisturizer; and protect with mineral sunscreen.

Daily Body Moisturizing: Apply your hand and body moisturizer liberally over your whole body before you leave the house.

Evening Facial Routine: Cleanse using Two-Step Cleanse and nourish with retinol, serum, and moisturizer.

Diet

Breakfast: Gluten-Free Flax Pancakes with Blackberry Cashew Cream (page 332); you can buy frozen gluten-free pancakes in a pinch.

Lunch: Kelp Noodle Salad (page 364)

Afternoon Snack: Rice cake with almond or apple butter

Dinner: Vegan Lasagna (pages 350–351) + green salad

Fitness

Cardio: Try a cardio routine that you've never done before. Do the new practice for at least 20 minutes, but make sure to do 40 minutes of cardio in all.

Morning ME Time

1. Brush your teeth.

2. Prepare and mindfully sip warm lemon or ginger water.

3. Practice your five-minute mini yoga routine.

4. Meditate while focusing on your breath and body for five to ten minutes. Also, focus on your general health today. Do you normally have the energy to do what you want to do? Do you feel revitalized after a night of sleep? Do you have any chronic pain? Remind yourself that meditation is a powerful technique that can help not only melt away stress but also increase your concentration and boost your immune system.

5. Conclude with the intention: *Today I will forgive myself for not being perfect.*

DAY 23

Beauty

Morning Facial Routine: Cleanse with brightening cleanser; nourish with serum, vitamin C, and moisturizer; and protect with mineral sunscreen.

Daily Body Moisturizing: Apply your hand and body moisturizer liberally over your whole body before you leave the house.

Evening Facial Routine: Cleanse using the Two-Step Cleanse and nourish with retinol, serum, and moisturizer.

Diet

Breakfast: Coconut Chia Pudding (page 330) or steel-cut oatmeal with sliced banana + Serenity Juice (page 325)

Lunch: Curried Waldorf Salad (page 360) + warm sprouted grain pita/wrap

Afternoon Snack: Rooty Fruity Smoothie (page 328)

Dinner: Quinoa and Black Bean Burger (page 349) + Cauliflower Mash (page 359)

Fitness

Cardio: Do 20 minutes of your choice of cardio.

Flexibility: Do 20 minutes of your choice of flexibility practice.

Morning ME Time

1. Brush your teeth.

2. Prepare and mindfully sip warm lemon or ginger water.

3. Practice your five-minute mini yoga routine.

4. Meditate while focusing on your breath and body for five to ten minutes.

5. Conclude with the intention: *Today I will let go of who I think I should be, and embrace who I am.*

DAY 24

Beauty

Dry Brushing: Bring this refreshing practice into your pre-shower routine today. See page 147 for more information.

Morning Facial Routine: Cleanse with brightening cleanser; nourish with serum, vitamin C, and moisturizer; and protect with mineral sunscreen.

Daily Body Moisturizing: Apply your hand and body moisturizer liberally over your whole body before you leave the house.

Evening Facial Routine: Cleanse using the Two-Step Cleanse and nourish with retinol, serum, and moisturizer. If you have a facial cleansing brush, use it this evening to remove Step 2 of your cleanse.

Diet

Breakfast: Sprouted grain or gluten-free toast with almond butter and sliced banana + Liver Cleanse Juice (page 324)

Lunch: Romaine lettuce with Chia Caesar Dressing (pages 359–360) and croutons

Afternoon Snack: Rice cake with almond or apple butter

Dinner: Veggie Hot Pot (pages 353–354)

Fitness

Cardio: Do 20 minutes of your choice of cardio.

Weight Training: Try a weight-training routine you've never done before. Do it for 20 minutes.

Morning ME Time

1. Brush your teeth.

2. Prepare and mindfully sip warm lemon or ginger water.

3. Practice your five-minute mini yoga routine.

4. Meditate while focusing on your breath and body for five to ten minutes.

5. Conclude with the intention: *Today I will plug in to the stillness deep within, no matter what life throws at me.*

DAY 25

Beauty

Morning Facial Routine: Cleanse with brightening cleanser; nourish with serum, vitamin C, and moisturizer; and protect with mineral sunscreen.

Daily Body Moisturizing: Apply your hand and body moisturizer liberally over your whole body before you leave the house.

Evening Facial Routine: Cleanse using the Two-Step Cleanse and nourish with retinol, serum, and moisturizer.

Diet

Breakfast: Coconut Quinoa Porridge (page 331) + The Flow Juice (page 323)

Lunch: Moroccan Beet Soup (page 339) + green side salad

Afternoon Snack: Apple or pear + handful of raw nuts and seeds

Dinner: Roasted Beet, Orange, and Hazelnut Salad (pages 365–366) + brown rice or quinoa

Fitness

Cardio: Do 40 minutes of your choice of cardio.

Morning ME Time

1. Brush your teeth.

2. Prepare and mindfully sip warm lemon or ginger water.

3. Practice your five-minute mini yoga routine.

4. Meditate while focusing on your breath and body for five to ten minutes. During today's meditation, take a moment to notice what happens to your breath when your mind wanders. Does it become shallower? Deeper? Faster? Realize that being connected with your breath helps you align at the deepest level with your physical self.

5. Conclude with the intention: *Today I will listen to my truth.*

In addition to your morning routine, today you will also do the following writing exercise:

Start Small, Dream Big: When I dreamed of writing my first book, *Gorgeously Green,* about living an earth-friendly life, I had big dreams. The ultimate dream of any new writer is to have Oprah Winfrey hold your book up to the world—it's kind of like winning an Oscar if you're an actor. However, I hadn't even written a word of my book at this point; I just had a dream. Like every vision and dream I've ever had, the key to achieving it was my willingness to start with the small steps that were right in front of me: if I hadn't sat in a chair, opened a new blank document on my computer, and written "Chapter 1," that book would never have been written. When people ask me how I got started, I just say that I wrote the first word (or I picked up the phone, or I wrote the e-mail). It's all about taking action despite your fears and putting one foot in front of the other while holding the vision loosely.

Set your timer today for three minutes and simply write about a dream you have and what might be holding you back. Don't let your pen stop until the timer goes off. Then write down three actions that you can take today toward achieving your dream—and *do them!*

DAY 26

Beauty

Morning Facial Routine: Cleanse with brightening cleanser; nourish with serum, vitamin C, and moisturizer; and protect with mineral sunscreen.

Daily Body Moisturizing: Apply your hand and body moisturizer liberally over your whole body before you leave the house.

Evening Facial Routine: Cleanse using the Two-Step Cleanse; peel; and nourish with retinol, serum, and moisturizer.

Peel 4: This is the last peel of the program. See page 280 for detailed information on doing the peel. If your skin is getting used to the peels, see if you can leave this one on for 20 minutes.

Diet

Breakfast: Gorgeously Green Queen Smoothie (page 327) + Bircher Muesli (page 329)

Lunch: Everything Salad

Afternoon Snack: Pipe Cleaner Smoothie (page 327)

Dinner: Vegan Pesto Millet Bowl (pages 351–352)

Fitness

Cardio: Do 20 minutes of your choice of cardio.

Flexibility: Try a flexibility practice you've never done before. Do it for 20 minutes.

Morning ME Time

1. Brush your teeth.

2. Prepare and mindfully sip warm lemon or ginger water.

3. Practice your five-minute mini yoga routine.

4. Meditate while focusing on your breath and body for five to ten minutes. Today, again you will focus on a particular aspect of your breath. With each breath, silently repeat the mantra *So'ham* (pronounced "so hum"), inhaling on *So* and exhaling on *Hum*. In Sanskrit, this mantra means, "I am that."

5.   Conclude with the intention: *Today I will watch for any negative or limiting thoughts that prevent me from living my true purpose, and I will let go of them and watch them drift off and dissipate into nothingness.*

DAY 27

Beauty

Morning Facial Routine: Cleanse with brightening cleanser; nourish with serum, vitamin C, and moisturizer; and protect with mineral sunscreen.

Daily Body Moisturizing: Apply your hand and body moisturizer liberally over your whole body before you leave the house.

Evening Facial Routine: Cleanse using the Two-Step Cleanse and nourish with retinol, serum, and moisturizer.

Diet

Breakfast: Super Crunch Granola (pages 334–335) with unsweetened, nondairy milk + Serenity Juice (page 325)

Lunch: Warm Quinoa and Butternut Squash Salad (pages 368–369)

Afternoon Snack: Countess Coconut Smoothie (page 326)

Dinner: Bok Choy and Ginger Curry (pages 341–342) + brown rice or quinoa

Fitness

Cardio: Do 20 minutes of your choice of cardio.

Weight Training: Do 20 minutes of your choice of weight training.

Morning ME Time

1. Brush your teeth.

2. Prepare and mindfully sip warm lemon or ginger water.

3. Practice your five-minute mini yoga routine.

4. Meditate while focusing on your breath and body for five to ten minutes.

5. Conclude with the intention: *Today I will remind myself throughout the day that my true purpose is simply to love.*

DAY 28

Beauty

Dry Brushing: Bring this refreshing practice into your pre-shower routine today. See page 147 for more information.

Morning Facial Routine: Cleanse with brightening cleanser; nourish with serum, vitamin C, and moisturizer; and protect with mineral sunscreen.

Daily Body Moisturizing: Apply your hand and body moisturizer liberally over your whole body before you leave the house.

Evening Facial Routine: Cleanse using the Two-Step Cleanse and nourish with retinol, serum, and moisturizer. If you have a facial cleansing brush, use it this evening to remove Step 2 of your cleanse.

Diet

Breakfast: Sprouted grain or gluten-free toast topped with almond butter and sliced banana + Gorgeously Clean Greens Juice (page 324)

Lunch: Creamy Butternut Squash Soup (page 337) + brown rice

Afternoon Snack: Rice cake with apple/cherry butter

Dinner: Macro Bowl (pages 345–346)

Fitness

Day of rest.

Morning ME Time

1. Brush your teeth.

2. Prepare and mindfully sip warm lemon or ginger water.

3. Practice your five-minute mini yoga routine.

4. Meditate while focusing on your breath and body for five to ten minutes.

5. Conclude with the intention: *Today I will let go of fighting my past and focus on building my future.*

In addition to your morning routine, today we will also do a writing exercise.

Whatever You Put Attention On Increases: I believe 100 percent in the spiritual principle that what you put your attention on increases. This is why I think it's imperative to write as many gratitude lists as you can. In my worst moments, my "thank-you" lists save my backside by stopping me from drifting into self-pity. Moreover, gratitude lists get me to focus on the things I love in my life—thus helping them increase. So grab your notebook and write the title "Thank You For" and set your timer for two minutes. Write out what you're grateful for, and do not let your pen stop until the timer goes off!

DAY 29

Beauty

Morning Facial Routine: Cleanse with brightening cleanser; nourish with serum, vitamin C, and moisturizer; and protect with mineral sunscreen.

Daily Body Moisturizing: Apply your hand and body moisturizer liberally over your whole body before you leave the house.

Evening Facial Routine: Cleanse using the Two-Step Cleanse and nourish with retinol, serum, and moisturizer.

Diet

Breakfast: Coconut Quinoa Porridge (page 331) + Liver Cleanse Juice (page 324)

Lunch: Apple/pear + Greek Salad (pages 362–363)

Afternoon Snack: Handful of Gorgeously Green Trail Mix (pages 361–362)

Dinner: Warm Lentil and Roasted Tomato Salad (pages 367–368)

Fitness

Cardio: Do 40 minutes of your choice of cardio.

Moning ME Time

1.   Brush your teeth.

2.   Prepare and mindfully sip warm lemon or ginger water.

3.   Practice your five-minute mini yoga routine.

4.   Meditate while focusing on your breath and body for five to ten minutes. Today, think a bit about how you interact with the world around you. Are you pessimistic? Do you keep people at a distance? Do you allow the world to affect you, or do you put up a hard outer wall? If you don't allow yourself to connect with the people and events around you, it's often easy to feel alone and miss out on some of the best experiences life has to offer.

5.   Conclude with the intention: *Today I will soften my hard edges and open to the light and beauty of the Divine.*

DAY 30

Beauty

Dry Brushing: Bring this refreshing practice into your pre-shower routine today. See page 147 for more information.

Morning Facial Routine: Cleanse with brightening cleanser; nourish with serum, vitamin C, and moisturizer; and protect with mineral sunscreen.

Daily Body Moisturizing: Apply your hand and body moisturizer liberally over your whole body before you leave the house.

Evening Facial Routine: Cleanse using the Two-Step Cleanse and nourish with retinol, serum, and moisturizer.

Diet

Breakfast: Ridiculously Healthy Muffin (page 334) or Chocolate Brownie Oatmeal (pages 329–330)

Lunch: Mock Tuna Salad Open-Faced Sandwich (pages 346–347)

Afternoon Snack: Apple/pear + handful Super Crunch Granola (pages 334–335)

Dinner: Creamy Vegan "Mac n' Cheese" (pages 344–345) + Alkalizing Salad (page 356)

Fitness

Congratulations! You've made it to the end of the 30 days. Today, let's close things out with a short cardio session and some exploration.

Cardio: Walk at a brisk pace for 20 minutes.

Exploration: Think about the ways of working out you have done over the last 30 days. Was there anything that you really loved? Anything that you hated? Take this opportunity to really listen to your body. This information can help you create a lifelong movement routine that will keep you feeling—and looking—your best.

Morning ME Time

1. Brush your teeth.

2. Prepare and mindfully sip warm lemon or ginger water.

3.   Practice your five-minute mini yoga routine.

4.   Meditate while focusing on your breath and body for five to ten minutes. Today, I recommend that you meditate on one of my favorite quotes from the late Maya Angelou, because it is filled with wisdom: "I've learned that people will forget what you said, people will forget what you did, but people will never forget how you made them feel."

5.   Conclude with the intention: *Today I will give freely of what I've been given, knowing that the Universe provides me with exactly what I need.*

Chapter 12

Food Recipes

JUICES

· ·

THE FLOW JUICE

This lively juice helps relieve water retention and bloating. It is great for helping with weight loss, too.

Serves 1

1 cucumber
1 pear
1 cup parsley
½ cup fresh mint
2 celery stalks
½ small fennel bulb

Process all ingredients through your juicer.

. . . .

GORGEOUSLY CLEAN GREENS JUICE

This delicious juice helps to boost your energy, immunity, and detoxification systems.

Serves 1

1 apple
½ small fennel bulb
½ cucumber
2 cups spinach
½ green bell pepper
1 stick celery
Handful sunflower seeds
4 macadamia nuts

Process all ingredients through your juicer. Strain if desired.

. . . .

LIVER CLEANSE JUICE

Apples help to sweeten this savory cocktail. It packs such a liver-detoxifying punch that you might want to drink at least one of these a week.

Serves 1

2 apples
2 cups spinach
2 cups dandelion leaves
2 cups broccoli florets
1 clove garlic
1 stalk celery
1 inch ginger root
1 teaspoon ground turmeric (or 1 inch turmeric root)

Process all ingredients through your juicer.

∙∙

SERENITY JUICE

This wonderful juice helps to not only calm your nervous system, but also balance your hormones.

Serves 1

2 medium carrots
1 apple
1 cup red grapes
1 inch ginger root
2 cups spinach
½ small fennel bulb
1 medium beet (with leaves)
1 stalk celery
½ sweet potato

Process all ingredients through your juicer.

∙∙

SPICY VEGETABLE COCKTAIL JUICE

This recipe is contributed by Tess Masters (aka The Blender Girl), who is the juice queen. This is a delicious lunchtime juice.

Serves 1

5 small organic tomatoes
2 stalks celery
2 green onions
1 handful kale leaves
⅓ cup flat-leaf parsley
⅓ cup cilantro
1 carrot
½ red bell pepper
½ lemon, peeled
2 cloves garlic
Pinch Celtic sea salt or Himalayan crystal salt
Smidge cayenne pepper (optional)

Process all ingredients through your juicer. Strain if desired.

SMOOTHIES

COUNTESS COCONUT SMOOTHIE

This smoothie is a delicious treat. It's perfect for an afternoon pick-me-up when you might ordinarily reach for a muffin or a cookie.

Serves 1

½ cup unsweetened almond milk
½ cup coconut water
1 tablespoon coconut meat or butter
1 tablespoon raw coconut oil
Handful raw almonds
2 tablespoons ground flaxseeds
2 dates, presoaked

Process all ingredients in your blender.

ENERGY BOOSTER SMOOTHIE

I often make this smoothie before hitting a hard-core yoga or Pilates class.

Serves 1

1 cup unsweetened almond milk
½ banana
½ cup frozen blueberries
1 tablespoon maca powder
Handful spinach leaves
1 tablespoon hemp protein powder
½ cup ice

Process all ingredients in your blender.

· ·

GORGEOUSLY GREEN QUEEN SMOOTHIE

This is my go-to morning smoothie. It's sweet and satisfying and gets me set for the day.

Serves 1

Handful raw kale leaves
Handful spinach leaves
Handful romaine leaves
½ banana
2 dates, presoaked
1 tablespoon goji berries
Handful raw walnuts
1 cup unsweetened rice milk
½ cup ice

Process all ingredients in your blender.

· ·

PIPE CLEANER SMOOTHIE

If I'm not as "regular" as I would like to be, I whip up a glass of this delicious smoothie, and it usually sets things straight.

Serves 1

8 ounces coconut water
1 tablespoon flaxseeds
Handful raw walnuts
1 tablespoon slippery elm powder*
1 teaspoon chia seeds, presoaked
1 apple or pear
Handful spinach leaves
2 dates, presoaked

Process all ingredients in your blender.

*You can find slippery elm powder at most good health-food stores and online.

ROOTY FRUITY SMOOTHIE

Beets are so great for cleansing the liver that if I feel like something a little more hearty than a beet juice, I whip up a glass of this smoothie.

Serves 1

¼ cup beet juice
¾ cup unsweetened rice milk
½ banana
Handful spinach leaves
1 tablespoon goji berries
1 tablespoon chia seeds (presoaked overnight)
2 dates
½ cup ice

Process all ingredients in your blender.

Smoothie Tips

- Presoak nuts, dates, and seeds before adding to your smoothie to make them easier to blend and digest.
- I like to add dates for sweetness, but if you want to reduce your sugar intake (or if you are diabetic), substitute with stevia drops or monk fruit powder.
- If you are new to supplements such as powdered greens or superfood powders, add them sparingly in the beginning (a half teaspoon of each) until you know that they work for you and your digestion.
- I love to add probiotics (gut-friendly microorganisms) to my smoothies. My first choice is a liquid probiotic, or powder. Since capsules can be hard to digest, I split them open if it's all I can find.

BREAKFAST

....

BIRCHER MUESLI

I love this traditional Swiss recipe. The great thing is that you don't have pots and pans to scrub out.

Serves 2

1 cup old-fashioned oats
2 tablespoons ground flaxseeds
2 tablespoons pumpkin seeds
2 tablespoons sunflower seeds
2 tablespoons sliced almonds or pecan pieces
2 apples
1 teaspoon lemon juice
1 cup plain or coconut yogurt
4 dates, pitted and chopped
Fresh berries or tropical fruits, depending on the season

The night before, place the oats in a bowl and cover them with filtered water (plus an extra inch of water). Place the seeds in a small bowl and cover with filtered water. Let both soak overnight.

In the morning, toast the nuts in a hot cast-iron pan. Peel and grate the apples and mix them into the soaked oats, then stir in the lemon juice. Add the nuts, seeds, and yogurt, and finally top with fresh fruit.

....

CHOCOLATE BROWNIE OATMEAL

This is a twist on traditional oatmeal and is so filling and satisfying in the winter months. The addition of raw cacao packs a potent antioxidant punch while delivering an irresistible chocolaty flavor.

Serves 2

1 cup old-fashioned oats
1 cup filtered water
1 cup unsweetened almond milk
2 teaspoons raw cacao powder
1 teaspoon coconut oil
2 teaspoons brown rice syrup
Handful walnuts, toasted

In a small saucepan, combine the oats, water, and almond milk. Simmer, uncovered, over low heat for 5 to 8 minutes, stirring continuously. Remove from the heat and stir in the cacao powder. Transfer the mixture to a bowl. Top with the coconut oil, brown rice syrup, and walnuts.

COCONUT CHIA PUDDING

This is extra easy to make the night before and is so creamy and delicious that you will just keep coming back for more.

Serves 1

1 cup unsweetened coconut milk
¼ teaspoon vanilla extract
1 tablespoon organic maple syrup*
¼ cup chia seeds
Fresh seasonal fruit or slivered almonds and goji berries

Combine the coconut milk, vanilla extract, maple syrup, and chia seeds in a glass container with an airtight lid. Place the mixture in the fridge. After about 30 minutes, stir it again, then replace the lid and leave it overnight. When you are ready to eat your pudding, spoon it into a bowl and top it with fruit or almonds and goji berries.

*You can use an alternate sweetener such as stevia or monk fruit powder, but I do like the nutty taste of the maple syrup.

COCONUT QUINOA PORRIDGE

This is such a great way to eat a high-protein grain such as quinoa.

Serves 2

1 cup quinoa
2 cups unsweetened coconut milk
4 to 6 dates, pitted and chopped
½ cup unsweetened coconut flakes
¼ teaspoon ground cinnamon
¼ teaspoon ground ginger
1 teaspoon raw virgin coconut oil (optional)
Seasonal fruit (optional)

Place the quinoa in a heavy-bottomed saucepan with the coconut milk and chopped dates. Bring to a boil. Cover and turn the heat to low; simmer until all the milk is absorbed, approximately 15 minutes. Remove from heat and stir in the coconut flakes and spices. Re-cover the pan and let the porridge sit for approximately 3 to 5 minutes. Spoon into bowls and top with coconut oil and/or fruit.

DATE PUREE

I use date puree as a healthy sweetener for baking and as a topping for oatmeal, yogurt, pancakes, and even muffins. Dates are packed with fiber and minerals, so they deliver a potent nutritional punch while adding a nutty sweetness to your dish.

8 dates, pitted
1½ cups filtered water
1 teaspoon vanilla extract

Place the dates and water in a heavy-bottomed saucepan. Bring the mixture to a boil. Then, turn down the heat and simmer gently for 15 minutes. Allow the mixture to cool before adding vanilla extract. Place the mixture in a high-speed blender and blend until smooth.

Your date puree will keep in the fridge in a sealed container for up to four days.

GLUTEN-FREE FLAX PANCAKES WITH BLACKBERRY CASHEW CREAM

I'm a bit pancake-crazy. I just love whipping up different kinds of batters and experimenting with toppings.

Serves 4 to 6

Pancakes

2 cups gluten-free baking/pancake mix*
3 tablespoons ground flaxseed
1 cup unsweetened almond milk
2 tablespoons coconut oil

Blackberry Cashew Cream

2 cups whole raw cashews
¾ cup filtered water
½ cup frozen blackberries
1 tablespoon agave nectar or Xylitol

Fruit Topping

2 large Granny Smith apples, peeled, cored, and cubed
1 tablespoon water
½ cup chopped and pitted dates

Note: Make the blackberry cashew cream and fruit topping for your pancakes ahead of time.

For the cream:

Cover the nuts with filtered water and soak overnight. In the morning, rinse the nuts well and place them in a high-speed blender. Add the ¾ cup filtered water and blend until thick and creamy. The cream should be the consistency of regular whipped cream. If it's too thick, add a little more water. When it has reached the desired consistency, add the berries and sweetener and blend for 30 seconds or until the cream has turned purple. Scoop the cream out into a glass container. Cover and chill for at least an hour. The cream will stay good for two days in a sealed container in your refrigerator.

For the fruit topping:

Place all the ingredients in a heavy saucepan over a low heat. Stir the mixture constantly until the apples are tender but retain their shape, approximately five minutes. Be careful not to overcook them.

For the pancakes:

Mix together the pancake mix, flaxseed, and almond milk. In a cast-iron frying pan, heat the coconut oil over high heat. When it's bubbling, add about 2 tablespoons of batter per pancake into the pan and fry until golden brown.

To serve, top the piping-hot pancakes with a dollop of cashew cream and a spoonful of warm fruit.

*Having tried almost every kind of gluten-free mix on the market, for me it's a toss-up between Pamela's and The Pure Pantry brands. The latter does a wonderful buckwheat pancake mix that's nutty and brown. My family, however, prefers Pamela's because it gives them more of a traditional pancake.

RAW COCONUT YOGURT

This yogurt is a delight! To me, it tastes like summer, plus it's creamy and satisfying. If you have trouble finding coconut meat and raw coconut water, check out the freezer section of the local health-food store or an Asian store.

Serves 4

2 cups young coconut meat, fresh or frozen
¼ cup raw coconut water or filtered water
¼ teaspoon probiotic powder or 2 capsules' worth of powder

Place all the ingredients in a high-speed blender and process until smooth. Pour the mixture into a large Mason jar (only fill to ¾ full) and leave overnight in a warm spot. (I leave mine in the oven with the light turned on, because it's always a little warm in there.) After 8 to 12 hours, remove from the warm spot, open carefully, and mix well to remove bubbles.

Store in the fridge for up to four days.

RIDICULOUSLY HEALTHY MUFFINS

I make a big batch of these and eat them for breakfast or as an afternoon snack. They also freeze really well, which means you can just take out one or two when desired.

Serves 6 to 8

3 tablespoons raw virgin coconut oil

1 small banana

3 organic eggs or 4¼ teaspoons Ener-G Egg Replacer plus 6 tablespoons water

¼ cup all-purpose gluten-free or quinoa flour

¼ cup almond meal

2 tablespoons ground flaxseeds

½ teaspoon baking powder

¼ teaspoon salt

1 teaspoon vanilla extract

1 teaspoon ground cinnamon

½ cup unsweetened coconut milk

½ cup pecans

Preheat the oven to 400 degrees F. In a large bowl, mix together all the ingredients. Pour the batter into a greased muffin pan or muffin cups. Bake for 18 to 20 minutes or until a toothpick comes out clean.

SUPER CRUNCH GRANOLA

I'm always tweaking my granola recipes to suit everyone in the family, but here is one that passed everyone's muster. My husband loves it with homemade almond milk, and my daughter gobbles it up topped with creamy Greek yogurt. Either way, I think this one's a winner.

Serves 6

2 cups rolled gluten-free oats

½ cup walnuts, chopped

½ cup raw sunflower seeds

½ cup raw almonds, chopped

½ cup pecans, halved

½ cup chia seeds, soaked overnight

1 teaspoon cinnamon

½ teaspoon sea salt

3 tablespoons raw virgin coconut oil

½ cup maple syrup

½ cup brown rice syrup

2 tablespoons water

1 tablespoon vanilla extract

½ cup goji berries

½ cup dried apricots, chopped

Preheat the oven to 300 degrees F. Mix all the dry ingredients together in a large bowl. Melt the coconut oil, syrups, water, and vanilla together in a small saucepan. When fully melted, mix it into the dry mixture.

Spread the granola over a parchment paper–lined baking sheet and bake for about 40 minutes, turning over the granola every 15 minutes and scooping the crispy bits from the sides of the pan into the middle. Try not to break up the clusters when you turn the granola. For the last 5 minutes of cooking, add the fruit.

Allow the granola to cool completely before spooning it into an airtight canister for storage in a warm, dry spot. Your granola should keep well for up to three weeks.

Goji Berries

Goji berries are rich in antioxidants, particularly carotenoids such as beta carotene and zeaxanthin. One of zeaxanthin's key roles is to protect the retina of the eye by absorbing blue light. In fact, increased intake of foods containing zeaxanthin may decrease the risk of developing age-related macular degeneration (AMD), the leading cause of vision loss and blindness in people over the age of 65.

SOUPS

CAULIFLOWER AND LEEK SOUP

This is a variation on the traditional potato-leek soup that I was raised with. This low-calorie soup is creamy and satisfying—and packed with healthy goodness.

Serves 4

3 tablespoons veggie broth

½ yellow onion, minced

2 leeks, chopped

3 garlic cloves, minced

Sea salt and pepper, to taste

1 tablespoon Bragg Liquid Aminos

4 cups vegetable broth

1 head organic cauliflower, chopped (whole, not just florets)

½ cup silken tofu

¼ cup fresh chives, chopped

Extra virgin olive oil

In a large stockpot, heat the veggie broth. Add the onion and leeks and gently "sauté" until tender (if it becomes too dry, add another tablespoon of veggie broth). Add the garlic, seasoning, Bragg Liquid Aminos, broth, and cauliflower. Bring to a boil, turn down heat, and simmer for 20 minutes or until the densest portion of the cauliflower is tender when pricked with a fork. Transfer the mixture to a high-speed blender, add the silken tofu, and blend until smooth. Gently reheat in a saucepan. Serve topped with fresh chives and a drizzle of olive oil.

CREAMY BUTTERNUT SQUASH SOUP

I make this soup year-round because it's hearty enough for a lunch or dinner when served with a scoop of nutty brown rice and a crunchy green salad. It's also really easy to make. Plus, it freezes beautifully for up to three months.

Serves 4

3 tablespoons veggie broth
½ yellow onion, chopped
1 leek, chopped
2 garlic cloves, minced
½ teaspoon ground cumin
½ teaspoon turmeric
¼ teaspoon nutmeg
2 cups butternut squash, cubed
3 cups vegetable broth
½ cup silken tofu

Heat the veggie broth in a heavy-bottomed stockpot. Add the onion, leek, and garlic and "sauté" until tender and transparent. Add the spices and mix well. Add the squash and vegetable broth. Cover and simmer for 25 minutes. Remove from heat. Stir in the silken tofu. Transfer the soup to a high-speed blender and blend until smooth.

HEARTY PROVENÇAL SOUP

This is one of my favorite go-to summer soups. It's hearty enough for a family dinner, and when served with either a side of quinoa or a warm, crusty loaf of bread, you're in for a treat. The spinach pesto topping is what elevates this soup beyond a regular veggie soup. I always make a big pot and freeze what I don't use that day.

Serves 4

Soup

3 tablespoons veggie broth
3 cloves garlic, finely chopped
1 sprig fresh thyme, leaves removed
3 medium carrots, peeled and finely chopped
2 stalks celery, finely chopped
1 yellow onion, finely chopped
½ medium zucchini, chopped
1 cup sliced brown mushrooms
¼ head Savoy cabbage, cored and thinly shredded
8 cups vegetable stock
One 15-ounce can cannellini beans
Sea salt and freshly ground black pepper, to taste

Pesto

2 cups fresh basil leaves
1 cup baby spinach leaves
2 cloves garlic, peeled and chopped
1 cup extra virgin olive oil
½ cup almonds, toasted
Kosher salt, to taste

In a large stockpot, heat the veggie broth and gently "sauté" all the veggies and herbs until they have softened, approximately 5 to 8 minutes. Make sure to stir constantly to avoid burning. Add the stock and the beans, and turn heat down to low. Cover the pan and simmer for 30 minutes.

Meanwhile, place the pesto ingredients in a high-speed blender and blend until smooth.

Ladle soup into bowls and top each with a generous spoonful of pesto.

· ·

MOROCCAN BEET SOUP

I love to cook with beets whenever I can because they are so incredibly nourishing. I grate them, juice them, and roast them. This recipe is exquisite because of the subtle flavors and beautiful, velvety texture. You will fall in love with it.

Serves 4

4 tablespoons olive oil
½ large yellow onion, sliced
1 teaspoon cumin seeds
1 teaspoon turmeric
2 garlic cloves, peeled and sliced
1½ pounds beets (about 6 medium beets), peeled and cubed
1 large potato, peeled and cubed
4½ cups vegetable stock
3 tablespoons red wine vinegar
1 small bunch parsley, roughly chopped
2 teaspoons sea salt
1 cup Greek yogurt, thinned with a little milk
Extra virgin olive oil

Heat the oil in a large, heavy saucepan and add the onion. Turn down to low and fry the onion for about 10 minutes until it is slightly browned. Add the cumin seeds, turmeric, and garlic and fry for 2 more minutes. Add the beets and potato, followed by the stock. Simmer for 20 minutes or until the cubes of potato are completely soft. Remove from heat and stir in the vinegar, half of the parsley, and the sea salt. Transfer to a food processor and blend until smooth. Return to saucepan and heat until very warm just prior to serving.

Serve in warmed bowls and top with a generous drizzle of yogurt, a sprinkle of parsley, and a few drops of olive oil.

MAINS

· ·

ASIAN MUSHROOM STIR FRY

I love making foods with Asian mushrooms, because they have so many health benefits, including immune and cardiovascular support, and they have been found to contain anticancer properties. Moreover, their smoky flavor is delectable in virtually any dish.

Serves 2

3 tablespoons veggie broth
3 tablespoons low-sodium tamari
½ yellow onion, minced
1 clove garlic, peeled and minced
10 to 12 shiitake mushrooms (if small, leave intact; if large, slice in halves)
1 maitake mushroom, broken apart
2 cups bean sprouts
1 head Swiss chard, stems and stalks removed, roughly chopped
2 tablespoons tamari or shoyu sauce

Heat the veggie broth and tamari in a stainless-steel sauté pan or wok, over low heat. Add the onion and garlic and "sauté" until soft, approximately 3 minutes. Add the mushrooms and 1 tablespoon of water, and turn the heat up to medium. Fry for about 5 minutes, continuously moving the mushrooms around to prevent them from sticking.

Add the bean sprouts, chard, tamari sauce, and one more tablespoon of water. Fry until the chard has wilted. Remove from heat and serve immediately.

BAKED TEMPEH WITH BALSAMIC GLAZE

Tempeh is a really healthy fermented soy food with a nutty texture and taste. I like to add a lot of flavor to my tempeh by marinating and glazing it. This is one of my favorite recipes.

Serves 2

½ cup balsamic vinegar (get the aged, syrupy stuff)
1 tablespoon maple syrup
1 tablespoon tamari sauce
½ teaspoon mixed dried Italian herbs
1 package of tempeh, sliced in half horizontally
2 teaspoons arrowroot or tapioca starch

Mix the vinegar, maple syrup, tamari sauce, and Italian herbs together in a shallow baking dish. Add the tempeh, coating it well on both sides. Cover the dish and marinate for two hours.

Heat a cast-iron, ridged grill pan. When the pan is smoking hot, add the tempeh slices to the pan and sear on both sides, approximately 1 minute per side. Mix the arrowroot starch into the leftover marinade and then add it to the pan. Let the marinade bubble while you gently stir it around the tempeh for 2 minutes.

Transfer the tempeh to a platter and spoon the marinade over the top of each slice.

BOK CHOY AND GINGER CURRY

This is a comforting curry that makes an incredibly satisfying dinner, full of all the flavors you need to assuage your taste buds.

Serves 2

1 tablespoon raw virgin coconut oil
1 medium yellow onion, minced

2 cloves garlic, peeled and minced

1 inch fresh ginger root, peeled and minced

1 teaspoon curry powder

1 teaspoon ground turmeric

2 heads bok choy, chopped into bite-size pieces

1 cup brown mushrooms, sliced

1 cup fresh bean sprouts

1 cup veggie stock or broth

½ cup coconut milk

2 cups baby spinach

Heat the coconut oil in a large, stainless-steel skillet. Add the onion and sauté until translucent. Add the garlic, ginger, and spices. Sauté for another minute. Add the bok choy, mushrooms, bean sprouts, veggie stock, and coconut milk. Cover the pan and simmer for 15 minutes. Turn off the heat. Add the spinach, replace the lid, and allow the spinach to wilt in the steam for a few minutes.

. . . .

BROWN RICE, ASPARAGUS, AND GREEN BEAN RISOTTO

Although I love the creaminess of Arborio rice, which is traditionally used in risotto, I wanted to see if a whole grain such as brown rice would work as well, because it's way healthier. It requires a little more cooking, but if you use organic, short-grain brown rice, you'll be able to create a creamy, hearty risotto.

Serves 4

4 to 5 cups vegetable stock or broth + 3 tablespoons for "sautéing"

1½ cups shiitake mushrooms, sliced

1 small yellow onion, minced

2 cloves garlic, peeled and minced

½ cup white wine

1 cup short-grain brown rice

Sea salt and pepper, to taste

Extra virgin olive oil

1 cup asparagus, chopped in inch-long pieces

1 cup chopped French green beans (in inch-long pieces)
Parma (vegan Parmesan cheese)

Place the stock in a saucepan and turn the heat on low. For making a risotto, the stock must be warm before you add it to the grain.

Heat 3 tablespoons veggie broth/stock in a large skillet and gently "sauté" the mushrooms until they are cooked through. Remove them from the pan and set them aside.

Add the onions to the pan and sauté until translucent, approximately 5 minutes. Add the garlic and sauté for another minute. Add the wine and sauté for two more minutes. Mix in the rice.

Begin to ladle the stock into the pan, stirring constantly. Wait until one ladle of broth is fully absorbed before adding the next. Be patient with the risotto; don't try to rush it by turning the heat up.

It will take 40 minutes for all the stock to be absorbed, by which time the grain will be chewy and perfectly al dente. Season your risotto with sea salt and pepper.

Meanwhile, steam the asparagus and green beans for 4 minutes or until they are bright green and al dente. Remove from heat and run under cold water to prevent them from cooking any further.

Once the stock is absorbed, immediately stir the mushrooms into the risotto.

Spoon the risotto into warmed bowls and drizzle with a generous amount of olive oil. Lay the asparagus and green beans on top of each bowl. Top with a little Parma.

CREAMY MUNG BEAN OR BLACK BEAN PASTA

If you've never tasted mung bean pasta, you are in for a treat. It usually comes in fettuccine-style ribbons. It is nutty and has a lovely, chewy texture. My husband and I are hooked on it because it is a protein-packed, gluten-free way to enjoy pasta.

Serves 4

1 cup raw cashews, presoaked overnight
1 cup water
1 clove garlic, peeled
2 teaspoons nutritional yeast
2 teaspoons tamari sauce
1 teaspoon lemon juice
2 teaspoons dulse flakes
½ cup oil-preserved sun-dried tomatoes
One package organic mung bean pasta*

Place all the ingredients except the pasta in a high-speed blender, and blend until smooth.

Cook the pasta according to the directions on the package. Drain, place back in the saucepan, and gently combine with the creamy sauce. Heat the mixture up over low heat, stirring continuously. Serve immediately.

*You can find these noodles in the international section at most health-food stores.

CREAMY VEGAN "MAC N' CHEESE"

This is a firm favorite of my daughter's. Thank goodness, because I had to wean her off the boxed stuff, which was no easy feat!

Serves 4

1 cup raw cashews, presoaked for at least 4 hours
1½ cups water
1 teaspoon sea salt
¼ teaspoon black pepper
1 teaspoon nutritional yeast
3 shallots, minced
2 cups baby spinach
8 to 10 ounces gluten-free macaroni

Preheat the oven to 375 degrees F.

Place the cashews, water, salt, pepper, and nutritional yeast in a high-speed blender and blend until smooth.

Place the shallots in a sauté pan with about ¼ cup of water and sauté over low heat until lightly browned. Add the spinach (and a little more water if needed), and wait for the spinach to wilt. Add the shallot mixture to the blender and blend until smooth.

Meanwhile, cook some gluten-free macaroni according to the directions on the box.

After draining the pasta, empty it into a casserole dish. Mix in the creamy sauce and bake for 20 to 30 minutes.

MACRO BOWL

This is almost my all-time favorite dinner. It is so simple and healthy that you can't go wrong.

Serves 2

Vegetables

1 cup quinoa
1½ cups water or vegetable broth
1 small sweet potato, peeled and cubed
1 daikon radish, chopped into 2-inch slices
3 cups spinach
1 cup wakame seaweed, soaked in warm water for 5 to 10 minutes and then cut into ribbons
1 cup black beans
1 avocado, sliced

Dressing

1 rounded tablespoon white or yellow miso
2 tablespoons seasoned rice vinegar
½ teaspoon grated fresh ginger
1 small clove garlic, peeled and minced
Pinch of paprika

2 tablespoons toasted sesame oil

2 tablespoons grape seed oil

2 tablespoons silken tofu

Combine all the dressing ingredients in a blender and blend until smooth. Set aside.

Combine the quinoa and water in a saucepan and bring to a boil. Lower the heat, cover, and simmer for 15 minutes.

Meanwhile, steam the sweet potato and daikon radish for about 10 minutes or until tender. Add the spinach into the steamer for the last minute of cooking.

Divide the quinoa, veggies, seaweed, and beans between two bowls. Drizzle the dressing on top, and finish with half a sliced avocado on each.

· ·

MOCK TUNA SALAD OPEN-FACED SANDWICH

I must say that I love tuna salad, but I really try to stay away because tuna can be loaded with mercury. This tasty salad is made with tempeh, and I love to serve it as an open-faced sandwich.

Serves 2

One 8-ounce package tempeh

2 scallions, chopped

2 stalks celery, diced

2 large cucumber pickles, diced

¼ cup vegan mayo

2 tablespoons dulse flakes

Sea salt and pepper, to taste

2 slices gluten-free or sprouted-grain bread

2 leaves romaine lettuce

Tomato slices (optional)

Fresh parsley (optional)

Boil the whole cake of tempeh for 10 minutes. Drain and leave it to cool.

Mix the scallions, celery, cucumber, mayo, dulse flakes, salt, and pepper in a medium bowl. Crumble the cooled cake of tempeh into the mayo mixture.

Toast the bread and top with a leaf of romaine lettuce and a couple of scoops of your tempeh salad. Dress with sliced tomato and/or chopped fresh parsley, if desired.

....

MOROCCAN STUFFED EGGPLANT

I love Moroccan spices, especially when they are combined with the caramelized flesh of eggplant. This dish makes use of the Quinoa-Millet Apricot Salad, so if you are planning ahead, you can make double the salad one day and cook this dish the next.

Serves 2

Main

1 large eggplant
2 cups Quinoa-Millet Apricot Salad (pages 364–365)
Cilantro (optional)
2 tablespoons Cashew Cream, Savory (page 262)

Marinade

2 cloves garlic, minced
1 teaspoon chili pepper flakes
1 teaspoon ground cumin
1 teaspoon ground coriander
1 teaspoon smoked paprika
2 teaspoons grated lemon zest
⅓ cup olive oil

Preheat the oven to 400 degrees F. Cut the eggplant in half and score the cut sides. Place them on a parchment paper–lined baking sheet. Mix the marinade ingredients together in a small bowl. Spoon the marinade on top of the cut side of each eggplant half. Place the eggplants in the oven for 45 minutes. When they are cooked, remove them from the oven and allow them to cool to room temperature.

Place each eggplant half on a plate, cut side up, and spoon a cup of Quinoa Salad onto each one. Top with chopped fresh cilantro and/or a little yogurt.

....

PECAN-STUFFED SHIITAKE MUSHROOMS

My favorite mushrooms to stuff are shiitake because of their smoky flavor and incredible health benefits. They have been found to be helpful in boosting the immune system and keeping the cardiovascular system in good shape. They are also an excellent source of iron.

Serves 4

12 to 16 medium shiitake mushrooms
3 tablespoons grape seed or olive oil + 1 tablespoon for brushing
1 teaspoon fenugreek seeds
1 medium onion, minced
2 cloves garlic, peeled and minced
1 small fennel bulb, finely chopped
4 ounces tempeh, finely chopped
2 tablespoons tamari sauce
1 cup chopped pecans
1 cup gluten-free breadcrumbs
Salt and pepper, to taste
12 to 16 teaspoons extra virgin olive oil
Flat-leaf parsley, chopped

Preheat oven to 375 degrees F. Remove the stalks from the mushrooms. Brush the bottom of each mushroom with a little grape seed oil and arrange them bottom-side down in a baking dish.

Heat the oil in a large skillet and add the fenugreek seeds. Sauté for a minute. Then add the onion, garlic, and fennel. Sauté over a medium heat, constantly stirring, until the onion and fennel are soft. Next, add the tempeh and sauté for 2 to 3 minutes more. Stir in the tamari. Then, add the pecans and breadcrumbs and sauté for another minute. Season well with sea salt and pepper.

Place 1 teaspoon olive oil into each mushroom. Spoon the vegetable mixture into the mushroom shells.

Cover with foil and bake for 15 minutes. Remove foil and bake for 10 more minutes.

Sprinkle with parsley before serving.

· ·

QUINOA AND BLACK BEAN BURGERS

These protein-packed burgers are a firm family favorite. Instead of serving them in buns, I serve the patty on a thick slice of tomato and top with veggie mayo (tarted up with some garlic and/or chipotle paste) and fresh basil leaves. They are perfect for a cookout.

Serves 6 to 8

3 tablespoons veggie broth
1 small yellow onion, chopped finely
8 oil-packed sun-dried tomatoes, finely chopped
4 oil-packed artichoke hearts, finely chopped
One 15-ounce can black beans, drained
2 cloves garlic, peeled and finely chopped
1½ cups cooked quinoa
1 teaspoon Italian seasoning
Sea salt and pepper, to taste
2 tablespoons grape seed or coconut oil

Heat the veggie broth in a skillet and add the onion. "Sauté" the onion until translucent, approximately 3 minutes. Add the sun-dried tomatoes, artichoke hearts, black beans, 1½ cups water, and garlic. Sauté, stirring constantly, for 4 more minutes. Remove from the heat and transfer to a food processor. Add the quinoa and seasoning. Process until the mixture has come together but is still a bit chunky. Create your patties, cover with parchment paper, and allow them to chill in the fridge for a few hours or overnight.

When you are ready to fry them, heat the oil in a cast-iron skillet. When the oil is sizzling, carefully drop the patties into the skillet and fry for about 3 minutes on each side or until brown and crispy. Serve immediately.

SPICY VEGGIE CHILI

I love to use cumin in my chili because it adds a sweetness and depth to the mingling flavors.

Serves 4 to 6

3 tablespoons veggie broth
1 large onion, chopped
4 cloves garlic, peeled and minced
1 teaspoon ground cumin
½ teaspoon ground cinnamon
1 teaspoon sea salt
One 28-ounce can organic chopped tomatoes
1 cup pinto beans
1 cup black beans
2 cups cubed butternut squash
2 cups cubed zucchini
2 teaspoons chili powder
1 chipotle pepper in adobo sauce, finely chopped (optional)*
1 cup fresh cilantro, chopped (optional)
Plain yogurt (optional)

Heat the veggie broth in a large skillet. Add onions and "sauté" until soft. Then add the garlic and spices and sauté for another minute. Transfer to a slow cooker. Add tomatoes, beans, and veggies. Stir well. Cook on a low setting for 6 to 8 hours. Garnish with cilantro and yogurt, if desired.

*Adding this pepper will seriously kick up the heat factor.

VEGAN LASAGNA (GLUTEN FREE)

I did a taste test with the family recently: I cooked one traditional lasagna and this recipe. I was convinced that my husband and daughter would prefer the traditional, but this one was the winner.

Serves 4

"Ricotta"

1½ cups raw cashews, soaked for a few hours
2 tablespoons lemon juice
2 tablespoons nutritional yeast
½ teaspoon salt
2 cloves garlic, peeled and minced
¼ cup water
4 tablespoons minced herbs (parsley, chives, and basil are best)

Lasagna

3 tablespoons veggie broth
3 large portobello mushrooms, sliced
2 cups baby spinach
1 large jar organic marinara sauce
About ½ packet of gluten-free, no-cook lasagna noodles
2 tablespoons vegan Parmesan

Preheat the oven to 375 degrees F.

Create the "ricotta" by blending all ingredients until smooth.

Heat the veggie broth in a large skillet and "sauté" the mushrooms until they are lightly browned. Set aside.

Grease a medium baking dish. Start with a layer of mushrooms. Cover this with a thin layer of spinach and then a layer of marinara sauce, then a layer of lasagna, and then a layer of the ricotta. Repeat until you've filled the pan or run out of ingredients.

Sprinkle the vegan Parmesan over the top and bake for 30 to 40 minutes or until it's bubbling and the edges are browned.

VEGAN PESTO MILLET BOWL

My husband and daughter can't get enough of this dish. It's simple comfort food at its best. Millet is a very healthy grain, which is packed with magnesium.

Serves 4

Polenta

1 cup millet, rinsed
1 teaspoon grape seed oil
2 cups water or veggie broth
½ teaspoon sea salt
1 tablespoon nutritional yeast
¼ tsp dried Italian herbs

Sauce

3 tablespoons veggie broth
1 medium onion, chopped
2 cloves garlic, minced
One 15-ounce can organic diced tomatoes

Topping

2 cups fresh basil leaves, plus additional for garnish
½ cup olive oil
1 clove garlic, peeled
½ cup pine nuts
½ teaspoon salt
2 cups baby spinach leaves
4 tablespoons Cashew Cream, Savory (page 261)
Handful of fresh basil leaves

Heat 1 teaspoon of grape seed oil in a heavy skillet, and toast millet (constantly stirring) until a nutty aroma is released (5–6 minutes). Transfer to a saucepan. Add the water or broth. Turn heat down to low, cover pan, and simmer until all liquid is absorbed (about 15 minutes). Stir in nutritional yeast and Italian seasoning.

To create the sauce, heat the veggie broth in a heavy saucepan and "sauté" the onions and garlic until soft. Add the tomatoes and simmer on a low heat for 15 minutes.

Meanwhile, place basil, olive oil, garlic, pine nuts, and salt in a high-speed blender and blend until thoroughly combined.

Steam the spinach.

Place a generous mound of millet in each bowl. Cover with a generous helping of the sauce, followed by a spoonful of spinach, 1 tablespoon of the basil mixture, and 1 tablespoon of cashew cream. Top with a couple of fresh basil leaves.

VEGGIE AND PORTOBELLO MUSHROOM CURRY

This is a great go-to in my house. Aside from the fact that I love a curry, this is a one-pot dish, which makes life very easy.

Serves 4

2 medium portobello mushrooms, cubed
1 large yellow onion, chopped
3 medium carrots, sliced
2 large sweet potatoes, peeled and cubed
2 cups vegetable broth
1 cup coconut milk
1 tablespoon lemon juice
1 teaspoon salt
1 tablespoon curry powder
1 teaspoon ground turmeric
2 tablespoons minced fresh ginger root
2 cloves garlic, peeled and minced
2 cups cauliflower florets
½ cup chopped cilantro

Add all the ingredients except the cilantro into your slow cooker and cook for 4 to 5 hours on a medium setting. Garnish with cilantro.

VEGGIE HOT POT

I make this simple veggie hot pot almost every week and use up whatever veggies I need to. It's so clean and simple, and yet exquisite because the taste of the veggies is elevated in this simple broth. Feel free to substitute with whatever veggies you need to use up.

Serves 4

1 inch ginger root, peeled
3 cloves garlic, peeled
½ cup mirin (Japanese cooking wine)
½ cup vegetable broth
1 yellow onion, peeled
1 head of broccoli
½ green cabbage
1 small bunch of watercress, trimmed
4 medium carrots
1 cluster of trumpet or enoki mushrooms
1 cup sugar snap or snow peas
½ bunch asparagus
8-ounce block firm tofu, cubed (optional)
One package buckwheat noodles
Handful of sesame seeds
Tamari sauce for seasoning

Ideally, you need a large, heavy-bottomed enamel pan or Dutch oven. Place the ginger, garlic, mirin, and broth in the pan. Place the whole onion in the center and arrange the veggies and tofu all around it. Simmer on a low heat for 12 to 15 minutes.

While the pot is simmering, cook the noodles according to package directions.

Divide the noodles between four bowls, then spoon the broth and veggies on top. Finally, sprinkle with sesame seeds and season to taste with the tamari sauce.

●●

VEGGIE TACOS

My family and I love tacos, so I found a way of making the taco "meat" filling out of vegan ingredients that would pass muster with my husband and daughter. This recipe was a home run!

Serves 2

"Meat"

1 cup green lentils
1 cup walnuts, toasted
½ cup oil-packed sun-dried tomatoes
1½ teaspoons smoked paprika
1 teaspoon ground chili powder
Sea salt and pepper, to taste

Avocado Cream

2 avocados
Juice of 1 lime
¼ cup silken tofu
Sea salt and pepper, to taste

Tacos

4 large romaine lettuce leaves*
1 red bell pepper, sliced thinly
½ red onion, sliced thinly
A handful of fresh cilantro

To make the "meat," cook the lentils in a pot of boiling water for 20 to 25 minutes or until soft. Drain and allow them to cool off. Once cool, place them in food processor with the other ingredients and pulse until the mixture resembles crumbles.

While the lentils are cooling, blend together the ingredients of the avocado cream until smooth.

When you are ready to serve, lay the romaine leaves out on two plates. Fill with the taco "meat" and top with pepper, onion, cilantro, and avocado cream.

*You can use corn taco shells, but I prefer to use crunchy lettuce.

SIDES AND SALADS

....

ALKALIZING SALAD

This crispy salad is so full of clean goodness and will help to alkalize your system. I eat a variation of it at least three times per week.

Serves 2

Salad

1 bunch dinosaur kale, washed, stalks removed, and finely shredded
1 bunch watercress, washed, stalks removed, and roughly chopped
2 stalks celery, finely chopped
4 large radishes, halved and sliced
2 cups alfalfa sprouts
1 cup unsulfured apricots, chopped

Dressing

½ avocado
3 tablespoons silken tofu
2 tablespoons extra virgin olive oil or flaxseed oil
3 tablespoons filtered water
1 tablespoon apple cider vinegar
1 teaspoon lemon juice
1 teaspoon raw honey
½ teaspoon sea salt

For the salad, simply combine all ingredients in a large bowl.

For the dressing, blend all the ingredients in a food processor or blender until smooth and creamy.

To serve, split salad into two dishes and top with 1 large tablespoon of dressing each. This dressing will keep for up to three days in a sealed container.

....

GREEN SALAD

I love a fresh, green salad. The key is to use a variety of different leaves (not from a bag). The crunch comes from a fresh head of lettuce. Dial up the flavor with tons of fresh herbs.

Serves 2

4 cups of mixed leaves (Romaine, Red Oak, Frissee etc)
1 cup fresh herbs, chopped (mint, basil, chives, parsley etc)
2 cups blanced (steamed for 1 minute) broccoli florets
2 Persian cucumbers, sliced
1 sliced apple or Kiwi
½ ripe avocado sliced

Dressing:

1tbsp olive oil
1/2tbsp lemon juice
2tsp Braggs Amino Acids

....

EVERYTHING SALAD

When I'm really hungry, I like to make an "Everything" salad, which basically means I raid my fridge/freezer and pantry in order to make a salad that is hearty and satisfying, and which uses up what might be hanging around in my crisper drawer. Here are some ideas: Lettuce, spinach, kale, cucumber, carrots, shaved beets, fennel, olives, mushrooms, chickpeas, edamame, baked tofu, marinated artichokes, sun dried tomatoes, nuts and seeds.

Dress your salad with loads of fresh lemon juice and a little good-quality olive oil.

ARTICHOKE-OLIVE HUMMUS

Everyone goes crazy for the artichoke-and-olive hummus at my farmers' market, but it's *so* easy to make!

Serves 4

One 15-ounce can organic garbanzo beans (chickpeas)
¼ cup lemon juice
½ cup raw tahini
1 small garlic clove, peeled
1 tablespoon extra virgin olive oil
½ teaspoon sea salt
½ teaspoon ground cumin
2 to 3 tablespoons water
3 oil-packed artichoke hearts
8 pitted Kalamata olives

Simply pop all the ingredients except the artichoke hearts and olives into a food processor and blend until smooth. Add the artichokes and olives and pulse until they are well chopped but not pureed.

Your hummus will keep in an airtight container in your fridge for up to one week.

BEET AND CARROT SLAW

I love a slaw with the sweet, earthy taste of raw beets. I make this in about two minutes by using the grater attachment on my food processor.

Serves 2

Slaw

2 large beets, peeled and grated
4 large carrots, peeled and grated
½ cup sunflower seeds
½ cup fresh flat-leaf parsley, chopped

Dressing

1 cup extra virgin olive oil
¼ cup apple cider vinegar
1 teaspoon Dijon mustard
1 teaspoon raw honey
Sea salt, to taste

In a large bowl, combine the slaw ingredients. In a separate bowl, whisk together the dressing ingredients. Add the dressing to the slaw and mix well.

CAULIFLOWER MASH

This is way healthier and more delicious than regular mashed potatoes. It's also easier to make!

Serves 4

1 large organic cauliflower, chopped (whole, not just florets)
2 tablespoons veggie broth
2 cloves garlic, peeled and minced
1 teaspoon lemon zest
Sea salt and freshly ground pepper, to taste

Steam the cauliflower for 15 minutes or until tender when a fork is inserted. Transfer to a high-speed blender or food processor. Add the other ingredients and blend until smooth.

CHIA CAESAR DRESSING

I love to toss this dressing on crunchy romaine leaves with crispy sourdough croutons.

Serves 2

½ cup extra virgin olive oil
1 tablespoon lemon juice

2 cloves garlic, peeled

1 teaspoon onion powder

1 teaspoon Dijon mustard

1 teaspoon vegetarian Worcestershire sauce

1 teaspoon chia seeds

In a blender, blend all the ingredients except the chia seeds. Transfer to serving jug or glass jar and mix in the chia seeds.

CURRIED WALDORF SALAD

This is my favorite fall and winter salad because I can make good use of the crunchy, organic apples that are abundant in the farmers' markets then. This salad is also filling and satisfying, especially when served with a warm, whole wheat pita.

Serves 2

Salad

1 unpeeled apple, diced into large chunks

1 cup thinly chopped celery

1 cup seedless grapes, halved

½ cup pecans, toasted

3 cups baby spinach

Dressing

½ cup plain yogurt

⅓ cup vegan mayo

1 teaspoon grated lemon zest

1 tablespoon fresh lemon juice

2 teaspoons curry powder

½ teaspoon agave nectar or honey

Combine all the salad ingredients in a large bowl. In a separate bowl, whisk together the dressing ingredients. Drizzle the dressing over the salad and toss carefully, making sure everything is well coated.

DANDELION, APPLE, AND CHICKPEA SALAD

I love using dandelion leaves because they are great for cleansing your liver, and who doesn't need a bit of a liver cleanse every now and again? Dandelion leaves, however, can be a bit bitter, so I like to sauté them and then pair them with the sweetness of a crisp apple. This salad takes a few minutes to throw together and makes a perfect fall lunch or dinner appetizer.

Serves 2 to 4

One 15-ounce can organic garbanzo beans (chickpeas)
2 tablespoons raw virgin coconut oil
1 large clove garlic, peeled and minced
¼ teaspoon red pepper flakes
2 cups dandelion leaves, washed and removed from stems
2 medium crisp apples, peeled, cored, and roughly chopped
Balsamic vinegar (make sure it's aged vinegar—as in the thick, syrupy stuff)
Sea salt and pepper, to taste

Rinse and drain the garbanzo beans. Heat the oil in a large skillet and add the garlic, red pepper flakes, and dandelion leaves. Sauté over a medium heat until the leaves have wilted. Remove from heat.

Arrange the garbanzo beans on a dish and top with the wilted greens. Top with the apple pieces and drizzle with balsamic vinegar. Season with sea salt and pepper.

GORGEOUSLY GREEN TRAIL MIX

This is my go-to trail mix. I always make a large batch and keep it in an airtight canister on my counter.

Serves 4

1 cup raw cashews
1 cup raw sunflower seeds
½ cup goji berries

½ cup cacao nibs
½ cup dried, unsweetened coconut flakes

Preheat the oven to 400 degrees F.

Soak the cashews and sunflower seeds for 20 minutes in separate bowls of 2 cups of water each.

Drain the cashews and sunflower seeds. Pat them dry and lay them on a parchment paper–lined baking sheet.

Place in the oven for 10 minutes or until they are just about to turn brown. Remove and allow them to cool.

When the nuts and seeds are completely cool, place them in a canister along with the other ingredients and mix well.

GREEK SALAD

I only make Greek salad when I can find really good organic tomatoes, because hothouse tomatoes in the winter months taste watery. In the summer, this salad is bursting with insane flavors and reminds me of sitting in a little Greek taverna.

Serves 4

Salad

6 large organic tomatoes, roughly chopped
6 organic Persian or regular cucumbers, roughly chopped
1 cup pitted Kalamata olives
½ red onion, thinly sliced
4 ounces feta or soy cheese, cubed

Dressing

1 cup extra virgin olive oil
Juice of 1 lemon
Pinch of dried oregano
Sea salt and cracked pepper, to taste

Combine all the salad ingredients in a large bowl. In a separate bowl, whisk together the dressing ingredients. Drizzle the dressing over the salad and toss carefully, making sure everything is well coated.

KALE AND SEAWEED SALAD

Many of the raw restaurants and delis in Los Angeles offer variations on this crunchy and nutritious salad, but they are soooooo expensive! I say, make your own every time.

Serves 2 to 4

Salad

¾ ounce dried wakame seaweed (soaked in warm water for 5 to 10 minutes, then cut into thin strips)
1 large bunch dinosaur kale, washed, removed from stems, and shredded
1 tablespoon sesame seeds
2 tablespoons pumpkin seeds, toasted (optional)

Dressing

1 tablespoon toasted sesame oil
3 tablespoons raw tahini
3 tablespoons lemon juice
2 tablespoons tamari
½ inch ginger, peeled and grated
1 garlic clove, peeled and minced

Rinse and drain the seaweed. Combine it with the kale in a large bowl. Place all the dressing ingredients in a high-speed blender and blend until smooth. Dress the salad and sprinkle with the sesame and pumpkin seeds.

KELP NOODLE SALAD

I've recently discovered kelp noodles, and I'm pretty smitten. I've seen them in Whole Foods for months now, but just passed them by, not really knowing what on earth I would do with them. Then I noticed what it said on the package: "Great in Salads." I wasn't entirely convinced, especially when I saw my husband's expression when he caught a glimpse of them, but I carried on regardless. The result was a divinely crunchy, light, and tasty salad. I'm hooked!

Serves 2

Salad

6 to 8 romaine leaves
One 12-ounce package kelp noodles
1 large carrot, peeled and cut into matchsticks
1 large Persian cucumber, cut into matchsticks
½ avocado, sliced
Handful cilantro, chopped

Dressing

¼ cup miso
2 tablespoons rice vinegar
2 tablespoons soy sauce
½ teaspoon minced fresh ginger
1 teaspoon raw honey

Wash and dry the lettuce leaves and arrange them on a plate. Rinse the kelp noodles under cold water and drain. Blend the dressing ingredients, adding a little water if it seems too thick. Dress the noodles and add the carrots and cucumber. Pile the noodles on top of the lettuce leaves and top with avocado and cilantro.

QUINOA-MILLET APRICOT SALAD

I love to mix healthy protein-packed grains, which is why I created this tasty and satisfying salad.

Serves 2

½ cup quinoa
½ cup millet
½ cup shelled pistachios
1 cup dried or fresh apricots, sliced
2 scallions, chopped finely
1 cup baked tofu, diced (optional)
½ cup olive oil
Juice of 1 lemon
¼ cup fresh cilantro, chopped
¼ cup fresh mint, chopped
Sea salt and pepper, to taste

Mix the grains together and rinse well. Bring 2 cups water to a boil in a heavy saucepan and add the grains. Reduce heat to medium, cover, and simmer for 15 to 20 minutes or until the water is absorbed. Remove from heat and let sit, covered, for 5 minutes. Chill the grains in the fridge for about 30 minutes.

While the grains are in the fridge, toast your pistachios in a dry cast-iron skillet for a few minutes. Be sure to keep moving them around the pan, or they will burn! When they seem gently toasted, remove, and allow them to cool.

Remove your grains from the fridge and transfer them to a large bowl, and add the pistachios and all the other ingredients. Make sure your salad is well tossed before serving.

This salad stays fresh in your fridge in an airtight container for up to three days.

ROASTED BEET, ORANGE, AND HAZELNUT SALAD

I could eat roasted beets almost every day of the week. And hazelnuts are so healthy that I wanted to find a way to incorporate them into a crunchy salad. When I combined them with the beets and succulent sweet oranges, they found their perfect mates.

Serves 2

Salad

4 to 5 medium beets, peeled and cut into bite-size wedges
1 medium orange
1 avocado, sliced
1 cup feta or crumbly goat cheese
½ cup hazelnuts, toasted in a hot oven for 10 minutes

Dressing

1 medium orange
1 tablespoon red wine vinegar
1 teaspoon honey
3 tablespoons extra virgin olive oil
Sea salt and pepper, to taste
½ teaspoon Dijon mustard
1 teaspoon cumin seeds, lightly crushed

Preheat the oven to 400 degrees F.

Place the beets in a roasting pan.

Grate the zest of one orange into a small bowl and squeeze the juice into another small bowl.

Whisk together the vinegar, honey, and olive oil and season with sea salt and pepper. Divide this mixure between two bowls. Whisk the mustard into one of the bowls and set aside. Whisk the cumin, orange zest, and orange juice into the other bowl and then pour this mixture over the beets. Make sure each wedge is well coated.

Lightly cover the roasting pan with foil before placing it in the oven for 50 minutes. Remove when done and leave to cool.

Peel the other orange and cut away all the pith. Using a sharp paring knife, cut the segments away from the dividing membranes.

When you are ready to assemble, carefully place the beets in a large bowl and add the orange segments. Top with the avocado, cheese crumbles, and toasted hazelnuts. Drizzle the mustard dressing over the salad, taking care not to toss or mix the salad, as you don't want everything to turn pink.

STEAMED GREEN VEGGIES

You obviously can't eat enough of these. Whether it's spinach, kale, or chard, just know that the more leafy greens you can get into your body, the better.

Serves 2

4 to 6 cups greens (my favorite is Swiss chard), stems and stalks removed, and roughly chopped
1 clove garlic, pressed in a garlic press
2 teaspoons tamari sauce

Place the greens in a heavy stainless-steel pan with a tight-fitting lid. Add about 2 tablespoons of water. Cover and place over a very low heat. Steam the greens for 3 to 4 minutes or until fully wilted. Remove from heat and drain off any excess water.

Place the greens in a bowl. Add garlic and tamari sauce.

WARM LENTIL AND ROASTED TOMATO SALAD

My mother taught me to make this salad because we both adore green lentils—they give me energy and fill me up.

Serves 2 to 4

Salad

2 cups cherry tomatoes, organic if possible
1 large red onion, peeled and cut into chunks
2 tablespoons olive oil
1 teaspoon ground cumin
1 teaspoon sea salt
2 cups green lentils
3 cups water
4 tablespoons Cashew Cream, Savory (see page 261)
¼ teaspoon chipotle paste*
1 avocado, sliced (optional)

Dressing

½ cup extra virgin olive oil
1 tablespoon red wine vinegar
Juice of 1 lime
1 teaspoon chopped parsley or cilantro
1 teaspoon honey
Salt and pepper, to taste

Preheat the oven to 375 degrees F.

Place the tomatoes and onions on a baking sheet, keeping them separate, and drizzle with the olive oil. Using your fingers, massage the oil in, then sprinkle with cumin and salt and place in the oven for 35 to 40 minutes or until everything is browned and slightly shriveled. Remove these from the oven and allow to cool for 10 minutes.

While the vegetables are roasting, place the lentils and the water in a heavy saucepan and bring to a boil. Boil for 25 minutes and then drain off any excess water. Allow to cool.

While the lentils cool, whisk together the dressing ingredients.

In a small bowl, mix the cashew cream and chipotle paste.

Spoon the lentils onto a platter and gently mix in the onions. Top with the tomatoes, taking care not to mix them in. Dress the salad and then drizzle the chipotle–cashew cream mix over the top. Top with avocado.

*I make my paste by blasting a can of chipotle chilis in adobo sauce in my blender. You can find this in the ethnic section in large grocery stores. Once you've made the puree, it will keep in an airtight container in your fridge for months.

WARM QUINOA AND BUTTERNUT SQUASH SALAD

This is one of my favorite winter supper dishes because it's hearty and so tasty. It keeps well for a couple of days and can be eaten cold or reheated.

Serves 2

Salad

2 cups butternut squash, cubed

1 tablespoon olive oil

1 cup quinoa (red quinoa, if possible)

2 cups vegetable stock

1 sprig rosemary

1 small bunch broccolini (or broccoli florets), chopped into bite-size pieces

1 Granny Smith apple, peeled, cored, and cubed

2 cups Swiss chard, stalks and veins removed, roughly chopped

½ cup slivered almonds

Dressing

1 cup orange juice

¼ cup raw honey

½ cup white balsamic vinegar

1 cup extra virgin olive oil

½ teaspoon salt

Reduce the orange juice down to ½ cup by simmering in a pan. Chill until cool. Mix with other dressing ingredients and set aside.

Preheat the oven to 400 degrees F. Sprinkle the butternut squash cubes with the olive oil, spread evenly on a baking sheet, and roast until tender, about 20 minutes.

Place the quinoa in a small saucepan with the stock and the rosemary. Bring it to a boil, then turn down the heat to low and simmer for 15 minutes or until the quinoa grains become translucent. When cooked, drain and toss in a little olive oil.

Blanch the broccolini by adding it to a pan of boiling water for 1 minute, then removing.

Sauté the apple, Swiss chard, and blanched broccolini.

In a small bowl, whisk together the dressing ingredients. Combine all the vegetables and the quinoa and mix with the dressing. Top with almonds.

Chapter 13

Skin Care Recipes

I've been making my own skin potions for years. Some are better than others, but, on the whole, if you have time, making your own is a great money-saver, and it's fun! Some of these are used in your 30-day program, but some are just included in case you might be interested in trying them out.

If you're having trouble finding any of the ingredients listed, please go to www.sophieuliano.com to see some recommendations about where to buy.

FACIAL RECIPES

KELP FACIAL SCRUB

Kelp is so great for your skin because it's very rich in minerals. I simply adore this dry facial scrub. Keep it in your shower and use it every morning.

8-ounce clean plastic jar
1 cup instant oatmeal
½ cup kelp powder
½ cup dried milk powder (optional if you are vegan)
2 teaspoons cornmeal

Place all the ingredients in a high-speed blender, and pulse until it becomes a fine powder. Pour into the jar.

When you are in the shower or at the sink, pour a little into the palm of your hand. Add enough water to make a paste, and gently massage in circular motions over your face, neck, and chest. Rinse off.

As long as you don't get water in your scrub, it will last for up to six months.

· ·

CARROT AND MANGO BUTTER CLEANSER

4-ounce glass jar, sterilized*
⅔ cup mango butter
¼ cup shea butter
4 teaspoons jojoba oil
2 teaspoons carrot seed oil
¼ teaspoon vitamin E oil
2 teaspoons beeswax pellets

Melt all the ingredients in a small metal bowl set over a saucepan of boiling water. Everything should melt after about 4 minutes.

Pour the mixture into the jar and allow it to cool before screwing on the lid. You can keep your butter cleanser in a cabinet for up to six months.

*You can sterilize this by putting it through a hot wash in your dishwasher or dunking it in a pan of just-boiled water.

GREEN TEA TONER

This is one of my favorite summer toners, because it's uplifting, refreshing, and filled with antioxidants. It's also insanely easy to make!

2-ounce glass bottle, sterilized*
1 organic green tea bag
1 organic peppermint tea bag
½ cup aloe vera juice

Steep the green tea and peppermint tea bags each in half a cup of boiling water for 10 minutes, and allow them to cool.

Pour ¼ cup of each infusion into a liquid-measuring cup and add the aloe vera juice. Pour the mixture into the bottle. Use the toner each morning and evening after cleansing and exfoliating. Keep refrigerated and use up within one month.

*You can sterilize this by putting it through a hot wash in your dishwasher or dunking in a pot of just-boiled water for a few seconds.

ANTIBACTERIAL TONER

Vinegar is antiseptic and dissolves fatty, oily deposits on the skin. This makes it perfect for toning. Apple cider vinegar is rich in vitamins and minerals, so it's perfect for this recipe.

1-ounce dark glass bottle, sterilized*
2 tablespoons organic apple cider vinegar
1 cup distilled water
2 drops rosemary essential oil
3 drops lavender essential oil

Mix together all ingredients and transfer them to the bottle. Keep refrigerated and use up within one month.

*You can sterilize this by putting it through a hot wash in your dishwasher or dunking in a pot of just-boiled water for a few seconds.

VITAMIN C SERUM

Vitamin C is one of the most powerful tried and tested antiaging ingredients. That being said, it's very unstable. As soon as it's added to a lotion or cream, it begins to oxidize, thus losing its efficacy. The best way you can get it onto your skin is to deliver it straight on in its dry powder form.

Small glass jar with airtight lid, sterilized*
1 tablespoon aloe vera gel
¼ teaspoon vitamin C powder**
1 teaspoon distilled water

Simply mix the ingredients together and seal in the jar. Keep this in a cool, dark spot and remake it once or twice a week, making sure you sterilize the container each time.

Apply this every morning over your face, neck, and chest after cleansing. If your skin is really sensitive, reduce the amount of vitamin C powder by half.

*You can sterilize this by putting it through a hot wash in your dishwasher or dunking in a pot of just-boiled water for a few seconds.

**I've been fiddling around and experimenting lately with my homemade vitamin C serums and was *thrilled* to find a powdered L-ascorbic acid that actually dissolves, because the particles are small enough. Until now, I was using edible powdered vitamin C, and it never dissolved completely. You can find this excellent powdered vitamin C L-ascorbic acid at Making Cosmetics (www.makingcosmetics.com).

EYE SERUMS

You're better off using a lighter oil for around the delicate eye area. Hazelnut oil is perfect, and it penetrates easily. If you are allergic to nuts, you can substitute with grape seed oil.

For women in their 20s and 30s

1-ounce dark glass bottle, sterilized*

4 tablespoons hazelnut oil

12 drops borage seed oil

6 drops German chamomile essential oil

6 drops carrot seed oil

For women in their 40s and beyond

1-ounce dark glass bottle, sterilized*

4 tablespoons hazelnut oil

1 teaspoon evening primrose oil

½ teaspoon borage seed oil

12 drops palma rosa essential oil

12 drops lavender essential oil

½ teaspoon vitamin E oil

14 drops carrot seed essential oil

Mix the ingredients together and use a small funnel to pour the mixture into the bottle. Gently apply the eye serum around the eye area, taking care not to get it in your eyes. Let it absorb for about 10 minutes and then gently wipe away any excess oil with a cotton swab.

Keep your eye serums in a cool, dark cabinet and use within one year.

*You can sterilize this by putting it through a hot wash in your dishwasher or dunking in a pot of just-boiled water for a few seconds.

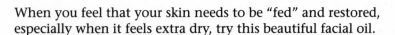

RESTORATIVE FACIAL OIL

When you feel that your skin needs to be "fed" and restored, especially when it feels extra dry, try this beautiful facial oil.

2-ounce dark glass bottle, sterilized*

1 tablespoon apricot oil

1 teaspoon rose hip seed oil

1 teaspoon macadamia nut oil

6 drops calendula essential oil

6 drops rose absolute essential oil

Mix all the ingredients in a small bowl or jug and use a funnel to transfer to the bottle.

Apply this at night two to three times a week. Use within one year.

*You can sterilize this by putting it through a hot wash in your dishwasher or dunking in a pot of just-boiled water for a few seconds.

•••

FACIAL OIL FOR BALANCING OILY OR PROBLEM SKIN

It's really important to remember that acne and oily skin are produced by overactive sebaceous glands. This overactivity can occur during times of hormonal change, such as puberty and postmenopause. Ironically, we are encouraged to scrub and clean our skin of any excess sebum when we have this skin condition. However, it's the overzealous cleaning that can lead to even more sebum production: the skin feels it isn't producing enough, so it then produces bucketloads to compensate. Fortunately, there are a number of essential oils that are great for balancing over-oily skin.

2-ounce dark glass bottle, sterilized*
4 tablespoons hazelnut or grape seed oil
16 drops juniper essential oil
20 drops geranium essential oil
20 drops lemon essential oil
4 drops rosemary essential oil

Mix all the ingredients and use a small funnel to pour into the bottle.

Apply this oil at night, and then blot your face with a tissue to remove any excess. Use within one year.

*You can sterilize this by putting it through a hot wash in your dishwasher or dunking in a pot of just-boiled water for a few seconds.

FACIAL OIL TREATMENTS FOR ROSACEA

Rosacea is an embarrassing condition that mostly begins after the age of 30. It presents itself as red, inflamed skin with pustules and pimples. There are many treatments for it, including antibiotics, but I've found that the following oils have helped a lot of my readers.

Morning Oil

1-ounce amber glass dropper bottle, sterilized*
4 tablespoons of sweet almond oil
30 drops of German chamomile essential oil
30 drops of parsley seed essential oil

Nighttime Oil

1-ounce amber glass dropper bottle, sterilized*
4 tablespoons sweet almond oil
10 drops galbanum essential oil
30 drops carrot seed essential oil
20 drops German chamomile essential oil
30 drops parsley seed essential oil

Mix the ingredients together and use a small funnel to pour each mixture into the bottle.

Shake each oil gently before using. Keep in a cool, dark spot for up to one year.

*You can sterilize this by putting it through a hot wash in your dishwasher or dunking in a pot of just-boiled water for a few seconds.

Home Treatment for Blackheads

If your blackheads are bad and you cannot afford to get an extraction facial, try this DIY facial, which is quite brilliant.

Fill a bowl with boiling water. Add 2 drops of lavender essential oil and quickly place a towel over it. Make an opening in the towel in which to insert your face, and allow your face to steam for 5 minutes.

Fill a sink with hot water and 3 teaspoons of apple cider vinegar. Rinse your face with this water. Wash your hands really well with clean water and rub a couple of drops of lavender oil between your fingers. Cover your "squeezing" fingers with facial tissue and use the sides of your fingers (*not* your nails) to gently squeeze your blackheads, taking care not to damage the surrounding skin. If a blackhead doesn't slip out relatively easily, leave it alone!

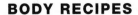

BODY RECIPES

Scrubs

....

GOOD MORNING COFFEE CELLULITE SCRUB

I love this scrub in my morning shower. The coffee contains caffeine and antioxidants, both of which are helpful in anticellulite treatments.

16-ounce Mason jar, sterilized*
1 cup brown sugar
1 cup grape seed oil
1 teaspoon pure vanilla extract
½ cup freshly ground coffee
10 drops grapefruit essential oil

Place the brown sugar in the jar. Pour the oil over it, and add the remaining ingredients. Stir well.

Once your jar has been opened and is sitting on the side of your bathtub or shower, you might get a little water in it as you scoop the goop. If you do, the shelf life will be greatly diminished because once you add water into the mix, bacteria can breed. I recommend trying to scoop out of the jar as far away from the shower as you can. If it does get a little water in it, you should use it up within one month. If you keep it dry, it will last for six months.

*You can sterilize this by putting it through a hot wash in your dishwasher or dunking in a pot of just-boiled water for a few seconds.

Be Careful!

Body scrubs can leave an oily residue on the floor of your shower or tub, which can be really dangerous in terms of slipping. I recommend wiping out your tub or shower with a vinegar-spritzed wad of paper towel after using a scrub or a bath oil.

LEMON EUCALYPTUS MUSCLE RELAXING SCRUB

I love this scrub after I've worked out hard because the Epsom salts help to release tight and tired muscles, and the eucalyptus is both refreshing and soothing.

16-ounce Mason jar, sterilized*
2 cups Epsom salts
1½ cups grape seed oil
2 tablespoons grated lemon zest
15 drops lemon essential oil
15 drops eucalyptus essential oil

Place the Epsom salts in the jar and add the oil. Use a teaspoon to stir in your remaining ingredients.

Once your jar has been opened and is sitting on the side of your bathtub or shower, you might get a little water in it as you scoop the goop. If you do, the shelf life will be greatly diminished because once you add water into the mix, bacteria can breed. I recommend trying to scoop out of the jar as far away from the shower as you can. If it does get a little water in it, you should use it up within one month. If you keep it dry, it will last for six months.

*You can sterilize this by putting it through a hot wash in your dishwasher or dunking in a pot of just-boiled water for a few seconds.

INDULGENT CHOCOLATE ROSE SUGAR SCRUB

This scrub is so yummy smelling that you'll want to gobble it up. The dried rose petals add an element of luxury to this sugar scrub, which makes it a perfect gift.

16-ounce Mason jar, sterilized*
2 cups brown sugar
2 cups sweet almond oil
2 tablespoons raw cacao powder
2 tablespoons dried rose petals**
10 drops geranium essential oil

Place the sugar in the jar and cover it with the oil. Use a teaspoon to gently stir in the remaining ingredients.

Once your jar has been opened and is sitting on the side of your bathtub or shower, you might get a little water in it as you scoop the goop. If you do, the shelf life will be greatly diminished because once you add water into the mix, bacteria can breed. I recommend trying to scoop out of the jar as far away from the shower as you can. If it does get a little water in it, you should use it up within one month. If you keep it dry, it will last for six months.

*You can sterilize this by putting it through a hot wash in your dishwasher or dunking in a pot of just-boiled water for a few seconds.

**If you buy dried rose petals in bulk, they will be almost small enough to toss straight into your scrub; however, I like to pulse mine a couple of times in a blender to make them a little smaller. Be careful not to over-grind them, because you still want to be able to see little pieces.

LIQUID HAND AND BODY SOAP

The advantage of making your own hand and body soap is that you can customize it. I like to use a simple base of liquid Castile soap and add the essential oil blends that I love.

16-ounce pump dispenser bottle
16 ounces liquid Castile soap
1 teaspoon aloe vera gel
1 teaspoon vegetable glycerin
¼ teaspoon peppermint pure essential oil
¼ teaspoon lavender pure essential oil

Whisk the ingredients together in a glass liquid-measuring cup, then transfer to the bottle using a funnel.

Use within three months.

NOURISHING BATH AND BODY OIL

This is a simple, beautiful oil that you can either add to your bath or massage into your body.

4-ounce dark glass bottle, sterilized*
4 tablespoons sweet almond oil
2 tablespoons apricot kernel oil
2 tablespoons avocado oil
10 drops frankincense essential oil
30 drops palma rosa essential oil
15 drops neroli essential oil
40 drops lavender essential oil

Mix all the ingredients together and use a funnel to pour into the bottle. You can use this directly on your skin or add about 2 teaspoons to your bath water.

Keep in a cool, dark place for up to one year.

*You can sterilize this by putting it through a hot wash in your dishwasher or dunking in a pot of just-boiled water for a few seconds.

ANTICELLULITE OIL

Although you can't totally get rid of cellulite, you can improve its appearance by using this wonderfully detoxifying oil after dry brushing (page 147) and showering. When your skin is still warm, massage this oil into areas of cellulite.

2-ounce dark glass bottle, sterilized*
1 ounce grape seed oil
5 drops black pepper essential oil
5 drops grapefruit essential oil
5 drops fennel essential oil
5 drops juniper berry essential oil

Mix all the ingredients together and use a funnel to put into the bottle.

Use this oil up to three days a week. Store it in a cool, dark place for up to one year.

*You can sterilize this by putting it through a hot wash in your dishwasher or dunking in a pot of just-boiled water for a few seconds.

ANTIAGING LOTION PUSH-UP BAR

I'm obsessed with these little push-up lotion bars. They are so easy to make (I promise), and each one is chock full of seriously antiaging oils, butters, and essential oils. They are wonderful for smoothing over your legs, arms, and stomach—anywhere that feels extra dry. Because of the amazing antiaging ingredients, it's a perfect stick for your chest, too. (You can use it on your face, but it's a little too greasy for me. I'd only recommend it if you have very dry facial skin.) It's *perfect* to take on vacation, because after you've been in the sun all day, your skin will drink it up.

5 push-up tubes
1 ounce beeswax pellets

4 ounces macadamia nut oil*
2½ ounces shea butter
1½ ounce cocoa butter
1 teaspoon sea buckthorn oil
20 drops frankincense essential oil
15 drops ylang ylang essential oil

Place all the ingredients except for the sea buckthorn oil and the essential oils in a small steel or glass bowl and place over a saucepan of boiling water (use a bain-marie if you have one).

Turn down the heat to medium and melt the oils while stirring with the end of a wooden spoon or a popsicle stick.

As soon as the oils and butters have melted, remove the bowl from the heat and quickly add the sea buckthorn oil and the essential oils. Pour the mixture into a pouring jug and fill the push-up tubes—you have to work quickly here because the waxes and butters will start to set pretty quickly.

Leave the tubes to cool for at least 2 hours.

Store the bars in a cool, dark place for up to six months.

*If you'd like to use something a little less expensive, you can substitute grape seed oil or sweet almond oil.

Tip: As soon as you are done pouring, use paper towels to wipe out the bowl and the pouring jug. Get as much off as you can, because it'll make them much easier to wash. Then hand wash with very hot water and dish soap. Don't put them in the dishwasher, because the wax residue will get baked on.

· ·

LEMONGRASS ANTIBACTERIAL DEODORANT

This is an outstanding deodorant paste that is my daily go-to.

2-ounce glass jar with airtight lid
2 tablespoons coconut oil
2 tablespoons shea butter

⅓ cup baking soda

¼ cup arrowroot powder

6 drops lemongrass pure essential oil

Place the coconut oil and the shea butter in a double boiler over low heat and stir until it has all melted. Remove from the heat and whisk in the baking soda and the arrowroot powder. Stir in the essential oil and then pour into the jar.

At room temperature, the deodorant will be soft; if you want it to be more solid, store it in the fridge.

Store in a cool, dark spot and use within six months.

GREEN TEA SUNSCREEN

After much experimentation, I finally came up with this winning formula and I'm sooooo excited to share the recipe with you. I wanted to make a sunscreen with natural oils and butters that really nourish your skin (and contain their own natural sunscreens). This creamy, moisturizing sunscreen smells amazing and won't leave your skin shiny or powdery.

4-ounce dark glass jar, sterilized*

1 organic green tea bag

1 tablespoon mango butter

1 tablespoon shea butter

1 tablespoon avocado oil

1 tablespoon jojoba oil

1 teaspoon beeswax pellets

½ teaspoon vitamin E oil

4 tablespoons green tea

4 teaspoons zinc oxide powder

6 drops ylang ylang essential oil

6 drops vanilla essential oil

Make the green tea by steeping the tea bag in half a cup of hot water for 5 minutes. For this, I recommend that you boil the water and leave it to cool for about 5 minutes before steeping.

Meanwhile, place the butters, oils, and beeswax in a small stainless-steel bowl over a saucepan of boiling water. Allow the butters and wax to melt completely and then remove from the heat. This should only take a couple of minutes.

Add 1 tablespoon of warm green tea to the oil mixture and whisk vigorously. Repeat until you have added 4 tablespoons of green tea. Next, add the zinc oxide and whisk *vigorously* to ensure that there are no lumps. Finally, whisk in the essential oils.

Pour the mixture into the jar and keep it in a cool, dark spot for up to one month or in the fridge for up to three months. When it is refrigerated, it will harden, so take it out a few hours prior to using.

Texture: You can play with the texture by adding more green tea if it feels too thick.

SPF: This cream has an approximate SPF of 20. Make sure you reapply at least every 2 hours, because it is not waterproof.

*You can sterilize this by putting it through a hot wash in your dishwasher or dunking in a pot of just-boiled water for a few seconds.

. . . .

HAND BALM FOR DRY OR CRACKED HANDS

I give this balm to my mother, who always forgets to use rubber gloves in the kitchen and gardening gloves in the garden!

16-ounce dark glass jar, sterilized*
½ cup cocoa butter
½ cup shea butter
½ cup mango butter
½ cup sunflower oil
1 tablespoon jojoba oil
15 drops of geranium essential oil
15 drops patchouli essential oil

Melt the butters and oils together in a double boiler over low heat, stirring to remove lumps. Remove from heat and wait until oils cool, but don't let them solidify. As they begin to get thicker, whisk vigorously into a fluffy cream. Add the essential oils and spoon into the jar.

Keep in a cool, dark spot for up to one year.

*You can sterilize this by putting it through a hot wash in your dishwasher or dunking in a pot of just-boiled water for a few seconds.

Hair Recipes

. . . .

COCONUT MILK SHAMPOO

If you are trying to avoid the harsh foaming agents in conventional shampoos, you might want to give this nourishing shampoo recipe a try. The coconut milk is so hydrating for your hair that you'll want to use it at least once a week.

1 washed-out shampoo bottle (8 to16 ounces is fine)
⅓ cup unsweetened coconut milk
⅓ cup aloe vera juice
⅓ cup liquid Castile soap
10 drops lavender essential oil

Simply mix the ingredients together in a small liquid-measuring cup and pour into your shampoo bottle. Shake well before using, and use within one month.

. . . .

HOT-OIL HAIR TREATMENT

This is my favorite hair conditioning treatment, and it smells amazing. It does wonders for my overly heat-treated hair.

3 teaspoons jojoba oil

3 teaspoons avocado oil

3 teaspoons evening primrose oil or sunflower oil

1 teaspoon lemon juice

5 drops geranium essential oil

5 drops lavender essential oil

2 teaspoons apple cider vinegar

2 cups warm water

Gently heat the oils in a small bowl placed over a saucepan of boiling water (or a bain-marie). Heat for a minute or so until just warm. Remove from heat and apply the still-warm oil to your hair, making sure you massage it into your scalp. Cover your hair with a plastic shower cap—the disposable ones that you get at hotels are best—and wait for an hour.

When you are ready to rinse off the treatment, mix the vinegar and water together. First rinse your hair well under the shower, then use the vinegar solution as a final rinse.

. . . .

HAIR FOOD BALM

This is the most amazing multipurpose product. It can be used as a styling balm to tame flyaways and split ends; it can also be used as a deep-conditioning treatment. Finally, it is amazing for African American braids and/or dreadlocks.

4-ounce opaque glass jar

1 tablespoon shea butter

1 tablespoon olive oil

1 tablespoon avocado oil

1 tablespoon kukui nut oil

1 tablespoon coconut oil

2 teaspoons beeswax pellets

2 teaspoons vegetable glycerin

½ teaspoon castor oil

1 teaspoon honey

1 teaspoon panthenol
20 drops lavender essential oil
15 drops grapefruit seed extract

Place all the butter, oils, and beeswax in a double boiler over low heat and stir until everything has melted. Remove from the heat and stir in the remaining ingredients. Pour into the jar and allow it to set.

Keep it in a cool, dark cabinet and use within six months.

Perfume

. . . .

SOPHIE'S "GORGEOUS" BLEND PERFUME

I have always loved making my own perfumes because I feel like a scientist in my own kitchen, whipping up and experimenting with various concoctions. Perfumes are very personal, so you may want to play with various essential oils until you find a blend that you love. Remember that when you stock up on essential oils, they may seem expensive at first blush, but each bottle will last you for up to two years— you only use a few drops per perfume.

1-ounce dark glass bottle (screw cap or dropper is fine), sterilized*
A small funnel
1 tablespoon jojoba oil
5 drops sweet orange essential oil
10 drops grapefruit essential oil
10 drops frankincense essential oil
8 drops neroli essential oil
5 drops rose absolute (you can substitute with the less expensive geranium, if you like)

Using the funnel, pour the jojoba oil into the bottle. Add the drops in the order listed. Screw on the cap and leave the oils to mingle for a week.

Do a little patch test to make sure you are not allergic to any of the oils. To do this, apply 3 drops to the skin of your inner wrist, cover it with a Band-Aid, and leave it for 12 hours. If all is well, feel free to use this perfume on your wrists, neck, temples, and hair when you want to feel sensuous and gorgeous!

Keep it in a cool, dark cabinet and use within one year.

*You can sterilize this by putting it through a hot wash in your dishwasher or dunking in a pot of just-boiled water for a few seconds.

CONCLUSION

This is the true joy in life, the being used for a purpose recognized by yourself as a mighty one . . . being a force of nature instead of a feverish selfish little clod of ailments and grievances complaining that the world will not devote itself to making you happy.

I am of the opinion that my life belongs to the whole community and as long as I live it is my privilege to do for it whatever I can. I want to be thoroughly used up when I die, for the harder I work, the more I live. I rejoice in life for its own sake.

Life is no "brief candle" to me. It is a sort of splendid torch which I have got hold of for the moment; and I want to make it burn as brightly as possible before handing it on to future generations.

George Bernard Shaw

This quote by George Bernard Shaw is one of my all-time favorites. It lives on my fridge. When I read it, it fills me with a renewed sense of energy, purpose, and drive because I am reminded that life *is* a privilege and that it's my responsibility to live it to the fullest. I don't want to be that person who spends her life complaining that people are not making her happy. I want to *give* rather than receive, and I absolutely want to make that "splendid" torch burn as brightly as I can before handing it on to my beautiful daughter.

No matter what our circumstances are, we all possess that spark of fire deep within—that spark that can fire up the torch we've been given to hold until we pass on. I encourage you to hold your torch up as high as you can, because its light will burn away fear and doubt—and will allow your inner beauty to shine . . . for good!

BIBLIOGRAPHY

"1,4-Dioxane." Toxnet, Toxicology Data Network. http://toxnet.nlm.nih.gov /cpdb/chempages/1%2C4-DIOXANE.html.

"13th Report on Carcinogens (RoC)." National Toxicology Program, U.S. Department of Health and Human Services (2014). ntp.niehs.nih.gov/ntp/roc/twelfth/ profiles/butylatedhydroxyanisole.pdf.

"2,6-di-tert-butyl-p-cresol (BHT)." *UNEP Publications.* www.inchem.org/documents /sids/sids/128370.pdf.

Abramowitz, N. "The Dangers of Chasing Youth: Regulating the Use of Nanoparticles in Anti-aging." *University of Illinois Journal of Law, Technology & Policy* 2008, no. 1 (Spring 2008): 199–221. jltp.uiuc.edu/archives/Abramowitz.pdf.

Agency for Toxic Substances and Disease Registry. www.atsdr.cdc.gov.

Berge, U., J. Behrens, and S. I. Rattan. "Sugar-Induced Premature Aging and Altered Differentiation in Human Epidermal Keratinocytes." *Biogerontology: Mechanisms and Intervention* 1100 (April 2007): 524–529. onlinelibrary.wiley.com/ doi/10.1196/annals.1395.058/abstract.

Burkhart, C. G., and C. N. Burkhart. "Dihydroxyacetone and Methods to Improve Its Performance as Artificial Tanner." *The Open Dermatology Journal* 3 (2009): 42–43. http://benthamopen.com/todj/articles/V003/42TODJ.pdf.

Camire, M. E. "Chemical Changes During Extrusion Cooking." *Advances in Experimental Medicine and Biology* 434 (1998): 109–121. http:/link.springer.com/chapter/10.1007/978-1-4899-1925-0_11.

Clapp, R. W., M. M. Jacobs, and E. L. Loechler. "Environmental and Occupational Causes of Cancer New Evidence, 2005–2007," *Review on Environmental Health* 23, no. 1 (January–March 2008): 1–37. www.ncbi.nlm.nih.gov/pmc/articles/ PMC2791455.

"Coconut Oil Diethanolomine Condensate." *IARC Monographs.* monographs.iarc. fr/ENG/Monographs/vol101/mono101-005.pdf.

Culton, D. A., et al. "Nontuberculous Mycobacterial Infection after Fractionated CO_2 Laser Resurfacing." *Emerging Infectious Diseases* 19, no. 3 (March 2013): 365–70. wwwnc.cdc.gov/eid/article/19/3/12-0880_article.htm.

Danby, F. W. "Nutrition and Aging Skin: Sugar and Glycation." *Clinics in Dermatology* 28, no. 4 (July–August 2010): 409–11. www.ncbi.nlm.nih.gov/ pubmed/20620757.

Davidson, R. J., et al. "Alterations in Brain and Immune Function Produced by Mindfulness Meditation." *Psychosomatic Medicine* 65, no. 4 (July–August 2003): 564–70. www.ncbi.nlm.nih.gov/pubmed/12883106.

"Depending on How Much and How Long, Light from Self-Luminous Tablet Computers Can Affect Evening Melatonin, Delaying Sleep." Lighting Research Center (August 21, 2012). www.lrc.rpi.edu/resources/newsroom/pr_story. asp?id=235#.VANvEEiEh1U.

Diamanti-Kandarakis, E., et al. "Endocrine-Disrupting Chemicals: An Endocrine Society Scientific Statement." *Endocrine Reviews* 30, no. 4 (June 2009): 293–342. www.endocrine.org/~/media/endosociety/Files/Publications/Scientific%20State-ments/EDC_Scientific_Statement.pdf.

Dodson, R., et al. "Endocrine Disruptors and Asthma-Associated Chemicals in Consumer Products." *Environmental Health Perspectives* 120, no. 7 (July 2012). http://www.silentspring.org/resource/fact-sheet-hormone-disruptors-and-asthma-associated-chemicals-consumer-products.

Dyer, D. G., et al. "Accumulation of Maillard Reaction Products in Skin Collagen in Diabetes and Aging." *The Journal of Clinical Investigation* 91, no. 6 (June 1993): 2463–2469. http://www.ncbi.nlm.nih.gov/pmc/articles/PMC443306/pdf/jcin-vest00055-0133.pdf.

"Electromagnetic Fields and Public Health: Mobile Phones." World Health Organization, Fact Sheet 193 (October 2014). www.who.int/mediacentre/factsheets/ fs193/en.

Etcoff, N., et al. "The Real Truth About Beauty: A Global Report." Dove (September 2004). www.clubofamsterdam.com/contentarticles/52%20Beauty/dove_white_paper_final.pdf.

"Final Amended Report on the Safety Assessment of Methylparaben, Ethylparaben, Propylparaben, Isopropylparaben, Butylparaben, Isobutylparaben, and

Benzylparaben as Used in Cosmetic Products." *International Journal of Toxicology* 27, suppl. 4 (2008): 1–82. www.ncbi.nlm.nih.gov/pubmed/19101832.

"Final Report on the Safety Assessment of Phenoxyethanol." *International Journal of Toxicology* 9, no. 2 (March/April 1990): 259–77. ijt.sagepub.com/content/9/2/259. abstract.

"Formaldehyde and Cancer Risks." National Cancer Institute at the National Institutes of Health. www.cancer.gov/cancertopics/factsheet/Risk/formaldehyde.

"Free Radicals May Be Good for You." *ScienceDaily* (March 1, 2011). www.sciencedaily.com/releases/2011/02/110228090404.htm.

Fruijtier-Pölloth, C. "Safety Assessment on Polyethylene Glycols (PEGs) and Their Derivatives as Used in Cosmetic Products." *Toxicology* 214, nos. 1–2 (October 15, 2005): 1–38. www.sciencedirect.com/science/article/pii/S0300483X05002696.

Fu, J. J. J., et al. "A Randomized, Controlled Comparative Study of the Wrinkle Reduction Benefits of a Cosmetic Niacinamide/Peptide/Retinyl Propionate Product Regimen vs. a Prescription 0.02% Tretinoin Product Regimen." *The British Journal of Dermatology* 162, no. 3 (March 2010): 647–54. www.ncbi.nlm.nih.gov/pmc/articles/PMC2841824.

Garth H Rauscher, G. H., D. Shore, and D. P. Sandler. "Hair Dye Use and Risk of Adult Acute Leukemia." *American Journal of Epidemiology* 160, no. 1 (2004): 19–25. aje.oxfordjournals.org/content/160/1/19.full.

Glaser, J. L., et al. "Elevated Serum Dehydroepiandrosterone Sulfate Levels in Practitioners of the Transcendental Meditation (TM) and TM-Sidhi Programs." *Journal of Behavioral Medicine* 15, no. 4 (August 1992): 327–41. www.ncbi.nlm.nih.gov/pubmed/1404349.

Goldberg, T., et al. "Advanced Glycoxidation End Products in Commonly Consumed Foods." *Journal of the American Dietetic Association* 104, no. 8 (August 2004): 1287–91. www.ncbi.nlm.nih.gov/pubmed/15281050.

Goldman, W. "Carcinogenicity of Coal-Tar Shampoo." *The Lancet* 345, no. 8945 (February 4, 1995): 326. www.thelancet.com/journals/lancet/article/PIIS0140-6736%2895%2990317-8/fulltext.

"Guidance on the Safety Assessment of Nanomaterials in Cosmetics." European Commission Scientific Committee on Consumer Safety (June 2012). ec.europa.eu/health/scientific_committees/consumer_safety/docs/sccs_s_005.pdf.

"Hairdressers and Work-Related Respiratory Disease." *Occupational Airways* 4, no. 2 (August 1998). www.ct.gov/dph/lib/dph/environmental_health/eoha/pdf/oa_aug_1998.pdf.

Huncharek, M., and B. Kupelnick. "Personal Use of Hair Dyes and the Risk of Bladder Cancer: Results of a Meta-Analysis." *Public Health Reports* 120 (January–February 2005): 31–38. www.ncbi.nlm.nih.gov/pmc/articles/PMC1497675/pdf/15736329.pdf.

Johnson, W. Jr., "Final Report on the Safety Assessment of PEG-25 Propylene Glycol Stearate, PEG-75 Propylene Glycol Stearate, PEG-120 Propylene Glycol Stearate, PEG-10 Propylene Glycol, PEG-8 Propylene Glycol Cocoate, and PEG-55 Propylene Glycol Oleate." *International Journal of Toxicology* 20, suppl. 4 (2001): 13–26. www.ncbi.nlm.nih.gov/pubmed/11800049.

Katz, D. L., and S. Meller. "Can We Say What Diet Is Best for Health?" *Annual Review of Public Health* 35 (March 2014): 83–103. www.annualreviews.org/doi/full/10.1146/annurev-publhealth-032013-182351.

Kooyers, T. J., and W. Westerhof. "Toxicology and Health Risks of Hydroquinone in Skin Lightening Formulas." *Journal of the European Academy of Dermatology and Venereology* 20, no. 7 (August 2006): 777–80. onlinelibrary.wiley.com/doi/10.1111/j.1468-3083.2005.01218.x/abstract.

Levin, J., and S. Momin. "How Much Do We Really Know about Our Favorite Cosmeceutical Ingredients?" *Journal of Clinical and Aesthetic Dermatology* 3, no. 2 (February 2010): 22–41. www.ncbi.nlm.nih.gov/pmc/articles/PMC2921764.

Liao, C., F. Liu, and K. Kannan. "Occurrence of and Dietary Exposure to Parabens in Foodstuffs from the United States." *Environmental Science and Technology* 47, no. 8 (April 16, 2013): 3918–25. www.ncbi.nlm.nih.gov/pubmed/23506043.

Lin, F.H., et al. "Ferulic Acid Stabilizes a Solution of Vitamins C and E and Doubles Its Photoprotection of Skin." *Journal of Investigative Dermatology* 125, no. 4 (October 2005): 826–32: www.nature.com/jid/journal/v125/n4/full/5603565a.html.

Liu, S., S. Katharine Hammond, and Ann Rojas-Cheatham. "Concentrations and Potential Health Risks of Metals in Lip Products." *Environmental Health Perspectives* 121, no. 6 (June 2013). ehp.niehs.nih.gov/1205518.

Mizutari, K., et al. "Photo-Enhanced Modification of Human Skin Elastin in Actinic Elastosis by N(carboxymethyl) lysine. One of the Glycation Products of the Maillard Reaction." *Journal of Investigative Dermatology* 108, no. 5 (May 1997): 797–802. www.ncbi.nlm.nih.gov/pubmed/9129235.

Morita, K., et al. "Migration of Keratinocytes Is Impaired on Glycated Collagen Type I." *Wound Repair and Regeneration* 13, no. 1 (January–February 2005): 93–101. www.ncbi.nlm.nih.gov/pubmed/15659041.

Mukherjee, S., et al. "Retinoids in the Treatment of Skin Aging: An Overview of Clinical Efficacy and Safety." *Clinical Interventions in Aging* 1, no. 4 (December 2006): 327–48. www.ncbi.nlm.nih.gov/pmc/articles/PMC2699641.

Nohynek, G., et al. "*Grey Goo* on the Skin? Nanotechnology, Cosmetic and Sunscreen Safety." *Critical Reviews in Toxicology* 37 (2007): 251–57. chmwww.rutgers.edu/~kyc/pdf/491/wilson/cosmetics1.pdf.

Omprakash, H. M., and S. C. Rajendran. "Botulinum Toxin Deaths: What Is the Fact?" *Journal of Cutaneous and Aesthetic Surgery* 1, no. 2 (July–December 2008): 95–97. www.ncbi.nlm.nih.gov/pmc/articles/PMC2840902.

"Opinion on Resorcinol." European Commission Scientific Committee on Consumer Safety (March 2010). ec.europa.eu/health/scientific_committees/consumer_safety/docs/sccs_o_015.pdf.

Politano, V. T., et al. "Uterotrophic Assay of Percutaneous Lavender Oil in Immature Female Rats." *International Journal of Toxicology* 32, no. 2 (March–April 2013): 123–9. www.researchgate.net/publication/235379940_Uterotrophic_Assay_of_Percutaneous_Lavender_Oil_in_Immature_Female_Rats.

Prusakiewicz, J. J, et al. "Parabens Inhibit Human Skin Estrogen Sulfotransferase Activity: Possible Link to Paraben Estrogenic Effects." *Toxicology* 233, no. 3 (April 11, 2007): 248–56.

Ramón, E., et al. "Primary Prevention of Cardiovascular Disease with a Mediterranean Diet." *The New England Journal of Medicine* 368 (2013): 1279–90. www.nejm.org/doi/full/10.1056/NEJMoa1200303?query=featured_home&#t=articleTop.

Raut, S. A., and R. A. Angus. "Triclosan Has Endocrine-Disrupting Effects in Male Western Mosquitofish, *Gambusia affinis*." *Environmental Toxicology and Chemistry* 29, no. 5 (June 2010): 1287–91. onlinelibrary.wiley.com/doi/10.1002/etc.150/abstract?deniedAccessCustomisedMessage=&userIsAuthenticated=false.

Rendon, Marta, et al. "Evidence and Considerations in the Application of Chemical Peels in Skin Disorders and Aesthetic Resurfacing." *The Journal of Clinical and Aesthetic Dermatology* 3, no. 7 (July 2010): 32–43. www.ncbi.nlm.nih.gov/pmc/articles/PMC2921757.

Roberts, M. J., et al. "DNA Damage by Carbonyl Stress in Human Skin Cells." *Mutation Research* 522, nos. 1–2 (January 28, 2003): 45–56. www.ncbi.nlm.nih.gov/pubmed/12517411.

Roberts, S.C., et al. "Female Facial Attractiveness Increases During the Fertile Phase of the Menstrual Cycle." *Proceedings of the Royal Society* 271, suppl. 5 (August 7, 2004): S270–2. dx.doi.org/10.1098/rsbl.2004.0174.

Routledge, E., et al. "Some Alkyl Hydroxy Benzoate Preservatives (Parabens) Are Estrogenic." *Toxicology and Applied Pharmacology* 153, no. 1 (November 1998): 12–19. www.sciencedirect.com/science/article/pii/S0041008X98985441.

Russell, R. "Sex, Beauty, and the Relative Luminance of Facial Features." *Perception* 32, no. 9 (2003): 1093–1107. http://www.perceptionweb.com/abstract.cgi?id=p5101.

Safer, J. "Thyroid Hormone Action on Skin." *Dermatoendocrinology* 3, no. 3 (July–September 2011): 211–5. www.ncbi.nlm.nih.gov/pmc/articles/PMC3219173.

Sikora, E., G. Scapagnini, and M. Barbagallo. "Curcumin, Inflammation, Ageing and Age-Related Diseases." *Immunity and Ageing* 7, no. 1 (2010). www.immunity-ageing.com/content/7/1/1.

Singh, G. "Recent Considerations in Nonsteroidal Anti-Inflammatory Drug Gastropathy." *The American Journal of Medicine* 105, no. 1B (July 27, 1998). 31S–38S: www.ncbi.nlm.nih.gov/pubmed/9715832.

Telang, P. S. "Vitamin C in Dermatology." *Indian Dermatology Online Journal* 4, no. 2 (April–June 2013): 143–6. www.ncbi.nlm.nih.gov/pmc/articles/PMC3673383/.

Thun, M. J., et al. "Hair Dye Use and Risk of Fatal Cancers in U.S. Women," *Journal of the National Cancer Institute* 86, no. 3 (1994): 210–15. jnci.oxfordjournals.org/content/86/3/210.

Tisserand, R. "Neither Lavender Oil nor Tea Tree Oil Can Be Linked to Breast Growth in Young Boys." roberttisserand.com/articles/TeaTreeAndLavenderNot-LinkedToGynecomastia.pdf.

Wozniak, M. and M. Murias. "Xenoestrogens: Endocrine Disrupting Compounds." *Ginekologia Polska* 79, no. 11 (November 2008): 785–90. www.ncbi.nlm.nih.gov/pubmed/19140503.

Yogianti, F., et al. "Inhibitory Effects of Dietary *Spirulina platensis* on UVB-Induced Skin Inflammatory Responses and Carcinogenesis." *Journal of Investigative Dermatology* 134 (2014): 2610–19. www.nature.com/jid/journal/v134/n10/full/jid2014188a.html.

Zeng, J., et al. "Evidence for Inactivation of Cysteine Proteases by Reactive Carbonyls via Glycation of Active Site Thiols." *The Biochemical Journal* 398, no. 2 (September 2006): 197–206. www.biochemj.org/bj/398/0197/3980197.pdf.

ACKNOWLEDGMENTS

When I write a proposal for a new book, it always feels as if it's a one-woman show and that it's all me, but four books in, I now know that the moment I get the green light, the "village" moves in, and my book is only as good as the "village" who support me.

In this case, I have been fortunate enough to be surrounded by a community of wise, strong, and beautiful women. Let me begin with literary agent extraordinaire, Sharon Bowers, whose humor, wisdom, and direction got me fired up before the first word of my book was written—Sharon, you are the best, and I am honored to have found you. Moving on to Tess Masters, a sister on this holistic journey, and a fire cracker who not guided me to where I needed to go with *Gorgeous for Good*, but who continues to inspire me with her passion and love for all things gorgeous and green (and all the colors in between). Kate Kerrigan—you are not only one of the funniest and most talented writers I know, but you are also so very generous friend—thank you for all your great advice and help in getting *Gorgeous for Good* off the ground.

Johanne Morris, manager extraordinaire—all I can say is that you deserve a medal for outstanding tolerance! Thank you for your weekly cheerleading, your inspiration, and for always thinking BIG. You are the best.

A huge "thank you" to Patty Gift at Hay House for inviting me into the Hay House community, which honestly feels like home. I am so happy to be where I belong, and to have been guided throughout this process by Laura Gray, who is the most soulful, gentle, intelligent, and funny editor I have ever worked with.

My gratitude also goes out to my amazing *Gorgeous for Good* team: Julia Wyson, Julia Towner, and Katharine Crnko.

A large part of my "village" is all of the amazing professionals who have not only helped me over the years, but been kind enough to take the time to contribute to my book: Emily Fritchey (aka The Skin Whisperer)—you are a unique and powerful voice in the holistic skin care community, and I am so grateful for all our hours of discussions about the passions we share. Dr. Julia Tatum Hunter, who I always turn to for her innate wisdom and thorough research—I am thrilled that you were available to answer all my many questions. Dr. Christiane Northrup, Dr. Rebecca Fitzgerald, Dr. David Kean, Dr. Richard Horowitz—I am fortunate to be surrounded by the best of the best, and I am deeply grateful that you all took the time out of your busy schedules to contribute your expertise to *Gorgeous for Good*.

Jack Guy, who has to be the best photographer on the planet—thank you for getting me over my fear of wearing little to no makeup for our photo shoot, and for giving me the courage to be natural and myself on that windy afternoon in Malibu. Alexis Seabrook is the illustrator who I always turn to because she is the best.

Finally, last but never least, the two beings that I hold most close to my heart: my husband, Joseph, and my beautiful daughter, Lola. It's not easy living with a writer on a deadline, and you both continue to not only put up with me hunched over my computer first thing in the morning to last thing at night, but also support me in every way you can. I am the luckiest girl on the planet to be blessed with you both.

ABOUT THE AUTHOR

New York Times best-selling author Sophie Uliano is a leading expert in the field of natural health and beauty who takes a down-to-earth approach to beauty, focusing on what's truly healthy. Her popular website—www.sophieuliano.com—brings together a community of like-minded women and provides in-depth articles, reviews, beauty picks, recipes, and more, covering the latest beauty trends. She has written three books: *Gorgeously Green, Do It Gorgeously,* and *The Gorgeously Green Diet.* Follow her on Facebook at facebook.com/gorgeouslygreen or on Twitter at twitter.com/sophieuliano.

Hay House Titles of Related Interest

We hope you enjoyed this Hay House book. If you'd like to receive our online catalog featuring additional information on Hay House books and products, or if you'd like to find out more about the Hay Foundation, please contact:

Hay House, Inc., P.O. Box 5100, Carlsbad, CA 92018-5100
(760) 431-7695 or (800) 654-5126
(760) 431-6948 (fax) or (800) 650-5115 (fax)
www.hayhouse.com® • www.hayfoundation.org

• • •

Published and distributed in Australia by: Hay House Australia Pty. Ltd.,
18/36 Ralph St., Alexandria NSW 2015
Phone: 612-9669-4299 • *Fax:* 612-9669-4144 • www.hayhouse.com.au

Published and distributed in the United Kingdom by: Hay House UK, Ltd.,
Astley House, 33 Notting Hill Gate, London W11 3JQ
Phone: 44-20-3675-2450 • *Fax:* 44-20-3675-2451 • www.hayhouse.co.uk

Published and distributed in the Republic of South Africa by: Hay House SA
(Pty), Ltd., P.O. Box 990, Witkoppen 2068
Phone/Fax: 27-11-467-8904 • www.hayhouse.co.za

Published in India by: Hay House Publishers India,
Muskaan Complex, Plot No. 3, B-2, Vasant Kunj, New Delhi 110 070
Phone: 91-11-4176-1620 • *Fax:* 91-11-4176-1630 • www.hayhouse.co.in

Distributed in Canada by: Raincoast Books,
2440 Viking Way, Richmond, B.C. V6V 1N2 •
Phone: 1-800-663-5714 • *Fax:* 1-800-565-3770 • www.raincoast.com

• • •

Take Your Soul on a Vacation

Visit www.HealYourLife.com® to regroup,
recharge, and reconnect with your own magnificence.
Featuring blogs, mind-body-spirit news, and
life-changing wisdom from Louise Hay and friends.

Visit www.HealYourLife.com today!

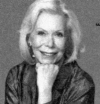
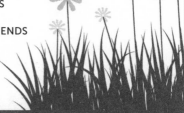